Cancer Treatment and Research

Volume 169

Series editor

Steven T. Rosen, Duarte, CA, USA

More information about this series at http://www.springer.com/series/5808

Aldo M. Roccaro · Irene M. Ghobrial
Editors

Plasma Cell Dyscrasias

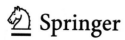 Springer

Editors
Aldo M. Roccaro
Department of Medical
   Oncology/Hematology
ASST Spedali Civili di Brescia
Brescia
Italy

Irene M. Ghobrial
Department of Medical Oncology
Dana-Farber Cancer Institute
Boston, MA
USA

ISSN 0927-3042   ISSN 2509-8497 (electronic)
Cancer Treatment and Research
ISBN 978-3-319-82078-1   ISBN 978-3-319-40320-5 (eBook)
DOI 10.1007/978-3-319-40320-5

Printed on acid-free paper

This Springer imprint is published by Springer Nature
The registered company is Springer International Publishing AG Switzerland

Contents

Part I
Monoclonal Gammopathy of Undetermined Significance and Smoldering Myeloma

MGUS and Smoldering Multiple Myeloma: Diagnosis and Epidemiology

María-Victoria Mateos and Ola Landgren

Abstract

Monoclonal gammopathy of undetermined significance (MHUS) is characterized by the presence of a serum M-protein less than 3 g/dL, less than 10 % clonal plasma cells in the bone marrow, and the absence of myeloma-defining event. Smoldering multiple myeloma (SMM) is an asymptomatic disorder characterized by the presence of ≥3 g/dL serum M-protein and/or 10–60 % bone marrow plasma cell infiltration with no myeloma-defining event. The risk of progression to multiple myeloma (MM) requiring therapy varies greatly for individual patients, but it is uniform and 1 % per year for MGUS, while higher (10 % per year) and not uniform for SMM patients. The definition of MM was recently revisited patients previously labeled as SMM with a very high risk of progression (80–90 % at 2 years) were included in the updated definition of MM requiring therapy. The standard of care is observation for MGUS patients and although this also applies for SMM, a recent randomized trial targeting high-risk SMM showed that early intervention was associated with better progression-free and overall survival. Biomarkers have become an integrated part of diagnostic criteria for MM requiring therapy, as well as clinical risk stratification of patients with SMM. This paper reviews and discusses clinical implications for MGUS and SMM patients.

Keywords

Multiple myeloma requiring therapy · Monoclonal gammopathy of undetermined significance · Smoldering myeloma

M.-V. Mateos (✉)
University Hospital of Salamanca/IBSAL, Paseo San Vicente, 58-182, 37007 Salamanca, Spain
e-mail: mvmateos@usal.es

O. Landgren
Myeloma Service, Memorial Sloan-Kettering Cancer Center, New York, USA

© Springer International Publishing Switzerland 2016
A.M. Roccaro and I.M. Ghobrial (eds.), *Plasma Cell Dyscrasias*,
Cancer Treatment and Research 169, DOI 10.1007/978-3-319-40320-5_1

1 Introduction

In 1978, Monoclonal gammopathy of undetermined significance (MGUS) was described by Kyle and Greipp and 2 years later, based on a series of six patients who met the criteria for multiple myeloma (MM) but whose disease did not have an aggressive course, the same authors coined the term smoldering multiple myeloma (SMM) [1]. In 2014, the International Myeloma Working Group (IMWG) updated the definition of multiple myeloma (MM) which in turn impacted the definition of both MGUS and SMM [2]. MGUS diagnosis requires the presence of <3 g/dL serum M-protein and <10 % bone marrow plasma cells with no hypercalcemia, renal failure, anemia, and bone lesions that can be attributed to the underlying plasma cell disorder. Indeed, SMM is now defined as a plasma cell disorder characterized by the presence of one or both of the features of ≥3 g/dL serum M-protein and 10–60 % bone marrow plasma cells (BMPCs), but with no evidence of myeloma-related symptomatology (hypercalcemia, renal insufficiency, anemia or bone lesions (CRAB)) or any other myeloma-defining event (MDE). According to this recent update, the definition of MM includes patients with BMPCs of 60 % or more, serum free light-chain (FLC) levels of ≥100, and those with two or more focal lesions of the skeleton as revealed by magnetic resonance imaging (MRI). Thus, the definition of MM requiring therapy has changed from symptoms to biomarkers. Kristinsson et al., through the Swedish Myeloma Registry, recently reported that 14 % of patients diagnosed with multiple myeloma indeed SMM, and, using the world population as a reference, estimated the age-standardized incidence of SMM to be 0.44 cases per 100,000 people [3]. The incidence of MGUS is higher than SMM and is present in roughly 3–4 % of the population over the age of 50 years [4].

2 Differential Diagnosis with Other Entities

Based on current diagnostic criteria, SMM is distinguished from monoclonal gammopathy of undetermined significance (MGUS) and MM requiring therapy (Table 1). Specifically, MGUS is characterized by a serum M-protein concentration of less than 3 g/dL, less than 10 % plasma cell infiltration in the bone marrow, and absence of CRAB criteria and absence of MDE [2]. Furthermore, MM requiring therapy is defined as follows: presence of one or more of the CRAB criteria and/or one of the MDE, in conjunction with 10 % or more clonal BMPC infiltration or biopsy-proven bony or extramedullary plasmacytoma. As per the criteria, presence of end-organ damage (i.e., CRAB criteria) needs to be correctly evaluated to distinguish myeloma-related symptomatology from some signs or symptoms that could otherwise be attributed to comorbidities or concomitant diseases [5].

Table 1 Differential diagnosis of MGUS, SMM and MM requiring therapy

Feature	MGUS	SMM	MM requiring therapy
Serum M-protein	<3 g/dL and	≥3 g/dL and/or	–
Clonal BMPC infiltration	<10 %	10–60 %	≥10 % or biopsy-proven plasmacytoma
Symptomatology	Absence of MDE*	Absence of MDE*	Presence of MDE*

*MDE includes (1) hypercalcemia: serum calcium > 0.25 mmol/L (>1 mg/dL) higher than the upper limit of normal or >2.75 mmol/L (>11 mg/dL); (2) renal insufficiency: serum creatinine >177 μmol/L (2 mg/dL) or creatinine clearance <40 ml/min; (3) anemia: hemoglobin value of >2 g/dL below the lower normal limit, or a hemoglobin value <10 g/dL; (4) bone lesions: one or more osteolytic lesion revealed by skeletal radiography, CT, or PET-CT or the presence of any one or more of the following biomarkers of malignancy: clonal bone marrow plasma cell percentage ≥60 %; involved/uninvolved serum free-light chain ratio ≥100; >1 focal lesions revealed by MRI studies

3 Diagnostic Work-up

Initial investigation of a patient with suspected MGUS or SMM should include the tests shown in Table 2, which are coincidental with those used for a correct diagnosis of MM requiring therapy [6]. As far as SMM is concerned, due to the

Table 2 Work-up for newly diagnosed MGUS and SMM patients

- Medical history and physical examination
- Hemogram
- Biochemical studies, including of creatinine and calcium levels; Beta2-microglobulin, LDH and albumin
- Protein studies
  - Total serum protein and serum electrophoresis (serum M-protein)
  - 24-h urine sample protein electrophoresis (urine M-protein)
  - Serum and urine immunofixation
- Serum free light-chain measurement (sFLC ratio)
- Bone marrow aspirate ± biopsy: infiltration by clonal plasma cells, flow cytometry and fluorescence in situ hybridization analysis*
- Skeletal survey, CT, or PET-CT*
- MRI of thoracic and lumbar spine and pelvis; ideally, whole-body MRI (only for SMM)

FLC free light chain; CT computed tomography; PET-CT ^18F-fluorodeoxyglucose (FDG) positron emission tomography (PET)/CT; MRI magnetic resonance imaging
*These assessments can be deferred in patient with low-risk MGUS (IgG type, monoclonal protein <1.5 g/dL, normal free light-chain ratio)

updated IMWG criteria for the diagnosis of MM, there are some specific assessments to which physicians have to pay attention in order to make correct diagnosis.

(1) With respect to the evaluation of bone disease, the IMWG recommends that— in addition to a conventional skeletal survey—[18]F-fluorodeoxyglucose (FDG) positron emission tomography (PET)/computed tomography (CT) and/or low-dose whole-body CT shall be conducted to rule our bone and/or bone marrow involvement. Specifically, the aim is to exclude presence of osteolytic bone lesions, currently defined by the presence of at least one lesion (≥5 mm) revealed by X-ray, CT, or PET-CT. In addition, whole-body MRI of the spine and pelvis (or, ideally, if available, whole-body MRI) is a required component of the initial work-up. It provides detailed information about bone marrow involvement and identifies potential focal lesions which have been found to predict a more rapid progression to MM requiring therapy. In 2010, Hillengass et al. reported that the presence of two or more focal lesions in the skeleton by whole-body MRI was associated with a significantly shorter median time to progression (TTP) to active disease of 13 months, compared with the period when no focal lesions were present [7]. Kastritis and colleagues replicated these observations based on a smaller group of patients who underwent spinal MRI and were followed up for a minimum of 2.5 years. In their study, the median TTP to symptomatic disease was 14 months when more than one focal lesion was present [8]. Therefore, if two or more focal lesions are detected by MRI, based on the most recent IMWG criteria (REF), such a patient is defined as having MM requiring therapy.

(2) With respect to bone marrow infiltration, the Mayo Clinic group evaluated BMPC infiltration in a cohort of 651 patients and found that 21 (3.2 %) had an extreme infiltration (≥60 %) [9]. This group of patients had a median TTP to active disease of 7.7 months, with a 95 % risk of progression at 2 years. This finding was subsequently validated in a study of 96 patients with SMM, in whom a median TTP of 15 months was reported for the group of patients with this extreme infiltration. In a third study, six of 121 patients (5 %) with SMM were found to have 60 % or more BMPC, and all progressed to MM within 2 years [10]. Therefore, based on the most recent IMWG criteria (REF), if 60 % or more of clonal plasma cell infiltration is present either in bone marrow aspirate or biopsy, the diagnosis is MM requiring therapy. Additional assessments, for example, by flow cytometry or by identifying cytogenetic abnormalities in SMM patients, are not required to confirm or rule out MM requiring therapy, but can help estimate the risk of progression from SMM to MM requiring therapy.

(3) With respect to the serum free light-chain (FLC) assay, Larsen et al. studied 586 patients with SMM to determine whether there was a threshold FLC ratio that predicted 85 % of progression risk at 2 years. They found a serum involved/uninvolved FLC ratio of at least 100 in 15 % of patients and a risk of progression to symptomatic disease of 72 % [11]. Similar results were obtained in a study by Kastritis and colleagues from the Greek Myeloma Group [12]. In their study of 96 SMM patients, 7 % had an involved/uninvolved FLC ratio of ≥100 and almost all progressed within 18 months. In a third study, the risk of progression within 2 years was 64 %. Consequently, if the involved/uninvolved ratio is ≥100,

and the involved FLC concentration is >10 mg/dL, based on the most recent IMWG criteria (REF), a patient fulfills the criteria for MM requiring therapy.

Once MM requiring therapy has been ruled out and a diagnosis of SMM has been made, considering the specific assessments mentioned above, the serum and urine M-component, hemoglobin, calcium, and creatinine levels should be reevaluated 2–3 months later to confirm the stability of these parameters. The subsequent follow-up involves the same evaluation but the frequency should be adapted on the basis of risk factors for progression to MM requiring therapy (see below).

Table 3 Smoldering MM: markers predicting progression to MM requiring therapy

Features for identifying high-risk MGUS patients

- Concentration of Serum M-protein:
  –M-protein of 2.5 g/dL $\longrightarrow$ 49 % risk of progression at 20 years
- Type of Serum M-protein:
  –Patients with IgM or IgA isotype, the risk is higher compared with IgG MGUS
- Bone Marrow Plasma Cells:
  –>5 % of plasma cell bone marrow infiltration
- Abnormal serum FLC ratio:
  –High risk of progression (Hazar ratio 3.5), independent of the concentration and type of serum M-protein.

Features for identifying high-risk SMM patients: 50 % at 2 years

- Tumor burden:
  –≥10 % clonal plasma cell bone marrow infiltration plus
  –≥3 g/dL of serum M-protein and
  –serum free light-chain ratio between 0.125 and 8
- Bence Jones proteinuria positive from 24-h urine sample
- Peripheral blood circulating plasma cells >5 × 10^6/L

- Immunophenotyping characterization and immunoparesis:
  –≥ 95 % of aberrant plasma cells by flow within the plasma cell bone marrow compartment plus
  –immunoparesis (>25 % decrease in one or both uninvolved immunoglobulins relative to the lowest normal value)

- Cytogenetic abnormalities:
  –Presence of t(4;14)
  –Presence of del17p
  –Gains of 1q24
  –Hyperdiploidy
  –Gene Expression Profiling risk score > −0.26

- Pattern of serum M-component evolution
  –Evolving type: if M-protein ≥ 3 g/dL, increase of at least 10 % within the first 6 months. If M-protein < 3 g/dL, annual increase of M-protein for 3 years
  –Increase in the M-protein to ≥3 g/dL over the 3 months since the previous determination

- Imaging assessments
  –MRI: Radiological progressive disease (MRI-PD) was defined as newly detected focal lesions (FLs) or increase in diameter of existing FL and a novel or progressive diffuse infiltration.
  –Positive PET/CT with no underlying osteolytic lesion

MRI magnetic resonance imaging; *PET-CT* ^{18}F-fluorodeoxyglucose (FDG) positron emission tomography (PET)/CT

4 Risk Factors Predicting Progression to MM Requiring Therapy

Patients diagnosed of MGUS have a low and uniform risk of progression to MM requiring therapy, 1 % per year [13]. However, most patients diagnosed with SMM will progress to MM requiring therapy and will need to start treatment. However, based on current criteria, SMM is not a uniform entity and once the diagnosis has been confirmed, the doctor should evaluate the risk of progression to MM requiring therapy with the aim to offer an appropriate, risk-based follow-up, and to optimize the management of the SMM patient. The average risk of progression from SMM to MM requiring therapy is about 10 % per year [14].

Several studies have proposed clinical predictors of progression from MGUS/SMM to MM requiring therapy. Although they are not exact by any means, such clinical markers are useful for physicians in that they provide a probability measure of progression (Table 3).

5 Management of MGUS and SMM Patients

Patients with MGUS should be tested again in 4–6 months since the suspicion of the diagnosis to exclude and evolving MM. The standard of care is not to treat unless MM or order plasma cell disorder is developed. The standard of care for the management of SMM patients has been observation until MM develops. However, several groups evaluated the role of early intervention in this group of patients using conventional and novel agents.

There have been different trials evaluating the role of early treatment with melphalan and prednisone (MP), or novel agents, such as thalidomide or even bisphosphonates.

None of these trials provided evidence favoring the early treatment of patients with SMM. However, they were conducted without considering the differences in the risk of progression to active disease, and while the high-risk subgroup of patients may have benefited, this could have been counterbalanced by the absence of benefit in low-risk patients. The Spanish Myeloma Group (GEM/Pethema) has conducted a phase III randomized trial in 119 SMM patients at high risk of progression to active disease (according to the Mayo and/or Spanish criteria) that compared early treatment with lenalidomide plus dexamethasone as induction followed by lenalidomide alone as maintenance versus observation. The primary end-point was TTP to symptomatic MM, and after a median follow-up of 40 months, the median TTP was significantly longer in patients in the early treatment group than in the observation arm (not reached vs. 21 months; hazard ratio, HR = 5.59; $p < 0.001$). Secondary end-points included response, OS and safety. The PR or better after induction was 82 %, including 14 % of cases of stringent complete response (sCR) plus CR, and after maintenance the sCR/CR rate increased to 26 %. The safety profile was acceptable and most of the adverse events reported were grade 1 or 2. The OS analysis showed that the 3-year survival rate was also higher for the group of patients who received early treatment with lenalidomide-based therapy (94 vs. 80 %; HR = 3.24; p = 0.03) [15]. A recent update of this trial confirmed the efficacy of early treatment in terms of TTP (HR = 6.21; 95 % CI: 3.1–12.7, p < 0.0001) and the benefit to OS was even more evident with longer follow-up (HR = 4.35, 95 % CI: 1.5–13.0, p = 0.008) [16]. This study showed for the first time the potential for changing the treatment paradigm for high-risk SMM patients based on the efficacy of early treatment in terms of TTP to active disease and of OS. Moreover, several trials currently underway are focusing on high-risk SMM patients using novel agents.

6 Managing MGUS and SMM Patients in Clinical Practice

Patients with low-risk MGUS may be reevaluated every 2 years, whereas those with high-risk MGUS should be followed annually for life or until they develop an unrelated condition that severely limits life expectancy. At the time of the follow-up examination, a careful history and physical examination should be performed, looking for symptoms or signs of one of the malignant disorders known to evolve from MGUS. The serum and urine M-protein values should be measured, as well as the complete blood count, calcium, and creatinine. Patients should always be told to obtain medical evaluation promptly if clinical symptoms occur.

Concerning SMM, given the extensive background to this disease described above, the first step in clinical practice is to identify the risk of progression to active disease for each newly diagnosed SMM patient. A key question is which risk model is the best to use for the purpose of estimating the risk of progression from SMM to MM requiring therapy. The Mayo Clinic and Spanish models enable initial risk stratification of SMM and, in fact, both were validated in a prospective trial. However, new risk models are emerging that incorporate new clinical and biological features [10, 14, 17–22] (Table 4). The components of these models are not identical, and, importantly, they are all probability models and not markers reflective of defined biological mechanisms directly related to progression (Table 3).

SMM patients should be classified as follows:

(1) SMM patients at low risk of progression who are characterized by the absence of the aforementioned high-risk factors (using the validated Mayo and Spanish risk models), with an estimated probability of progression at 5 years of only 8 %. Patients in this group behave similarly to MGUS-like patients and should be followed annually.

(2) The second group includes SMM patients at intermediate risk of progression and they only display some of the aforementioned high-risk factors. They have a risk of progression at 5 years of 42 %, and they must be followed up every 6 months.

Table 4 Risk models for the stratification of SMM

Risk model	Risk of progression to MM	
Mayo Clinic • ≥10 % clonal PCBM infiltration • ≥3 g/dL of serum M-protein • Serum FLC ratio between <0.125 or >8	1 risk factor 2 risk factors 3 risk factors	**Median TTP** 10 years 5 years 1.9 years
Spanish Myeloma • ≥95 % of aberrant PCs by MFC • Immunoparesis	No risk factor 1 risk factor 2 risk factors	**Median TTP** NR 6 years 1.9 years
Heidelberg • Tumor mass using the Mayo Model • t(4;14), del17p, or +1q	T-mass low + CA low risk T-mass low + CA high risk T-mass high + CA low risk T-mass high + CA high risk	**3-year TTP** 15 % 42 % 64 % 55 %
SWOG • Serum M-protein ≥ 2 g/dL • Involved FLC > 25 mg/dL • GEP risk score > −0.26	No risk factor 1 risk factor ≥ 2 risk factors	**2-year TTP** 30 % 29 % 71 %
Penn • ≥40 % clonal PCBM infiltration • sFLC ratio ≥ 50 • Albumin ≤ 3.5 mg/dL	No risk factor 1 risk factor ≥2 risk factors	**2-year TTP** 16 % 44 % 81 %
Japanese • Beta 2-microglobulin ≥ 2.5 mg/L • M-protein increment rate > 1 mg/dL/day	2 risk factors	**2-year TTP** 67.5 %
Czech and Heidelberg • Immunoparesis • Serum M-protein ≥ 2.3 g/dL • Involved/uninvolved sFLC > 30	No risk factor 1 risk factor 2 risk factors 3 risk factors	**2-year TTP** 5.3 % 7.5 % 44.8 % 81.3 %
Barcelona • Evolving pattern = 2 points • Serum M-protein ≥ 3 g/dL = 1 point • Immunoparesis = 1 point	0 points 1 point 2 points 3 points	**2-year TTP** 2.4 % 31 % 52 % 80 %

(3) The third group includes high-risk SMM patients classified on the basis of one of the risk models mentioned above. Half of them will progress during the 2 years following diagnosis. These groups of patients need a close follow-up every 2–3 months. Key questions are whether this high-risk group should be treated, and how they should be treated. Although the Spanish trial showed significant benefit from the early treatment in high-risk SMM patients, there are some limitations that prevent the results being generally applicable at present; these may be resolved when the results of the ongoing clinical trials become available. In our opinion, the best approach for high-risk SMM is to refer them to centers that specialize in anti-myeloma therapy and offer them participation in clinical trials [23].

Financial disclosures:
María-Victoria Mateos has received payment from Celgene Corporation for the presentation of lectures and participation on advisory boards. Ola Landgren has received payment for giving scientific lectures at seminars sponsored by Celgene, Onyx, Millennium, and BMS.

References

1. Kyle RA, Greipp PR (1980) Smoldering multiple myeloma. N Engl J Med 302(24):1347–1349. doi:10.1056/NEJM198006123022405
2. Rajkumar SV, Dimopoulos MA, Palumbo A, Blade J, Merlini G, Mateos MV, Kumar S, Hillengass J, Kastritis E, Richardson P, Landgren O, Paiva B, Dispenzieri A, Weiss B, LeLeu X, Zweegman S, Lonial S, Rosinol L, Zamagni E, Jagannath S, Sezer O, Kristinsson SY, Caers J, Usmani SZ, Lahuerta JJ, Johnsen HE, Beksac M, Cavo M, Goldschmidt H, Terpos E, Kyle RA, Anderson KC, Durie BG, Miguel JF (2014) International myeloma working group updated criteria for the diagnosis of multiple myeloma. Lancet Oncol 15(12):e538–548. doi:10.1016/s1470-2045(14)70442-5
3. Kristinsson SY, Holmberg E, Blimark C (2013) Treatment for high-risk smoldering myeloma. N Engl J Med 369(18):1762–1763. doi:10.1056/NEJMc1310911#SA1
4. Kyle RA, San-Miguel JF, Mateos MV, Rajkumar SV (2014) Monoclonal gammopathy of undetermined significance and smoldering multiple myeloma. Hematol Oncol Clin North Am 28(5):775–790. doi:10.1016/j.hoc.2014.06.005
5. Blade J, Dimopoulos M, Rosinol L, Rajkumar SV, Kyle RA (2010) Smoldering (asymptomatic) multiple myeloma: current diagnostic criteria, new predictors of outcome, and follow-up recommendations. J Clin Oncol 28(4):690–697. doi:JCO.2009.22.2257 [pii] 10.1200/JCO.2009.22.2257 [doi]
6. Dimopoulos M, Kyle R, Fermand JP, Rajkumar SV, San Miguel J, Chanan-Khan A, Ludwig H, Joshua D, Mehta J, Gertz M, Avet-Loiseau H, Beksac M, Anderson KC, Moreau P, Singhal S, Goldschmidt H, Boccadoro M, Kumar S, Giralt S, Munshi NC, Jagannath S (2011) Consensus recommendations for standard investigative workup: report of the international myeloma workshop consensus panel 3. Blood 117(18):4701–4705. doi:10.1182/blood-2010-10-299529
7. Hillengass J, Fechtner K, Weber MA, Bauerle T, Ayyaz S, Heiss C, Hielscher T, Moehler TM, Egerer G, Neben K, Ho AD, Kauczor HU, Delorme S, Goldschmidt H (2010) Prognostic significance of focal lesions in whole-body magnetic resonance imaging in patients with asymptomatic multiple myeloma. J Clin Oncol 28(9):1606–1610. doi:10.1200/JCO.2009.25.5356
8. Kastritis E, Moulopoulos LA, Terpos E, Koutoulidis V, Dimopoulos MA (2014) The prognostic importance of the presence of more than one focal lesion in spine MRI of patients with asymptomatic (smoldering) multiple myeloma. Leukemia 28(12):2402–2403. doi:10.1038/leu.2014.230
9. Rajkumar SV, Larson D, Kyle RA (2011) Diagnosis of smoldering multiple myeloma. N Engl J Med 365(5):474–475. doi:10.1056/NEJMc1106428
10. Waxman AJ, Mick R, Garfall AL, Cohen A, Vogl DT, Stadtmauer EA, Weiss BM (2014) Classifying ultra-high risk smoldering myeloma. Leukemia. doi:10.1038/leu.2014.313
11. Larsen JT, Kumar SK, Dispenzieri A, Kyle RA, Katzmann JA, Rajkumar SV (2013) Serum free light chain ratio as a biomarker for high-risk smoldering multiple myeloma. Leukemia 27(4):941–946. doi:10.1038/leu.2012.296
12. Kastritis E, Terpos E, Moulopoulos L, Spyropoulou-Vlachou M, Kanellias N, Eleftherakis-Papaiakovou E, Gkotzamanidou M, Migkou M, Gavriatopoulou M, Roussou M, Tasidou A, Dimopoulos MA (2013) Extensive bone marrow infiltration and

abnormal free light chain ratio identifies patients with asymptomatic myeloma at high risk for progression to symptomatic disease. Leukemia 27(4):947–953. doi:10.1038/leu.2012.309

13. Kyle RA, Durie BG, Rajkumar SV, Landgren O, Blade J, Merlini G, Kroger N, Einsele H, Vesole DH, Dimopoulos M, San Miguel J, Avet-Loiseau H, Hajek R, Chen WM, Anderson KC, Ludwig H, Sonneveld P, Pavlovsky S, Palumbo A, Richardson PG, Barlogie B, Greipp P, Vescio R, Turesson I, Westin J, Boccadoro M (2010) Monoclonal gammopathy of undetermined significance (MGUS) and smoldering (asymptomatic) multiple myeloma: IMWG consensus perspectives risk factors for progression and guidelines for monitoring and management. Leukemia 24(6):1121–1127. doi:10.1038/leu.2010.60

14. Kyle RA, Remstein ED, Therneau TM, Dispenzieri A, Kurtin PJ, Hodnefield JM, Larson DR, Plevak MF, Jelinek DF, Fonseca R, Melton LJ, 3rd, Rajkumar SV (2007) Clinical course and prognosis of smoldering (asymptomatic) multiple myeloma. N Engl J Med 356(25):2582–2590. doi:356/25/2582 [pii] 10.1056/NEJMoa070389 [doi]

15. Mateos MV, Hernandez MT, Giraldo P, de la Rubia J, de Arriba F, Lopez Corral L, Rosinol L, Paiva B, Palomera L, Bargay J, Oriol A, Prosper F, Lopez J, Olavarria E, Quintana N, Garcia JL, Blade J, Lahuerta JJ, San Miguel JF (2013) Lenalidomide plus dexamethasone for high-risk smoldering multiple myeloma. N Engl J Med 369(5):438–447. doi:10.1056/NEJMoa1300439

16. Mateos M-V, Hernandez MT, Giraldo P, De La Rubia J, de Arriba F, López-Corral L, Rosiñol L, Paiva B, Palomera L, Bargay J, Oriol A, Prosper F, López J, Olavarría E, Quintana N, García JL, Blade J, Lahuerta JJ, San Miguel JF (2014) Long term follow-up on the tretament of high risk smoldering myeloma with lenalidomide plus low dose Dex (Rd) (phase III spanish trial): persistent benefit in overall survival. Blood 124(21):3465–3465

17. Perez-Persona E, Mateo G, Garcia-Sanz R, Mateos MV, de Las Heras N, de Coca AG, Hernandez JM, Galende J, Martin-Nunez G, Barez A, Alonso JM, Martin A, Lopez-Berges C, Orfao A, San Miguel JF, Vidriales MB (2010) Risk of progression in smouldering myeloma and monoclonal gammopathies of unknown significance: comparative analysis of the evolution of monoclonal component and multiparameter flow cytometry of bone marrow plasma cells. Br J Haematol 148(1):110–114. doi:BJH7929 [pii] 10.1111/j.1365-2141.2009.07929.x [doi]

18. Neben K, Jauch A, Hielscher T, Hillengass J, Lehners N, Seckinger A, Granzow M, Raab MS, Ho AD, Goldschmidt H, Hose D (2013) Progression in smoldering myeloma is independently determined by the chromosomal abnormalities del(17p), t(4;14), gain 1q, hyperdiploidy, and tumor load. J Clin Oncol 31(34):4325–4332. doi:10.1200/jco.2012.48.4923

19. Dhodapkar MV, Sexton R, Waheed S, Usmani S, Papanikolaou X, Nair B, Petty N, Shaughnessy JD Jr, Hoering A, Crowley J, Orlowski RZ, Barlogie B (2014) Clinical, genomic, and imaging predictors of myeloma progression from asymptomatic monoclonal gammopathies (SWOG S0120). Blood 123(1):78–85. doi:10.1182/blood-2013-07-515239

20. Muta T, Iida S, Matsue K, Sunami K, Isoda J, Harada N, Saburi Y, Okamura S, Kumagae K, Watanabe J, Kuroda J, Aoki K, Ogawa R, Miyamoto T, Akashi K, Takamatsu Y (2014) Predictive significance of serum beta 2-microglobulin levels and M-protein velocity for symptomatic progression of smoldering multiple myeloma. Blood 124(21):3379–3379

21. Hajek R, Sandecka V, Seckinger A, Spicka I, Scudla V, Gregora E, Radocha J, Brozova L, Jarkovsky J, Rihova L, Mikulasova A, Starostka D, Walterova L, Adamova D, Kessler P, Brejcha M, Vonke I, Obernauerova J, Valentova K, Adam Z, Minarik J, Straub J, Gumulec J, Ho AD, Hillengass J, Goldschmidt H, Maisnar V, Hose D (2014) Prediction of progression of smouldering into therapy requiring multiple myeloma by easily accessible clinical factors [in 527 Patients]. Blood 124(21):2071–2071

22. Fernández de Larrea C, Isola I, Cibeira MT, Rosiñol L, Calvo X, Tovar N, Elena M, Magnano L, Aróstegui JI, Rozman M, Yagüe J, Bladé J (2014) Smoldering multiple myeloma: impact of the evolving pattern on early progression. Blood 124(21):3363–3363

23. Mateos MV, San Miguel JF (2013) New approaches to smoldering myeloma. Curr Hematol Malig Rep. doi:10.1007/s11899-013-0174-1

Part II
Multiple Myeloma

Vision Statement for Multiple Myeloma: Future Directions

Kenneth C. Anderson

Abstract

There has been great progress in the management and patient outcome in multiple myeloma due to the use of novel agents including immunomodulatory drugs and proteasome inhibitors; nonetheless, novel agents remain an urgent need. The three promising Achilles heels or vulnerabilities to be targetted in novel therapies include: protein degradation by the ubiquitin proteasome or aggresome pathways; restoring autologous antimyeloma immunity; and targeting aberrant biology resulting from constitutive and ongoing DNA damage in tumour cells. Scientifically based therapies targeting these vulnerabilities used early in the disease course, ie smouldering multiple myeloma, have the potential to significantly alter the natural history and transform myeloma into a chronic and potentially curable disease.

Keywords

Multiple myeloma · Targetted therapies · Immune therapies · Protein degradation

1 Introduction

Advances in biology, genomics, epigenetics, and immunity have transformed our understanding of the etiology and pathogenesis of multiple myeloma, allowing for delineation of those mechanisms both intrinsic to the tumor cell and in the host

K.C. Anderson (✉)
Jerome Lipper Multiple Myeloma Center, Dana-Farber Cancer Institute,
Harvard Medical School, Boston, USA
e-mail: kenneth_anderson@dfci.harvard.edu

© Springer International Publishing Switzerland 2016
A.M. Roccaro and I.M. Ghobrial (eds.), *Plasma Cell Dyscrasias*,
Cancer Treatment and Research 169, DOI 10.1007/978-3-319-40320-5_2

whereby monoclonal gammopathy of undetermined significance progresses to smoldering multiple myeloma and to active myeloma. Within myeloma, an unprecedented level of genetic heterogeneity and genomic instability has been defined, as well as clonal evolution underlying progression of disease [6, 33, 36]. The parallel development of in vitro and in vivo models of myeloma in its bone marrow milieu has facilitated the identification of mechanisms mediating myeloma cell homing to the bone marrow, growth, survival, and drug resistance, as well as egress to extramedullary sites [26, 28]. Taken together, these advances have allowed for the identification and targeting of Achilles heals or vulnerabilities in myeloma, directly leading to a transformation in therapeutic efficacy and patient outcome [4, 5, 12]. In the future, we will treat earlier in the disease course, at a time when patients are asymptomatic, to prevent the development of active disease using well-tolerated drug combination therapies targeting these Achilles heals. Myeloma will then be transformed to a chronic illness and ultimate cure.

2   Excess Protein Production

The first example of an Achilles heal in myeloma is due to their synthesis of excess monoclonal protein, which can either be degraded via the proteasomal or aggresomal cascade or secreted [25]. The development of the proteasome inhibitor Bortezomib demonstrated that primarily targeting the constitutive chymotryptic activity could achieve clinical responses in relapsed refractory myeloma, and it is now a standard component of initial and maintenance treatments. Furthermore, delineation of its mechanism of action has shown that it targets the tumor cell, tumor-host interaction, as well as bone marrow milieu and accessory cells [24]. Importantly, preclinical studies have informed the rational use of combination therapies, such as bortezomib with lenalidomide to trigger both intrinsic and extrinsic apoptotic signaling [38].

Bortezomib has already provided the framework for the development of second generation proteasome inhibitors carfilzomib [45, 46, 49], ixazomib [10, 30, 39], and marizomib [7, 9, 15], and also led to ongoing current efforts to target the ubiquitin proteasome cascade upstream of the proteasome with inhibitors of deubiquitylating enzymes [11, 48] or of the proteasome ubiquitin receptor to overcome proteasome inhibitor resistance. These preclinical and clinical studies have validated targeting the ubiquitin proteasome cascade for therapeutic application in myeloma.

When the proteasomal degradation pathway is inhibited, there is a compensatory upregulation of the aggresomal degradation pathway [25]. The latter can be blocked by either pan histone deacetylase inhibitors [17, 43] or by histone deacetylase six selective inhibitors [44], since the ubiquitinated misfolded protein binds to histone deacetylase 6, which in turn binds to the dynein tubulin carrier complex, thereby shuttling the protein load to the aggresome for its degradation. Already broad class I/II histone deacetylase inhibitors vorinostat [17] and panobinostat [43] have been combined with bortezomib to block the aggresomal and proteasomal degradation of protein, respectively. While the response rates and progression free survival are prolonged with combination therapy, side effects of the broad acting histone deacetylase inhibitors preclude their use for long-term benefit. Ricolinostat is a histone deacetylase 6 selective inhibitor with a more favorable tolerability profile [44] and therefore can be readily combined with proteasome inhibitors to allow for long-term blockade of both aggresomal and proteasomal degradation pathways.

3   The Host Immunosuppressive Environment

A second Achilles heal in myeloma is the immunosuppressive environment in the host. In this case, targeting the vulnerability consists of strategies to restore host anti-myeloma immunity. There are five strategies, which when combined will markedly improve patient outcome: immunomodulatory drugs, monoclonal antibodies, checkpoint inhibitors, vaccines, and cellular therapies.

Lenalidomide and other immunomodulatory drugs target cereblon [29, 35] and trigger the degradation of alios and ikaros gene products, thereby upregulating transcription of interleukin 2 and interferon gamma genes [18]. They upregulate cytolytic T cell, natural killer cell, and natural killer cell-T cell anti-MM immunity, while at the same time inhibiting aberrant increased regulatory T cell function in myeloma [20, 23]. Lenalidomide is now incorporated into initial, salvage, and maintenance therapies worldwide.

The search for therapeutic monoclonal antibodies in myeloma has been ongoing for decades, and is now coming to fruition. For example, elotuzumab targets SLAMF-7 on the multiple myeloma surface, mediating complement dependent and antibody dependent cellular cytotoxicity [47]. This antibody also targets natural killer cells and enhances their activity. Although single agent clinical trials of elotuzumab saturated SLAMF-7 sites on tumor cells, only stable disease and no clinical responses were observed. Importantly, preclinical studies showed that lenalidomide augments antibody dependent cellular cytotoxicity [47], and combination lenalidomide elotuzumab therapy of relapsed myeloma has markedly prolonged progression free survival in patients with relapsed myeloma [34, 40], providing the basis for its regulatory approval.

The second antibody example is anti-CD38 monoclonal antibodies daratumumab [16, 31] and SAR650984 [27]. CD38 was originally described as T 10 antigen expressed on activated T, B, natural killer, myeloid, and monocytoid cells, as well as endothelial cells and hematopoietic progenitor cells. Due to its broad expression, it was not developed therapeutically based on fears that there may not be an acceptable therapeutic window or index. Remarkably, anti-CD38 monoclonal antibody daratumumab achieves responses as a single agent in relapsed refractory myeloma; and as with elotuzumab, the combination of daratumumab with lenalidomide markedly augments clinical response.

Checkpoint inhibitors are the third immune targeted treatment approach in myeloma. Myeloma cells express PD-L1, as do plasmacytoid dendritic cells [8, 37] and myeloid-derived suppressor cells [21, 22] which both promote myeloma cell growth and drug resistance as well as downregulate host immune response. T, natural killer, and natural killer-T cells in myeloma express PD-1. Checkpoint blockade with anti-PD-L1 monoclonal antibody may therefore have broader effects than anti-PD-1 monoclonal antibody. Recent preclinical data shows that lenalidomide downregulates PD-L1 on myeloma cells, plasmacytoid dendritic cells, and myeloid derived suppressor cells; as well as downregulates PD-1 expression on immune effector T, natural killer, and T-natural killer cells [22]. Importantly, the combination of checkpoint inhibitors and lenalidomide markedly augments cytolytic response, another example of combination immune therapies.

The fourth example of immune therapies is vaccines. In myeloma two examples are peptide-based vaccines being evaluated to prevent progression of patients with smoldering multiple myeloma to active myeloma [1–3]; and myeloma-dendritic cell-based vaccines now in clinical trials to treat minimal residual disease post autologous stem cell transplant and improve patient outcome [41, 42]. In both cases, vaccines have achieved immune responses in patients against their own myeloma cells. The addition of lenalidomide in preclinical studies can augment this response [22], and the combination of vaccine with lenalidomide strategy is currently under evaluation in both settings. Moreover, checkpoint inhibitor therapy can similarly augment response to vaccination [3], setting the stage for combination vaccine, lenalidomide, and checkpoint inhibitor clinical trials, with the goal of achieving central and effector memory cell autologous anti-myeloma immunity.

Finally, adoptive cellular therapies represent a fifth immune strategy, exemplified by CART cells. The strategy of genetically activating host T cells to target tumor specific antigens, expanding them ex vivo, and transfusing them back to the patient has already achieved remarkable responses in leukemias and lymphomas. In myeloma, the optimal antigens are not defined; BCMA, SLAMF-7, and CD19 are among those under evaluation. A single patient with high-risk relapsed myeloma refractory to all known therapies has recently achieved a molecular complete response after CD19 CART therapy [19]. As a further example of combination therapy, she is receiving lenalidomide to prevent T cell exhaustion.

Thus the second Achilles heal in patients with myeloma is immunosuppression, which can be overcome by these and other related strategies. The ability in particular to achieve memory cell immunity in patients against their own myeloma is very promising, given the ability of host immunity to potently, selectively, and adaptively target ongoing genomic evolution underlying myeloma progression.

4   Genomic Abnormalities

The third Achilles heal in myeloma is predicated upon genomic analyses [6, 32, 33, 36]. To date, profiling of myeloma genomics and epigenomics has revealed a very heterogeneous and complex baseline status, with many abnormalities and multiple clones even at diagnosis. Moreover, further genomic and epigenomic changes and clonal evolution underlie relapse of disease. Ongoing attempts are targeting abnormalities with targeted single or combination agents; however, the lack of predominant abnormalities in myeloma, coupled with the genomic instability and evolution, represents a major obstacle to these approaches. However, genomic and epigenomic patient profiling analyses can identify those critical pathways which can then be targeted to abrogate aberrant biology.

The first example stems from our recent genomic study showing that a subset of patients with myeloma, leukemia, and lymphoma has decreased copy number and expression of YAP-1 [13]. In myeloma cells with constitutive genomic instability and DNA damage, a DNA damage response is initiated in which ABL-1 binds to nuclear YAP-1, thereby triggering p73-mediated apoptosis of damaged cells in a p53-independent process. Restoration of YAP-1 in vitro or in vivo can restore this apoptotic signaling and response. Importantly, YAP-1 expression is inhibited in these tumor cells by increased expression of STK4; and conversely, genetic depletion of STK4 can upregulate YAP-1 and related p73-mediated apoptosis. Efforts are ongoing at present to develop therapeutic STK4 inhibitors to treat this subset of patients.

A second example of a genomically-based Achilles heal is in those patient whose myeloma expresses very high levels of c-Myc [14]. In this patient subset, there are two processes that represent vulnerabilities to be targeted. First, there is a DNA damage response ongoing which can be targeted, i.e., with ATR inhibitors. Second, there is an abundance of reactive oxygen species, which can be further increased pharmacologically. We have shown that either inhibiting ATR or augmenting reactive oxygen species can trigger apoptosis in this subset of myeloma, and that the combination induces synergistic cytotoxicity.

These examples therefore utilize genomic studies to define critical pathways for therapeutic targeting.

5   Summary and Future Directions

There has been a paradigm shift in the treatment and outcome of myeloma based upon improved understanding of the biology of the myeloma cell in the host bone marrow microenvironment. Already increasing genomic and epigenomic understanding in myeloma has identified Achilles heals to target therapeutically. Importantly, multiple strategies for restoring host anti-myeloma immunity represent overcoming an additional Achilles heal in the host. Ultimately, combination targeted and immune therapies used early in the disease course offer the real potential for long-term disease-free survival and cure.

References

1. Bae J, Smith R, Daley J et al (2012) Myeloma-specific multiple peptides able to generate cytotoxic T lymphocytes: a potential therapeutic application in multiple myeloma and other plasma cell disorders. Clin Cancer Res 17:4850–4860
2. Bae J, Rao P, Voskertchian A et al (2015) A multiepitope of XBP-1, CD138, and CS1 peptides induces myeloma-specific cytotoxic T lymphocytes in T cells of smoldering myeloma patients. Leukemia 29:218–229

3. Bae J, Keskin D, Cowens K et al (in press) Lenalidomide polarizes Th1 specific anti-tumor response and expands XBP-1 antigen-specific central memory CD3 + CD8 + T cells against various solid tumors. Leukemia

4. Bianchi G, Richardson PR, Anderson KC (2014) Best treatment strategies in high-risk multiple myeloma: navigating a gray area. J Clin Oncol 32:2125–2132

5. Bianchi G, Richardson PG, Anderson KC (2015) Promising therapies in multiple myeloma. Blood 16:300–310

6. Bolli N, Avet-Loiseau H, Wedge DC et al (2014) Heterogeneity of somatic mutations, clonal architecture and genomic evolution in multiple myeloma. Nat Commun 5:2997

7. Chauhan D, Catley L, Li G et al (2005) A novel orally active proteasome inhibitor induces apoptosis in multiple myeloma cells with mechanisms distinct from Bortezomib. Cancer Cell 8:407–419

8. Chauhan D, Singh AV, Brahmandam M et al (2009) Functional interaction of plasmacytoid dendritic cells with multiple myeloma cells: a novel therapeutic target. Cancer Cell 16:309–323

9. Chauhan D, Singh A, Richardson P et al (2009) Combination of novel proteasome inhibitor NPI-0052 and lenalidomide trigger in vivo synergistic cytotoxicity in multiple myeloma. Blood 115:834–845

10. Chauhan D, Tian Z, Zhou B et al (2011) In vitro and in vivo selective antitumor activity of a novel orally bioavailable proteasome inhibitor MLN9708 against multiple myeloma cells. Clin Cancer Res 17:5311–5321

11. Chauhan D, Tian Z, Nicolson B et al (2012) A novel small molecule inhibitor of ubiquitin-specific protease-7 induces apoptosis in multiple myeloma cells and overcomes bortezomib resistance. Cancer Cell 22:345–358

12. Cottini F, Anderson KC (2015) Novel therapeutic targets in multiple myeloma. Clin Adv Hematol Oncol 13:236–248

13. Cottini F, Hideshima T, Xu C et al (2014) Rescue of YAP1 triggers DNA damage-induced apoptosis in hematological cancers. Nat Med 20:599–606

14. Cottini F, Hideshima T, Suzuki R et al (2015) Synthetic lethal approaches exploiting DNA damage in aggressive myeloma. Cancer Discov 5:972–87

15. Das DS, Ray A, Song Y et al (2015) Synergistic anti-myeloma activity of a proteasome inhibitor marizomib and immunomodulatory drug pomalidomide. Br J Haematol 171:798–812

16. de Weers M, Yu-Tzu Tai, van der Veer MS et al (2011) Daratumumab, a novel therapeutic human CD38 monoclonal antibody, induces killing of multiple myeloma and other hematological tumors. J Immunol 186:1840–1848

17. Dimopoulos M, Jagannath S, Yoon S-Y et al (2013) Vantage 088: an international, multicenter, randomized double-blind study of vorinostat (MK-0683) or placebo in combination with bortezomib in patients with multiple myeloma. Lancet Oncol 14:1129–1140

18. Gandhi AK, Kang J, Havens CG et al (2014) Immunomodulatory agents lenalidomide and pomalidomide co-stimulate T cells by inducing degradation of T cell repressors Ikaros and Aiolos via modulation of the E3 ubiquitin ligase complex CRL4(CRBN.). Br J Haematol 164:811–821

19. Garfall AL, Maus MV, Hwang WT et al (2015) Chimeric antigen receptor T cells against CD19 for multiple myeloma. N Engl J Med 373:1040–1047

20. Gorgun G, Calabrese E, Soydan E et al (2010) Immunomodulatory effects of lenalidomide and pomalidmide on interaction of tumor and bone marrow accessory cells in multiple myleoma. Blood 116:3227–3237

21. Gorgun G, Whitehill G, Anderson JL et al (2012) Tumor promoting immune suppressive myeloid derived suppressor cells in multiple myeloma microenvironment. Blood 121:2975–2987

22. Gorgun G, Samur MK, Cowens KB et al (2015) Lenalidomide enhances immune checkpoint blockade induced immune response in multiple myeloma. Clin Cancer Res 21:4607–18

23. Hideshima T, Chauhan D, Shima Y et al (2000) Thalidomide and its analogues overcome drug resistance of human multiple myeloma cells to conventional therapy. Blood 96:2943–2950
24. Hideshima T, Richardson P, Chauhan D et al (2001) The proteasome inhibitor PS-341 inhibits growth, induces apoptosis, and overcomes drug resistance in human multiple myeloma cells. Cancer Res 61:3071–3076
25. Hideshima T, Bradner J, Wong J et al (2005) Small molecule inhibition of proteasome and aggresome function induces synergistic anti-tumor activity in multiple myeloma. Proc Natl Acad Sci 102:8567–8572
26. Hideshima T, Mitsiades C, Tonon G et al (2007) Understanding multiple myeloma pathogenesis and the role of bone marrow microenvironment to identify new therapeutic targets. Nat Rev Cancer 7:585–598
27. Jiang H, Acharya C, An G et al (2016) SAR650984 directly induces multiple myeloma cell death via lysosomal-associated and apopototic pathways, which is further enhanced by pomalidomide. Leukemia 30:399–408
28. Kawano Y, Moschetta M, Manier S et al (2015) Targeting the bone marrow microenvironment in multiple myeloma. Immunol Rev 263:160–172
29. Kronke J, Udeshi ND, Narla A et al (2014) Lenalidomide causes selective degradation of IKZF1 and IKZF3 in multiple myeloma cells. Science 343:301–305
30. Kumar SK, Bensinger WI, Zimmerman TM et al (2014) Phase 1 study of weekly dosing with the investigational oral proteasome inhibitor ixazomib in relapsed/refractory multiple myeloma. Blood 124:1047–1055
31. Laubach JP, Tai YT, Richardson PG, Anderson KC (2014) Daratumumab granted breakthrough drug status. Expert Opin Investig Drugs 23:445–452
32. Lichter DI, Danaee H, Pickard MD et al (2012) Sequence analysis of β-subunit genes of the 20S proteasome in patients with relapsed multiple myeloma treated with bortezomib or dexamethasone. Blood 120:4513–4516
33. Lohr JG, Stojanov P, Carter SL et al (2014) Widespread genetic heterogeneity in multiple myeloma: implications for targeted therapy. Cancer Cell 25:1–10
34. Lonial S, Dimopoulos Palumbo A et al (2015) Elotuzumab therapy for relapsed or refractory multiple myeloma. N Engl J Med 373:621–631
35. Lu G, Middleton RE, Sun H et al (2014) The myeloma drug lenalidomide promotes the cereblon-dependent destruction of Ikaros proteins. Science 343(6168):305–309
36. Rashid N, Sperling A, Bolli N, Wedge D, Van Loo P, Tai Y-T, Shammas M, Fulciniti M, Smur M, Richardson P, Magrangeas F, Minvielle S, Futreal P, Anderson K, Avet-Loiseau H, Campbell P, Parmigiani G, Munshi N (2014) Differential and limited expression of mutant alleles in multiple myeloma. Blood 124:3110–3117
37. Ray A, Das DS, Song Y, Richardson P, Chauhan D, Anderson KC (2015) Targeting PD1-PDL1 in immune checkpoint in plasmacytoid dendritic cell interactions with T cells, natural killer cells, and multiple myeloma cells. Leukemia 29: 1441–1444
38. Richardson PG, Weller E, Lonial S et al (2010) Lenalidomide, bortezomib, and dexamethasone combination therapy in patients with newly-diagnosed multiple myeloma. Blood 116:679–686
39. Richardson PG, Moreau P, Laubach JP et al (2015) The investigational proteasome inhibitor ixazomib for the treatment of multiple myeloma. Future Oncol 11:1153–1168
40. Richardson PG, Jagannath S, Moreau P et al (2015) Elotuzumab in combination with lenalidomide and dexamethasone in patients with relapsed multiple myeloma: final results from the 1703 phase 1b/2, open-label, randomized study. Lancet Oncol 2:e516–27
41. Rosenblatt J, Vasir B, Uhl L et al (2011) Vaccination with DC/tumor fusion cells results in cellular and humoral anti-tumor immune responses in patients with multiple myeloma. Blood 117:393–402
42. Rosenblatt J, Avivi I, Vasir B et al (2013) Vaccination with dendritic cell/tumor fusions following autologous stem cell transplant induces immunologic and clinical responses in multiple myeloma patients. Clin Cancer Res 19:3640–3648

43. San Miguel JF, Richardson PG, Gunther A et al (2013) A Phase Ib study of panobinostat and bortezomib in relapsed or relapsed and refractory multiple myeloma. J Clin Oncol 31:3696–3703
44. Santo A, Hideshima T, Li-Jen Kung A et al (2012) Preclinical activity, pharmacodynamic and pharmacokinetic properties of a selective HDAC6 inhibitor, ACY-1215, in combination with bortezomib in multiple myeloma. Blood 119:2579–2589
45. Siegel DS, Martin T, Wang M et al (2012) A phase 2 study of single-agent carfilzomib in patients with relapsed and refractory multiple myeloma. Blood 120:2817–2825
46. Stewart AK, Rajkumar SV, Dimopoulos MA et al (2015) Carfilzomib, lenalidomide, and dexamethasone for relapsed multiple myeloma. N Engl J Med 372:142–152
47. Tai Y-T, Dillon M, Song W et al (2008) Anti-CS-1 humanized monoclonal antibody HuLuc63 inhibits myeloma cell adhesion and induces antibody-dependent cellular cytotoxicity in the bone marrow milieu. Blood 112:1329–1337
48. Ze Tian, D'Arcy P, Wang X et al (2014) A novel small molecule inhibitor of deubiquitylating enzyme USP14 and UCHL5 induces apoptosis in myeloma cells and overcomes bortezomib resistance. Blood 123:706–716
49. Vij R, Wang M, Kaufman JL et al (2012) An open-label, single-arm, phase 2 (PX-171-004) study of single-agent carfilzomib in bortezomib-naive patients with relapsed and/or refractory multiple myeloma. Blood 119:5661–5670

Genomic Aberrations in Multiple Myeloma

Salomon Manier, Karma Salem, Siobhan V. Glavey, Aldo M. Roccaro and Irene M. Ghobrial

Abstract

Multiple myeloma (MM) is a genetically complex disease. The past few years have seen an evolution in cancer research with the emergence of next-generation sequencing (NGS), enabling high throughput sequencing of tumors—including whole exome, whole genome, RNA, and single-cell sequencing as well as genome-wide association study (GWAS). A few inherited variants have been described, counting for some cases of familial disease. Hierarchically, primary events in MM can be divided into hyperdiploid (HDR) and nonhyperdiploid subtypes. HRD tumors are characterized by trisomy of chromosomes 3, 5, 7, 9, 11, 15, 19, and/or 21. Non-HRD tumors harbor IGH translocations, mainly t(4;14), t(6;14), t(11;14), t(14;16), and t(14;20). Secondary events participate to the tumor progression and consist in secondary translocation involving *MYC*, copy number variations (CNV) and somatic mutations (such as mutations in KRAS, NRAS, BRAF, P53). Moreover, the dissection of clonal heterogeneity helps to understand the evolution of the disease. The following review provides a comprehensive review of the genomic landscape in MM.

S. Manier · K. Salem · S.V. Glavey · A.M. Roccaro · I.M. Ghobrial (✉)
Medical Oncology, Dana-Farber Cancer Institute, Harvard Medical School, Boston, USA
e-mail: irene_ghobrial@dfci.harvard.edu

S. Manier
Department of Hematology, Lille Hospital University, Lille, France

A.M. Roccaro
Department of Hematology, CREA Laboratory, ASST-Spedali Civili di Brescia, Brescia, BS, Italy

© Springer International Publishing Switzerland 2016
A.M. Roccaro and I.M. Ghobrial (eds.), *Plasma Cell Dyscrasias*,
Cancer Treatment and Research 169, DOI 10.1007/978-3-319-40320-5_3

Keywords
Genomics · Next-generation sequencing · Myeloma · Clonal evolution

1 Introduction

Multiple myeloma (MM) is a genetically complex and heterogeneous disease resulting from a multiple genomic events leading to tumor development and progression. Uncovering and dissecting true driver events in MM might provide rational for new potential targets and therapeutic option in the disease. All MM are preceded by a monoclonal gammopathy of undetermined significance (MGUS) and smoldering myeloma (SMM). This model of the disease provides a framework to understand the genomic hierarchy in MM. Events found at MGUS stages are likely to be primary events and involved in tumor development, in contrary, events present at the MM stage and absent in MGUS are likely to be secondary events leading to tumor progression. Similarly, the study of clonal heterogeneity—defining clonal or subclonal genomic events helps also to dissect the phylogeny of tumors. Hierarchically, primary events are usually divided into hyperdiploid (HDR) and non-hyperdiploid subtypes. HRD tumors are characterized by trisomy of chromosomes 3, 5, 7, 9, 11, 15, 19, and/or 21. Non-HRD tumors harbor IGH translocations, mainly t(4;14), t(6;14), t(11;14), t(14;16), and t(14;20). Secondary events are required for tumor progression. Most of the copy number variations (CNV), *MYC* translocations and somatic mutations in MAPK, NFkB, and DNA repair pathways are only seen at MM stages and not in premalignant stages—so potential secondary events. However, the distinction between driver and passenger events is a current challenge to interpret correctly the genomic landscape of MM.

2 Inherited Variants

Although lifestyle or environmental exposures have not been consistently linked to the incidence of MM, there seems to be a two to fourfold elevated risk of MM in relatives of individuals with the disease [1]. This has been postulated to be a consequence of the co-inheritance of multiple low-risk variants. Investigating these families further and performing genome-wide association studies (GWAS) on large patient populations, three genetic loci were associated with a modest but increased risk of developing MM. These include 3p22.1 (rs1052501, in ULK4), 7p15.3 (rs4487645, surrounding by DNAH11 and CDCA7L) and 2p23.3 (rs6746082, surrounding by DNMT3A and DTNB) [2]. A follow-up study by the same group, including 4,692 individuals with MM and 10,990 controls, revealed four new loci: 3q26.2 (rs10936599, surrounding by MYNN and TERC), 6p21.33 (rs2285803 in PSORS1C2), 17p11.2 (rs4273077 in TNFRSF13B) and 22q13.1 (rs877529 in CBX7) [3]. These seven identified loci provide further evidence for an inherited genetic susceptibility to MM and reportedly account for ~ 13 % of the familial risk of MM. The complete functional role of each of these candidate genes remains to be elucidated. The authors found no association between genotypes and the expression level of their genes. Interestingly, in another GWAS study, the same team identified a strong association between the variant rs603965, responsible for c807G > A polymorphism in *CCND1* and the translocation t(11;14)(q13;q32), in which CCND1 is placed under the control of the immunoglobulin heavy (IGH) chain enhancer [4]. In this model, a constitutive genetic factor is associated with risk of a specific chromosomal translocation. Based on these initial studies, it is likely that more susceptibility loci will be identified in the future and possibly correlated to specific MM subtypes. For example, it has been largely reported that African-Americans have a higher risk of developing MM than Caucasians; however, no potential genetic variants have been identified to date [5]. Moreover, uncovering the functional role of these 7 SNPs significantly associated with MM might help to advance our understanding of MM oncogenesis.

3 Chromosomal Translocations

In MM, the large majority of chromosomal translocations involve chromosome 14, and specifically the IGH locus on 14q32.33, placing a partner gene under the control of the IGH enhancer. These translocations are generated by abnormal class switch recombination (CSR) events and are usually present in all clonal cells. They are also detectable in monoclonal gammopathy of unknown significance (MGUS), consistent with their early development in MM oncogenesis. Five major chromosomal partners—t(4;14), t(6;14), t(11;14), t(14;16), and t(14;20)—seem to impart a selective advantage to the clone by up regulating expression of specific oncogenes— *MMSET* and *FGFR3, CCND3, CCND1, MAF,* and *MAFB*, respectively [6]. It is likely that all these translocations lead to deregulation in the cell cycle G1/S transition, which has been described as a key early molecular abnormality in MM. This can be direct through t(11;14) and t(6;14) deregulating CCND1 and CCND3, respectively [7, 8]. In t(14;16), this is modulated through MAF which up regulates CCND2 by directly binding to its promoter [9] while in t(4;14), the exact mechanism is still uncertain but the translocation of FGFR3 and MMSET to the IGH enhancer is known to also up regulate CCND2 [6]. Recently, mutations involving the *MYC* locus have been identified in MM.

Translocation (4;14) is observed in about 15 % of MM cases [10] and has been associated with an adverse prognosis in a variety of clinical settings [11–14]. The juxtaposition results in deregulation in the expression of FGFR3 and MMSET/WHSC1 [15]. The breakpoints all reside between FGFR3 and MMSET resulting in overexpression of FGFR3 in 70 % of the cases and MMSET in all cases [16–18]. MMSET is a methyl-transferase protein, whose up regulation leads to the methylation of histone H3K36, thus regulates expression of several genes [19]. MMSET has been shown also to regulate histone H4K20 methylation and recruit 53BP1 at DNA damage sites [20]. FGFR3 is a tyrosine kinase receptor oncogene activated by mutations in several solid tumor types. Notably, FGFR3 is up regulated in only 70 % of patients with the translocation because of an unbalanced translocation with loss of the telomeric part of chromosome 4, bearing FGFR3 [12, 17, 21]. This suggests that MMSET is the main molecular target of the translocation. Interestingly, despite the poor prognosis associated with t(4;14), a survival advantage in these patients has been demonstrated through early treatment with the proteasome inhibitor Bortezomib [22, 23].

Translocation (6;14) is a rare translocation present in only about 2 % of MM patients [10] and results in the direct up regulation of *CCND3* via juxtaposition to the *IGH* enhancers [8, 11]. The breakpoints are all located 5' of the gene [16]. The overall prognostic impact of this translocation is neutral [24].

Translocation (11;14) is the most frequent translocation cited as being present in about 15–20 % of patients with MM [7]. Normally B cells express cyclin D2 and D3 but not D1. However, due to the translocation juxtaposing *CCND1* to the *IGH* enhancer, its expression is deregulated. The breakpoints seem to be located 5' of *CCND1* [16]. In terms of prognosis, this translocation is considered as neutral, however, Walker et al. recently showed that in 10 % of t(11;14) a *CCND1* mutation co-occurs and the combination is associated with a poor prognosis when compared with non-mutated t(11;14) patients [25].

Translocation (14;16) is estimated to be present in about 5–10 % of patients with MM and results in the overexpression of the *MAF* oncogene splice variant c-MAF, a transcription factor which up regulates a number of genes, including *CCND2* by binding directly to its promoter [9, 26]. Breakpoints are located 3' of *MAF* within the last exon of *WWOX*, a known tumor suppressor [16]. Though t(14;16) was associated with a poor prognosis in a number of clinical series [13, 27], a more recent retrospective multivariable analysis on 1003 newly diagnosed MM patients showed t(14;16) is not associated with a poor prognosis [27].

Translocation (14;20) is present in about 1 % of patients and is the rarest translocation of the major five. It results in up regulation of the *MAF* gene paralog *MAFB*. According to microarray studies, *MAFB* overexpression results in a similar gene expression profile (GEP) as that seen with *c-MAF* [11], implying common downstream targets including CCND2. The translocation is associated with a poor prognosis when present in MM but interestingly correlates to long-term stable disease when found in precursor conditions like MGUS and smoldering MM (SMM) [28]. This suggests that the translocation itself is not responsible for the poor prognosis but additional genetic events are likely required to accumulate imparting this negative prognosis.

MYC translocations have been recently identified in a cohort of 463 whole exome sequencing including extra baits on the *MYC* locus. MYC translocations were found in 85 patients (18.4 %). Partner genes include *IGH, IGL* and *IGK* loci, as well as *FAM46C, FOXO3, BMP6* and rarely *XBP1, TXNDC5, CCND1,* and *CCND3*. These translocations lead to significant overexpression of *MYC*, probably resulting from juxtaposition of super-enhancers surrounding the partner gene to *MYC* locus. *MYC* translocations are associated with a poor outcome [25].

4 Hyperdiploidy

Hyperdiploidy (HRD) is defined as a number of chromosomes between 48 and 74. HRD MM are characterized by multiple chromosomal gains, preferentially trisomy of chromosomes 3, 5, 7, 9, 11, 15, 19, and 21 [29]. The mechanism underlying this is not known but one hypothesis suggests that the gain of multiple whole chromosomes occurs during a single catastrophic mitosis rather than through the serial gain of chromosomes over time [30]. Nearly half of MGUS and MM tumors are hyperdiploid. Only a few HRD tumors have a co-existing primary IgH translocation—about 10 % of the cases—whereas non-HRD tumors usually have an IgH translocation [31]. Interestingly, in case with coexistent HRD and IGH translocations, HRD may precede IGH translocations in a proportion of patients, as revealed by single-cell sequencing analysis [32]. In terms of signaling pathways, HRD tumors display biological heterogeneity. Some harbor high expression of proliferation-associated genes while others are characterized by genes involved in tumor necrosis factor/nuclear factor-κB (TNF/NFκB) signaling pathway [33]. HRD is associated with a more favorable outcome in general [34], however, coexistent adverse cytogenetic lesions (del 17p, t(4;14) and gain of 1q) shorten survival in MM patients with HDR tumors [32].

5 Copy Number Variations

Copy number variations (CNVs) represent a common feature of MM and are thought to be secondary events, involved in tumor progression. CNVs result from gain and loss of DNA at both a focal level or of an entire chromosome arm. Similarly to single nucleotide mutations, CNVs are probably both driver and passenger events. Highly frequent and recurrent CNVs are likely to be driver, suggesting that the minimal amplified or deleted regions contain important genes involved in the development and progression of MM [35–39].

1q Gain: Duplication of the long arm of chromosome 1 is present in 35–40 % of patients [36, 40–43]. This is known to have an adverse effect on overall survival [44]. Gain of 1q21, detected with a specific probe for *CKS1B*, is an independent prognostic factor and remains when other adverse cytogenetic lesions that frequently coexist are removed [36, 44]. Though the relevant genes on 1q have not yet been fully explored, a minimally amplified region was identified between 1q21.1 and 1q23.3 containing 679 genes. Among these candidate oncogenes are *CKS1B*, *ANP32E*, *BCL9*, and *PDZK1* [36, 44, 45]. Of these genes, *ANP32E*, a protein phosphatase 2A inhibitor involved in chromatin remodeling and transcriptional regulation is of particular interest and has been shown to be independently associated with shortened survival [36]. These findings reinforce the role of gain of 1q in MM pathogenesis and suggest that patients with this type of CNV may benefit from specific inhibitors of these candidate genes and pathways that have been identified.

1p Deletion: Deletions of 1p are observed in approximately 30 % of MM patients and are associated with poor prognosis [36, 46, 47]. Two regions of the 1p arm are of interest in MM pathogenesis when deleted: 1p12 and 1p32.3. 1p12 contains the candidate tumor suppressor gene *FAM46C* whose expression has been correlated to that of ribosomal proteins and eukaryotic initiation/elongation factors involved in protein translation [48]. This gene has been shown to be frequently mutated in MM and has been independently correlated with a poor prognosis [36, 42, 46, 48]. Region 1p32.3 may be hemi- and homozygously deleted and contains the two target genes *CDKN2C* and *FAF1*. *CDKN2C* is a cyclin-dependent kinase 4 inhibitor involved in negative regulation of the cell cycle, whereas *FAF1* encodes a protein involved in initiation and enhancement of apoptosis through the Fas pathway. Deletion 1p is associated with adverse overall survival [49].

13q Deletion: Monosomy of the long arm of chromosome 13 is present in about 45–50 % of patients and is commonly associated with nonhyperdiploid tumors [24, 50–52]. In approximately 85 % of cases, deletion of chromosome 13 constitutes a monosomy or loss of the q arm, whereas in the remaining 15 % various interstitial deletions occur [50, 53]. Chromosome 13 has been extensively investigated as a prognostic factor and as a location of tumor suppressor genes. The minimally deleted region lies between 13q14.11–13q14.3 and contains 68 genes including *RB1*, *EBPL*, *RNASEH2B*, *RCBTB2*, and the microRNA miR-16-1 and miR-15a [36]. Molecular studies have shown that the tumor suppressor gene *RB1* is significantly under expressed in these deletions and may result in inferior negative cell cycle regulation [36]. Establishing the prognostic significance of deletion 13 is challenging because it is frequently associated with other high risk cytogenetic lesions such as t(4;14) [43]. As such, the historic link between deletion 13 and poor prognosis is a surrogate of its association with high-risk lesions.

17p Deletion: Most of chromosome 17 deletions are hemizygous and of the whole p arm, a genetic event observed in around 10 % of newly diagnosed MM cases with the frequency increasing in later stages of the disease [13, 54]. The minimally deleted region includes the tumor suppressor gene *TP53*. While cases without del(17p) have a rate of *TP53* mutation that is <1 %, cases with the deletion show a higher rate of mutation at 25–37 % [55]—suggesting that mono-allelic 17p deletion contributes to the disruption of the remaining allele. The *TP53* gene, which has been mapped to 17p13, is known to function as a transcriptional regulator influencing cell cycle arrest, DNA repair, and apoptosis in response to DNA damage. Loss of 17p is associated with an adverse overall survival [36]. The deletion is also linked to an aggressive disease phenotype, a greater degree of extra-medullary disease, and shortened survival [13, 24, 56].

6 Somatic Mutations

The generalization of next-generation sequencing a few years ago has enabled high throughput whole exome sequencing in several cancers, including MM. The frequency of somatic mutations in MM is at the median across cancer types, with an average of 1.6 mutations per Mb, as compare to less than 0.5/Mb in pediatric cancer, such as rhabdoid tumor or Ewing sarcoma, and about 10/Mb in melanoma and lung cancer [57]. In 2011, Chapman et al. reported whole genome sequencing (WGS) of 23 patients and whole exome sequencing (WES) of 16 patients with MM [48]. By comparing sequences from each tumor to its corresponding normal germline sample, researchers were able to identify tumor-specific mutations. Significantly mutated genes included three that were previously reported as being implicated in MM: *KRAS*, *NRAS*, and *TP53* as well as two newly described genes *FAM46C* and *DIS3*.

Several new oncogenic mechanisms were suggested by the pattern of somatic mutations across this data set. Nearly, half the patients showed mutations of genes involved in protein translation. One of these is the *DIS3* gene, also known as *RRP44*, which encodes a highly conserved RNA exonuclease and serves as the catalytic component of the exosome complex involved in regulating the processing and abundance of all RNA species [58, 59]. *DIS3* mutations, postulated to be loss of function, cluster in the enzyme's catalytic pocket and lead to the deregulation of protein translation as an oncogenic mechanism. Another significantly mutated gene, *FAM46C*, is less well characterized but thought to be functionally related to the regulation of translation.

The same team next reported a massively parallel sequencing of 203 patients with MM—including the 38 patients previously studied [60]. Beyond the five significantly mutated genes previously described, Lohr et al. identified another six significantly mutated genes (*BRAF*, *TRAF3*, *PRDM1*, *CYLD*, *RB1*, and *ACTG1*). Overall in this study, 65 % of the patients had mutations in one or more of the 11 recurrently mutated genes.

Similarly to *KRAS* and *NRAS*, *BRAF* is a known oncogene playing a role in regulating the MAP kinase pathway. Strikingly, mutations in *KRAS*, *NRAS*, and *BRAF* can be both clonal and subclonal. However, if mutations in these genes sometimes coexist in the same tumor, they are almost never simultaneously clonal indicating that they probably rarely occur in the same clone but rather in different subclones. In contrast, *KRAS* and *DIS3* mutations are reported to be often simultaneously clonal and therefore probably co-occurring in the same clone.

TRAF3 and *CYLD* are part of the NFkB pathway—which is also the case for 9 other mutated genes of significance in this cohort (*BTRC*, *CARD11*, *IKBKB*, *MAP3K1*, *MAP3K14*, *RIPK4*, *TLR4*, and *TNFRSF1A*)—reaffirming the central role of the NFkB pathway in MM.

Another significantly mutated gene is *PRDM1* (also called *BLIMP1*), a transcription factor involved in plasma cell differentiation. Loss of function mutations of *BLIMP1* occurs in diffuse large B cell lymphoma [61, 62]. The oncogene *IRF4*, a transcriptional regulator of *PRDM1* was also frequently mutated in addition to mutations seen in *PRDM1* itself.

Almost concomitantly, Bolli et al. reported a WES and copy number analysis of 84 MM samples [63]. They identified two new recurrently mutated genes, *SP140* and *LTB*. *SP140* is a lymphoid restricted homolog of *SP100* that encodes a nuclear body protein implicated in antigen response of mature B cells, and is truncated in several cases. *LTB*, a type II membrane protein of the TNF family involved in lymphoid development, also harbor truncated mutations.

Finally, Boyle et al. reported a WES of 463 patients enrolled in a large UK phase III clinical trial (ASH 2015, abstract #637), bringing the list to 15 significantly mutated genes, comprising *KRAS*, *NRAS*, *TP53*, *FAM46C*, *DIS3*, *BRAF*, *HIST1H1E*, *RB1*, *EGR1*, *TRAF3*, *LTB*, *CYLD*, *IFR4*, *MAX*, and *FGFR3*. Interestingly, mutations in RAS (43 % of the cases) and NFkB (17 % of the cases) are prognostically neutral. In contrast, mutations in *CCND1* and the DNA repair pathway (*TP53*, *ATM*, *ATR*, and *ZFHX4*) are associated with a negative impact on survival in contrast to those in *IRF4* and *EGR1* that are associated with a favorable overall survival.

The identification of driver mutations in MM holds great promise for personalized medicine, whereby patients with particular mutations would be treated with the appropriate targeted therapy. However, if the mutation is present in only a fraction of the cells, one might doubt whether such targeted therapy would be clinically efficacious.

7 Clonal Heterogeneity in Multiple Myeloma

In addition to the genetic complexity in MM, intra-clonal heterogeneity has emerged as a further level of complexity. Analyzing clonal heterogeneity by WES, Lohr et al. report that most patients harbor at least three detectable subclones with some having as many as seven, thus reaffirming that MM tumors are highly heterogeneous. Their finding that tumors contain on average at least five subclones is even an underestimation of the clonal diversity in MM as their method only allowed for the detection of subclones representing at least 10 % of the entire tumor sample [60].

It has become clear that following disease initiation, the steps necessary for MM development do not occur through a linear fashion but rather via branching, nonlinear pathways as proposed by Darwin in explaining the evolution of species. This idea is based on the notion that mutations occur randomly and are selected and propagated based on the clonal survival advantage that they confer [64, 65]. A phenomenon of parallel evolution whereby independent but not far-related clones might acquire similar mutations conferring important growth or survival advantages. This is revealed in single-cell level studies showing the same genetic pathway (RAS/MAPK) altered more than once within the same tumor but in divergent clones evolving separately [66]. In a series of t(11;14) MM, evidence for the persistence of the earliest MM progenitor cell clone was found with two cases characterized by the presence of a subclone carrying t(11;14) as the sole abnormality validating that this translocation is an early event in myeloma pathogenesis [66]. The clonal diversity is present at all the stages of the disease. Although less genetically complex than MM, the premalignant stages MGUS and SMM harbor clonal heterogeneity [67]. By studying sequential samples of SMM and overt MM, it was shown that the predominant clone of MM is already present at the SMM stage.

8 Conclusion

MM is genetically complex and heterogeneous disease, combining primary events, secondary events and clonal diversity, leading to tumor development and progression from MGUS to late stages of MM. It is likely that many driver events need to co-occur for MM development and progression. This genomic complexity is a challenge toward the cure of MM. In the past few years, a tremendous amount of information has been revealed by next-generation sequencing of MM tumors. If we have at present a good comprehension of the genomic landscape in MM at presentation, the near future should provide some insights regarding premalignant stages and resistance to treatment.

References

1. Altieri A, Chen B, Bermejo JL, Castro F, Hemminki K (2006) Familial risks and temporal incidence trends of multiple myeloma. Eur J Cancer 42(11):1661–1670
2. Broderick P, Chubb D, Johnson DC et al (2012) Common variation at 3p22.1 and 7p15.3 influences multiple myeloma risk. Nat Genet 44(1):58–61
3. Chubb D, Weinhold N, Broderick P et al (2013) Common variation at 3q26.2, 6p21.33, 17p11.2 and 22q13.1 influences multiple myeloma risk. Nat Genet 45(10):1221–1225
4. Weinhold N, Johnson DC, Chubb D et al (2013) The CCND1 c.870G > A polymorphism is a risk factor for t(11;14)(q13;q32) multiple myeloma. Nat Genet 45(5):522–525
5. Landgren O, Graubard BI, Katzmann JA et al (2014) Racial disparities in the prevalence of monoclonal gammopathies: a population-based study of 12,482 persons from the national health and nutritional examination survey. Leukemia 28(7):1537–1542
6. Bergsagel PL, Kuehl WM, Zhan F, Sawyer J, Barlogie B, Shaughnessy J Jr (2005) Cyclin D dysregulation: an early and unifying pathogenic event in multiple myeloma. Blood 106 (1):296–303
7. Chesi M, Bergsagel PL, Brents LA, Smith CM, Gerhard DS, Kuehl WM (1996) Dysregulation of cyclin D1 by translocation into an IgH gamma switch region in two multiple myeloma cell lines. Blood 88(2):674–681
8. Shaughnessy J Jr, Gabrea A, Qi Y et al (2001) Cyclin D3 at 6p21 is dysregulated by recurrent chromosomal translocations to immunoglobulin loci in multiple myeloma. Blood 98(1):217–223
9. Hurt EM, Wiestner A, Rosenwald A et al (2004) Overexpression of c-maf is a frequent oncogenic event in multiple myeloma that promotes proliferation and pathological interactions with bone marrow stroma. Cancer Cell 5(2):191–199
10. Prideaux SM, Conway O'Brien E, Chevassut TJ (2014) The genetic architecture of multiple myeloma. Adv Hematol 2014:864058
11. Zhan F, Huang Y, Colla S et al (2006) The molecular classification of multiple myeloma. Blood 108(6):2020–2028
12. Keats JJ, Reiman T, Maxwell CA et al (2003) In multiple myeloma, t(4;14)(p16;q32) is an adverse prognostic factor irrespective of FGFR3 expression. Blood 101(4):1520–1529
13. Fonseca R, Blood E, Rue M et al (2003) Clinical and biologic implications of recurrent genomic aberrations in myeloma. Blood 101(11):4569–4575
14. Chang H, Sloan S, Li D et al (2004) The t(4;14) is associated with poor prognosis in myeloma patients undergoing autologous stem cell transplant. Br J Haematol 125(1):64–68
15. Chesi M, Nardini E, Lim RS, Smith KD, Kuehl WM, Bergsagel PL (1998) The t(4;14) translocation in myeloma dysregulates both FGFR3 and a novel gene, MMSET, resulting in IgH/MMSET hybrid transcripts. Blood 92(9):3025–3034

16. Walker BA, Wardell CP, Johnson DC et al (2013) Characterization of IGH locus breakpoints in multiple myeloma indicates a subset of translocations appear to occur in pregerminal center B cells. Blood 121(17):3413–3419
17. Santra M, Zhan F, Tian E, Barlogie B, Shaughnessy J Jr (2003) A subset of multiple myeloma harboring the t(4;14)(p16;q32) translocation lacks FGFR3 expression but maintains an IGH/MMSET fusion transcript. Blood 101(6):2374–2376
18. Keats JJ, Maxwell CA, Taylor BJ et al (2005) Overexpression of transcripts originating from the MMSET locus characterizes all t(4;14)(p16;q32)-positive multiple myeloma patients. Blood 105(10):4060–4069
19. Martinez-Garcia E, Popovic R, Min DJ et al (2011) The MMSET histone methyl transferase switches global histone methylation and alters gene expression in t(4;14) multiple myeloma cells. Blood 117(1):211–220
20. Pei H, Zhang L, Luo K et al (2011) MMSET regulates histone H4K20 methylation and 53BP1 accumulation at DNA damage sites. Nature 470(7332):124–128
21. Hebraud B, Magrangeas F, Cleynen A et al (2015) Role of additional chromosomal changes in the prognostic value of t(4;14) and del(17p) in multiple myeloma: the IFM experience. Blood 125(13):2095–2100
22. San Miguel JF, Schlag R, Khuageva NK et al (2008) Bortezomib plus melphalan and prednisone for initial treatment of multiple myeloma. N Engl J Med 359(9):906–917
23. Avet-Loiseau H, Leleu X, Roussel M et al (2010) Bortezomib plus dexamethasone induction improves outcome of patients with t(4;14) myeloma but not outcome of patients with del(17p). J Clin Oncol 28(30):4630–4634
24. Avet-Loiseau H, Attal M, Moreau P et al (2007) Genetic abnormalities and survival in multiple myeloma: the experience of the Intergroupe Francophone du Myelome. Blood 109 (8):3489–3495
25. Walker BA, Wardell CP, Murison A et al (2015) APOBEC family mutational signatures are associated with poor prognosis translocations in multiple myeloma. Nat commun 6:6997
26. Hanamura I, Iida S, Akano Y et al (2001) Ectopic expression of MAFB gene in human myeloma cells carrying (14;20)(q32;q11) chromosomal translocations. Jpn J Cancer Res Gann 92(6):638–644
27. Ross FM, Ibrahim AH, Vilain-Holmes A et al (2005) Age has a profound effect on the incidence and significance of chromosome abnormalities in myeloma. Leukemia 19(9):1634–1642
28. Ross FM, Chiecchio L, Dagrada G et al (2010) The t(14;20) is a poor prognostic factor in myeloma but is associated with long-term stable disease in monoclonal gammopathies of undetermined significance. Haematologica 95(7):1221–1225
29. Smadja NV, Fruchart C, Isnard F et al (1998) Chromosomal analysis in multiple myeloma: cytogenetic evidence of two different diseases. Leukemia 12(6):960–969
30. Onodera N, McCabe NR, Rubin CM (1992) Formation of a hyperdiploid karyotype in childhood acute lymphoblastic leukemia. Blood 80(1):203–208
31. Fonseca R, Debes-Marun CS, Picken EB et al (2003) The recurrent IgH translocations are highly associated with nonhyperdiploid variant multiple myeloma. Blood 102(7):2562–2567
32. Pawlyn C, Melchor L, Murison A et al (2015) Coexistent hyperdiploidy does not abrogate poor prognosis in myeloma with adverse cytogenetics and may precede IGH translocations. Blood 125(5):831–840
33. Chng WJ, Kumar S, Vanwier S et al (2007) Molecular dissection of hyperdiploid multiple myeloma by gene expression profiling. Cancer Res 67(7):2982–2989
34. Smadja NV, Bastard C, Brigaudeau C, Leroux D, Fruchart C (2001) Groupe Francais de Cytogenetique H. Hypodiploidy is a major prognostic factor in multiple myeloma. Blood 98 (7):2229–2238
35. Carrasco DR, Tonon G, Huang Y et al (2006) High-resolution genomic profiles define distinct clinico-pathogenetic subgroups of multiple myeloma patients. Cancer Cell 9(4):313–325

36. Walker BA, Leone PE, Chiecchio L et al (2010) A compendium of myeloma-associated chromosomal copy number abnormalities and their prognostic value. Blood 116(15):e56–65
37. Walker BA, Leone PE, Jenner MW et al (2006) Integration of global SNP-based mapping and expression arrays reveals key regions, mechanisms, and genes important in the pathogenesis of multiple myeloma. Blood 108(5):1733–1743
38. Annunziata CM, Davis RE, Demchenko Y et al (2007) Frequent engagement of the classical and alternative NF-kappaB pathways by diverse genetic abnormalities in multiple myeloma. Cancer Cell 12(2):115–130
39. Keats JJ, Fonseca R, Chesi M et al (2007) Promiscuous mutations activate the noncanonical NF-kappaB pathway in multiple myeloma. Cancer Cell 12(2):131–144
40. Hanamura I, Stewart JP, Huang Y et al (2006) Frequent gain of chromosome band 1q21 in plasma-cell dyscrasias detected by fluorescence in situ hybridization: incidence increases from MGUS to relapsed myeloma and is related to prognosis and disease progression following tandem stem-cell transplantation. Blood 108(5):1724–1732
41. Boyd KD, Ross FM, Chiecchio L et al (2012) A novel prognostic model in myeloma based on co-segregating adverse FISH lesions and the ISS: analysis of patients treated in the MRC Myeloma IX trial. Leukemia 26(2):349–355
42. Chang H, Qi X, Jiang A, Xu W, Young T, Reece D (2010) 1p21 deletions are strongly associated with 1q21 gains and are an independent adverse prognostic factor for the outcome of high-dose chemotherapy in patients with multiple myeloma. Bone Marrow Transplant 45 (1):117–121
43. Fonseca R, Bergsagel PL, Drach J et al (2009) International myeloma working group molecular classification of multiple myeloma: spotlight review. Leukemia 23(12):2210–2221
44. Shaughnessy J (2005) Amplification and overexpression of CKS1B at chromosome band 1q21 is associated with reduced levels of p27Kip1 and an aggressive clinical course in multiple myeloma. Hematology 10(Suppl 1):117–126
45. Shi L, Wang S, Zangari M et al (2010) Over-expression of CKS1B activates both MEK/ERK and JAK/STAT3 signaling pathways and promotes myeloma cell drug-resistance. Oncotarget 1(1):22–33
46. Boyd KD, Ross FM, Walker BA et al (2011) Mapping of chromosome 1p deletions in myeloma identifies FAM46C at 1p12 and CDKN2C at 1p32.3 as being genes in regions associated with adverse survival. Clin Cancer Res Official J Am Assoc Cancer Res 17 (24):7776–7784
47. Chang H, Jiang A, Qi C, Trieu Y, Chen C, Reece D (2010) Impact of genomic aberrations including chromosome 1 abnormalities on the outcome of patients with relapsed or refractory multiple myeloma treated with lenalidomide and dexamethasone. Leuk lymphoma 51 (11):2084–2091
48. Chapman MA, Lawrence MS, Keats JJ et al (2011) Initial genome sequencing and analysis of multiple myeloma. Nature 471(7339):467–472
49. Leone PE, Walker BA, Jenner MW et al (2008) Deletions of CDKN2C in multiple myeloma: biological and clinical implications. Clin Cancer Res Official J Am Assoc Cancer Res 14 (19):6033–6041
50. Fonseca R, Oken MM, Harrington D et al (2001) Deletions of chromosome 13 in multiple myeloma identified by interphase FISH usually denote large deletions of the q arm or monosomy. Leukemia 15(6):981–986
51. Avet-Loiseau H, Li JY, Morineau N et al (1999) Monosomy 13 is associated with the transition of monoclonal gammopathy of undetermined significance to multiple myeloma. Intergroupe Francophone du Myelome. Blood 94(8):2583–2589
52. Chiecchio L, Protheroe RK, Ibrahim AH et al (2006) Deletion of chromosome 13 detected by conventional cytogenetics is a critical prognostic factor in myeloma. Leukemia 20 (9):1610–1617

53. Avet-Louseau H, Daviet A, Sauner S, Bataille R (2000) Intergroupe Francophone du M. Chromosome 13 abnormalities in multiple myeloma are mostly monosomy 13. Br J Haematol 111(4):1116–1117
54. Tiedemann RE, Gonzalez-Paz N, Kyle RA et al (2008) Genetic aberrations and survival in plasma cell leukemia. Leukemia 22(5):1044–1052
55. Lode L, Eveillard M, Trichet V et al (2010) Mutations in TP53 are exclusively associated with del(17p) in multiple myeloma. Haematologica 95(11):1973–1976
56. Drach J, Ackermann J, Fritz E et al (1998) Presence of a p53 gene deletion in patients with multiple myeloma predicts for short survival after conventional-dose chemotherapy. Blood 92 (3):802–809
57. Lawrence MS, Stojanov P, Polak P et al (2013) Mutational heterogeneity in cancer and the search for new cancer-associated genes. Nature 499(7457):214–218
58. Dziembowski A, Lorentzen E, Conti E, Seraphin B (2007) A single subunit, Dis3, is essentially responsible for yeast exosome core activity. Nat Struct Mol Biol 14(1):15–22
59. Schmid M, Jensen TH (2008) The exosome: a multipurpose RNA-decay machine. Trends Biochem Sci 33(10):501–510
60. Lohr JG, Stojanov P, Carter SL et al (2014) Widespread genetic heterogeneity in multiple myeloma: implications for targeted therapy. Cancer Cell 25(1):91–101
61. Tam W, Gomez M, Chadburn A, Lee JW, Chan WC, Knowles DM (2006) Mutational analysis of PRDM1 indicates a tumor-suppressor role in diffuse large B-cell lymphomas. Blood 107 (10):4090–4100
62. Pasqualucci L, Compagno M, Houldsworth J et al (2006) Inactivation of the PRDM1/BLIMP1 gene in diffuse large B cell lymphoma. J Exp Med 203(2):311–317
63. Bolli N, Avet-Loiseau H, Wedge DC et al (2014) Heterogeneity of genomic evolution and mutational profiles in multiple myeloma. Nat Commun 5:2997
64. Anderson K, Lutz C, van Delft FW et al (2011) Genetic variegation of clonal architecture and propagating cells in leukaemia. Nature 469(7330):356–361
65. Bahlis NJ (2012) Darwinian evolution and tiding clones in multiple myeloma. Blood 120 (5):927–928
66. Melchor L, Brioli A, Wardell CP et al (2014) Single-cell genetic analysis reveals the composition of initiating clones and phylogenetic patterns of branching and parallel evolution in myeloma. Leukemia 28(8):1705–1715
67. Walker BA, Wardell CP, Melchor L et al (2014) Intraclonal heterogeneity is a critical early event in the development of myeloma and precedes the development of clinical symptoms. Leukemia 28(2):384–390

Epigenetics in Multiple Myeloma

Siobhan V. Glavey, Salomon Manier, Antonio Sacco,
Karma Salem, Yawara Kawano, Juliette Bouyssou,
Irene M. Ghobrial and Aldo M. Roccaro

Abstract

Multiple myeloma is characterized by clonal proliferation of plasma cells within the bone marrow resulting in anemia, lytic bone lesions, hypercalcemia, and renal impairment. Despite advanced in our understanding of this complex disease in recent years, it is still considered an incurable malignancy. This is, in part, due to the highly heterogenous genomic and phenotypic nature of the disease, which is to date incompletely understood. It is clear that a deeper level of knowledge of the biological events underlying the development of these diseases is needed to identify new targets and generate effective novel therapies. MicroRNAs (miRNAs), which are single strand, 20-nucleotide, noncoding RNA's, are key regulators of gene expression and have been reported to exert transcriptional control in multiple myeloma. miRNAs are now recognized to play a role in many key areas such as cellular proliferation, differentiation, apoptosis and stress response. Substantial advances have been made in recent years in terms of our understanding of the biological role of miRNAs in a diverse range of hematological and solid malignancues, In multiple myeloma these advances have yielded new information of prognostic and diagnostic relevance which have helped to shed light on epigenetic regulation in this disease.

Keywords

Epigenetics · Methylation · DNA acetylation · miRNA

S.V. Glavey · S. Manier · A. Sacco · K. Salem · Y. Kawano · J. Bouyssou · I.M. Ghobrial ·
A.M. Roccaro (✉)
Harvard Medical School, Dana-Farber Cancer Institute, Boston, MA, USA
e-mail: aldomaria.roccaro@asst-spedalicivili.it

A.M. Roccaro
Department of Hematology, CREA Laboratory, ASST-Spedali Civili di Brescia,
Brescia, BS, Italy

A.M. Roccaro and I.M. Ghobrial (eds.), *Plasma Cell Dyscrasias*,
Cancer Treatment and Research 169, DOI 10.1007/978-3-319-40320-5_4

1   Genetic Aberration in Multiple Myeloma

Multiple myeloma (MM) is a cytogenetically heterogenous clonal plasma cell disorder preceded by an asymptomatic premalignant stage termed monoclonal gammopathy of undetermined significance "MGUS" [1, 2]. In 2012, 21,700 new MM cases were diagnosed in the United States, accounting for approximately 10 % of all hematological malignancies [3]. MGUS is present in approximately 3 % of the population over 50 years of age, which progresses to MM at a rate of 1 % per year on average [4, 5]. MM as opposed to MGUS is characterized by greater than 10 % plasma cells in the bone marrow and evidence of end organ damage (renal failure, anemia, lytic bone lesions and hypercalcemia). Despite major advances in the last decade in the treatment of MM, it is still considered an incurable disease. The clinical outcome for patients with MM is considerably heterogeneous and depends on a complex interplay of several variables including age, performance status, cytogenetics, and the biological features of the responsible clone.

MM is known to arise from plasma cells, which bear somatic mutations in the variable regions of the immunoglobulin genes following germinal center transit. Alone these cells have a low proliferative rate, and it is thought that precursor cells are responsible for the malignant proliferation of these cells [6]. These abnormal precursor B-cells likely originate in the lymph nodes and migrate to the bone marrow where a microenvironment exists to support their terminal differentiation.

In both MM and MGUS there is evidence of significant acquired chromosomal abnormalities. Two distinct patterns of genetic aberration are recognized, hyperdiploidy with increased numbers of trisomies, and chromosomal translocations in non-hyperdiploid patients [5]. These translocations can lead to deregulation of cyclins and oncogenes, such as FGFR3, MMSET, and MAF. The most frequently involved loci for IgH translocations are 11q13 (*CCND1*) in 15 %, 4p16 (*FGFR3/MMSET*) in 15 %, and 16q23 (*MAF*) in 5 % of cases [7].With progression from MGUS to MM and progression of the MM itself, secondary hits are seen, including chromosomal loss (e.g., 1p deletion, 13q deletion, and 17p deletion with loss of TP53), chromosomal amplification (e.g., 1q), new chromosomal rearrangements (e.g., involving MYC) and mutations (e.g., TP53, KRAS, NRAS, and FGFR3). Knowledge of the genetic events that underlie disease progression in MM is incomplete.

Nevertheless, specific chromosomal abnormalities, such as 17p deletion and 1q amplification are associated with particularly poor prognosis and increased incidence of extramedullary disease. Genetics and epigenetics are inherently linked and in this chapter we will focus on the epigenetics as a mechanism of regulation in this genomically complex disease. There are three main common epigenetic mechanisms that are thought to play a role in MM; aberrant DNA methylation, histone modifications, and noncoding RNA (miRNA) expression.

1.1 DNA Methylation in MM

The methylation of cytosine in the CpG (cytosine-phosphodiester bond-guanine) dinucleotide is the epigenetic mechanism that is most completely understood. DNA methylation occurs at cytosine residues on CpG islands, which are specific genomic regions containing a high frequency of CpG sites [8]. Most CpG islands are located in the proximal promoter regions of genes and are usually methylated in tumor cells, mediating gene silencing [9]. DNA methyltransferases (DNMTs) catalyze the transformation of cytosine to 5-methylcytosine. DNMT's themselves are regulated by noncoding RNAs and interplay between these two mechanisms of epigenetic modification are complex.

Gene promotor site DNA hypermethylation is the predominant mechanism of epigenetic regulation that serves to silence tumor suppressor genes in a wide variety of malignancies [10]. Studies in MM have shown variable DNA methylation patterns with identification of focal hypermethylation patterns in in aggressive subtypes [11]. Like in other malignancies genome wide studies in MM have revealed genome wide hypomethylation with gene specific promoter hypermethylation [12, 13]. In one study methylation subgroups were defined by translocations and hyperdiploidy, with t(4;14) myeloma having the greatest impact on DNA methylation [12]. The mechanism of altered methylation in MM is not fully understood, it is known that expression of DNMT1 is higher in MM plasma cells when compared to their normal counterparts. The concept of stage specific methylation has been explored in several studies and overall it is thought that DNA methylation changes significantly with disease progression [12]. Alterations in methylation may be an early event in myelomagenesis with abberant methylation in MGUS occurring primarily in CpG islands, wheras in MM it seems to occur outside of these regions [13]. Prognostic information arising from the study of epigenetics in MM includes the finding that DMMT3A has been shown to be aberrantly hypermethylated and underexpressed in MM where it is associated with an inferior overall survival [13].

1.2 miRNAs and Cancer

MicroRNAs (miRNAs) are a class of small noncoding RNAs that are implicated in a wide variety of cellular processes, many of which directly contribute to carcinogenesis. This includes regulation of key elements related to cell differentiation, proliferation, apoptosis, and stress response mechanisms. miRNAs are short 20–22 nucleotide RNA molecules that function as negative regulators of gene expression in eukaryotic organisms. miRNA mediated gene silencing pathways play essential roles in cell development, differentiation, proliferation, death, chromosome structure, and virus resistance [14–16]. The hypothesis that miRNAs may play an important role in cancer arose from the discovery that these noncoding RNA's are frequently present in the regions of the genome where cancer related genes such as oncogenes (OG) and tumor suppressor genes (TSG's) are encoded. Further large-scale miRNome analysis of several solid tumors revealed a set of commonly over expressed miRNAs with predicted targets of TSG's and OG's [17].

2   miRNA Synthesis and Function

Most of our current understanding of epigenetic regulation in MGUS and MM stems from studies that have revealed alterations in miRNA expression in these conditions. An understanding of miRNA regulation requires knowledge of the synthesis of these noncoding RNAs, which is outlined here in brief.

The synthesis of miRNA starts with transcription of miRNA genes by RNA polymerase II, which generates long capped, and polyadenylated primary precursor (pri-miRNA). Each pri-miRNA is subsequently processed in the nucleus by a microprocessor complex, which consists of two RNA III endonucleases, Drosha and Dicer, and the dsRNA-binding protein DGCR8/Pasha. The resultant precursor miRNA (pre-miRNA), which is approximately 70-nucleotides in length, is transported to the cytoplasm by exportin 5. Following this the pre-miRNA is cleaved by Dicer, which is an RNase III type endonuclease, to a 20-nucleotide miRNA duplex. The mature miRNA strand of the duplex, along with the Argonaute protein Ago 2, is further assembled into a ribonucleoprotein complex known as RISC, while the other strand is typically degraded. The mature miRNA in complex with RISC is able to recognize its target mRNA's by scanning cellular mRNA. This is accomplished most often via recognition of complementary sequences between the 3' untranslated region (3' UTR) of the mRNA and the 5' end of the miRNA, however, miRNAs have also been shown to bind to the 5' UTR and in the coding sequence of the target mRNA [18]. Typically the result is that the bound mRNA remains untranslated, or less often, is degraded. In both cases the result is a decreased expression of the protein encoded by the target mRNA. miRNAs are highly efficient at gene manipulation as a single miRNA can bind multiple genes and therefore have a plethora of effects on cell biology.

3   miRNA's in Blood Cancers

There are many examples of the role of miRNAs as oncogenes in hematological malignancies—the miR-17-92 cluster, which is transactivated by the c-myc oncogene, produces lymphomagenesis in murine models, miR-155 induces leukemia in transgenic murine models and miR-21, which targets TSG's like PTEN1, is implicated in a variety of neoplasms including MM [19–22].

miRNAs were definitively implicated for the first time in hematological malignancies when it was discovered that in chronic lymphocytic leukemia (CLL) the miR-15a/16-1 structure acts as a TSG by targeting the anti-apoptotic gene BCL-2 [23]. miRNAs have also been shown to have diagnostic and prognostic value in hematological malignancies and therefore miRNA profiling has recently been carried out in plasma cell diseases in order to further elucidate their role [24, 25].

4 Epigenetic Regulation in MGUS

Primary cytogenetic abnormalities are thought to play a major role in the development of MGUS and accumulation of further abnormalities occurs as a driving force in the progression to MM. The majority of MGUS cases are thought to be either driven by hyperdiploidy or aberrant translocation events that affect the immunoglobulin heavy chain (IgH) locus on chromosome 14q32 during class switching (non-hyperdiploid MGUS). The further progression from MGUS to MM is thought to occur as a result of a "second-hit" affecting critical cell cycle regulator genes and OG's such as RAS, p53, NF-kB and others. Understanding the primary differences between the normal plasma cell and that of MGUS could reveal early time point targets that might help prevent the development of the abnormal clone in at risk populations. Recently, due to knowledge gained about the role of miRNAs in cancer, studies evaluating changes in expression during the development of MGUS have been carried out.

A comprehensive study carried out by Pichiorri et al. [26] used miRNA microarrays and quantitative RT-PCR to characterize the miRNA expression in MM cell lines and CD138+ bone marrow plasma cells from patients with MM, MGUS and normal donors, allowing a disease progression profile to be assembled. Forty-eight miRNAs were found to be significantly deregulated in MGUS compared to healthy CD138+ plasma cells, the majority of these were upregulated, with only 7 miRNAs found to be downregulated. The most significantly upregulated miRNAs in MGUS were miR-21, miR-181a, and the oncogenic cluster miR-106b-25 [27]. Chi et al. compared MGUS patient plasma cells to that of healthy controls and MM patients and found that the MGUS cells had an miRNA profile that was more similar to MM than that of a normal plasma cell. Overall 39 miRNAs were deregulated in MGUS cells compared to healthy controls, 28 miRNAs were upregulated and 11 downregulated. Upregulated miRNAs in MGUS included miR-21, miR222, and miR-342 [28].

5 Epigenetic Regulation in MM

Recent studies have pointed toward modulation of enzymes regulating DNA methylation or histone modification as target for miRNAs [29, 30]. Acetylation of histones is a mode of fine control of transcriptional regulation that has been found to be deregulated in many cancers. Hypoacetylation of histones results in a condensed chromatin and reduced gene transcription, with the opposite true of hyperacetylation. The balance is carefully regulated by histone deacetylases (HDAC's) and histone acetyltransferases (HAT's), in cancer and increases in levels of HDAC's can lead to enhanced gene transcription. Aberrant DNA hypermethylation has been proposed to influence the expression of tumor suppressor genes such as SOCS-1 and E-cadherin, in MM cell lines and patients. In the same study hypermethylation at the CpG island promotor site of cyclin dependent kinase inhibitor 2A (CDKN2A) was demonstrated in MM and correlated with a poor prognosis if present at diagnosis [31]. Recently it was effectively demonstrated by Amodio et al. that miRNA manipulation can directly affect the methylation profile of MM cells. In this study miR-29b was shown to target DNMT3A and DNMT3B in MM cells resulting in the downregulation of these genes. Furthermore, an in vivo model, miR-29b mimics produced reduction in tumor growth in an MM xenograft mouse model and demonstrated an ability to overcome the protective effects of BMSC's in an in vivo bone marrow microenvironmental model [32].

Of note, a recent study investigating the effect of methylation on miRNA regulation demonstrated hypermethylation-dependent inhibition of miR-152, -10b-5p, and -34c-3p, which exerts a putative tumor suppressive role in MM [11]. Gain of function studies of these specific miRNAs led to induction of apoptosis and inhibition of proliferation as well as downregulation of putative oncogene targets of these miRNAs such as DNMT1, E2F3, BTRC, and MYCBP. These findings provide the rationale for epigenetic therapeutic approaches in subgroups of MM [11].

Therefore, it is apparent that miRNA targeted therapies have a potential application in MM and as more knowledge accumulates it is likely this will be case.

6 Epigentic Regulation in MGUS Progression

Although the cytogenetic abnormalities that contribute to the pathogenesis of MM have been characterized as the result of genomic studies, the sequence of events that leads to MM development, progression, and ultimately drug resistance is not clear. One such study by Shaughnessy et al. in 2007 produced a validated gene expression model of high risk MM which has been useful in identifying key players in this disease [33]. However, despite these advances and the discovery of "gene signatures" much remains to be explained about the development and progression of MM. Therefore the mechanisms of regulation of key genes in MM pathogenesis have been investigated, including the potential role of miRNAs in this process. Efforts to elucidate the miRNA profile of MM have revealed that there are a number of specific miRNAs that may be playing a role in MM. When comparing CD138+ cells from MM patients to healthy controls Pichiorri et al. found 37 miRNAs to be upregulated along with an equal number of downregulated miRNAs. Similar to MGUS, miR-21 and the cluster miR-106a-92 were also found to be upregulated in MM, however, in addition, upregulation of miR-32 and the Oncomir-1 cluster miR-17-92 was also present which could indicate a possible role in the progression from MGUS to MM [26]. miR-21 was previously implicated in the oncogenic potential of STAT3 in MM where miR-21 induction by STAT3 represents an important survival stimulus for MM cells [34].

Roccaro et al. further defined the deregulation of miRNAs in MM while also elucidating the functional role of specific miRNAs by investigating their target genes [35]. In this study miRNA expression patterns in MM were profiled in CD138+ cells from patients with relapsed/refractory MM in comparison to CD138+ cells isolated from healthy donor bone marrow and MM cell lines. A specific miRNA signature characterizing the disease was identified which was kept with previous studies. Seven miRNAs were found to have specific differential expression patterns between relapsed/refractory MM patients and healthy subjects. Increases in miRNA-222/-221/-382/-181a/-181b were demonstrated along with decreased expression of miRNA-15a and 16. The latter two miRNAs are located on chromosome 13 which when deleted in MM [(del (13)] is associated with reduced survival [36]. miRNA 15a and 16 have previously been reported to have decreased expression in hematological malignancies [23, 37].

Interestingly, it was also demonstrated that miRNA-15a and 16-1 were completely absent in MM patients harboring the 13q deletion. Furthermore, miRNA-15a and 16 regulate the proliferation of MM cells in vitro and in vivo along with being responsible for changes in cell cycle regulatory proteins resulting in G1 arrest. Reduced BCL2, a known target of miRNA-15a and 16, may induce G1 arrest in MM cells which is known to be the case in other malignancies. Other predicted targets of miRNA-15a and 16 found in this study include members of the AKT serine/threonine kinase family (AKT3) along with ribosomal protein S6 and MAP kinases. The impact of miRNA-15a and 16 on these signaling cascades was evaluated in this study and it demonstrated altered proliferation of MM induced by miRNA-15a and 16 was indeed mediated via inhibition of AKT3, ribosomal protein S6, MAP kinases and NF-Kb activator MAP3KIP3. miRNA-15a and -16 inhibit MAP3KIP3 in MM cells, which results in negative regulation of NF-kB signaling via TAK1. As NF-kB activation plays a pivotal role in cell growth and survival, both in MM and other plasma cell dyscrasias, it follows that reduced expression of inhibitors of this pathway may have an important biological role in these diseases [38–41]. Other studies implicating miRNAs in MM disease progression and prognosis include that by Zhou et al. where whole genome microarray analysis of CD138+ cells from newly diagnosed MM patients was used to perform an integrative analysis of both miRNA expression profiles and protein coding gene expression profiles. This revealed global increases in miRNA expression in high-risk disease [42].

Other predicted targets of the miRNAs which were found to be decreased in MM include important cell cycle regulators such as RAS, RET, cyclin D1, cyclin D2, and cyclin E along with pro-angiogenic genes such as bFGF and VEGF. It was shown in this study that MM cell-triggered endothelial cell growth and proliferation in vitro was inhibited by miRNA-15a and 16. VEGF plays a crucial role as a pro-angiogenic cytokine in MM [43], miRNA 15a and 16 are capable of reducing VEGF secretion from MM cells which is likely one of the mechanisms that contributes to their anti-MM activity. Targeting of VEGF by miRNA-15a and 16 has also been confirmed in other studies where inhibition of miR-15a and 16 resulted in reduced angiogenesis in nude mice [44].

Several other studies have confirmed miRNA deregulation in MM and have yielded important information regarding potential mRNA targets. The miR17-92 cluster plays a role in normal B-cell development and its deficiency leads to BCL2-like 11 apoptosis facilitator gene (BIM) over expression inhibiting B-cell development past the pro-B stage [45]. It has been hypothesized that this TSG and others are negatively regulated by increased miR-17-92 cluster expression in MM cells contributing to disease development and progression [27]. Consistent with these findings a study by Chi et al. also found miR-21 to be upregulated in both MM and MGUS as were all seven miRNAs encoded by the miR-17-92 cluster [28]. Unno et al. also reported the upregulation of the miR-17-92 cluster along with miR-106b-25 when comparing MM patient plasma cells and cell lines to healthy controls. Also noted in the study was the upregulation of miR-193b-365 which was not previously reported in hematological malignancies [46], however, has been reported to be upregulated in endometrial and breast cancers [47, 48].

Key regulators of miRNAs have also been found to be altered in MM. Argonaut-2 (AGO2), a master regulator of miRNA activity and B-cell differentiation [49, 50], was found to be upregulated in MM and associated with high-risk disease which supports the hypothesis that miRNA deregulation might be an important mechanism in MM pathobiology [33]. Depletion of AGO2, which effects the processing of miRNAs, is associated with apoptosis induction in MM cells inferring that the miRNAs influenced by this gene may be important players in this disease. Other miRNA processors that have been implicated in MM biology include Dicer which is expressed at higher levels in MGUS than in smoldering or full blown MM. Higher levels of Dicer are associated with improved progression free survival in MM possibly due to impaired miRNA functions [51]. IL-6 is a potent growth factor for MM cells [52]. SOCS1 is a negative regulator of IL-6 and is itself the target of miR-19a/b which leads to its downregulation in MM. Treatment of MM cell lines with miR-19a/b led to reduced MM tumor burden in mice [26] Targeting of the STAT3/IL-6 pathway in MM by miR-19a/b was demonstrated in MM cells [26].

7   miRNAs as Regulators of p53 Activity in MM

As previously mentioned, p53 is a critical TSG in MM and miRNAs that alter the expression of this gene are likely to serve as important prognostic targets in this and other neoplasms. miR-106-25 and miR-32 have the common target of PCAF which is a positive regulator of p53 [53]. Pichiorri et al. postulated that downregulation of PCAF could lead to inhibition of p53 via its histone acetylate function [27]. Other miRNAs that may play a role in p53 modulation in MM include miR-192, 194 and 215 which are downregulated in some cases of MM and can be activated by p53 to then modulate the expression of mouse double minute 2 (MDM2). Overexpression of MDM2 results in excessive inhibition of p53 with consequent loss of its TSG function [54]. miRNA 106a/b, miR-20b and mir-17-5 target Cyclin Dependent Kinase Inhibitor 1A (CDKN1A1) which functions as a regulator of cell cycle progression at G1. The expression of this gene is tightly controlled by the tumor suppressor protein p53, through which this protein mediates p53-dependent cell cycle G1 phase arrest in response to a variety of stress stimuli. Increasing CDKN1A1 gene expression induced by histone deacetylase inhibitors in MM cell lines results in apoptosis [55].

7.1   Histone Modifications in MM

Histones are ubiquitous proteins found in all eukaryotic cells that form the nucleosome as octamers. Each histone octamer consists of a pair of H2A, H2B, H3, and H4, which are tightly conformed around 147 bp of DNA. Positioning of nucleosomes is an epigenetic modification in itself that can regulate gene expression. Post translational modifications of histones occurs via a variety of mechanisms including deamination, phosphorylation, methylation, ubiquitination, and sumoylation all of which can alter the interaction of DNA with histones and this regulate gene expression [56, 57]. As mentioned previously, acetylation and deacetylation are carried out by histone acetyltransferase (HATs) and histone deacetylases (HDACs), respectively. Due to the role of HDACS in regulation of gene expression HDAC inhibitors have emerged as novel therapeutic agents for cancers, including MM. Mechanisms of action whereby HDAC inhibitors trigger anti-MM activities have not yet been fully characterized [58]. Vorinostat and panabinostat are the most widely studied HDAC inhibitors in MM. Vorinostat directly interacts with the catalytic site of HDACs and inhibits their enzymatic activity [58]. Inhibition of HDAC activity by vorinostat results in alteration of gene expression in various cancer cell lines, including MM [59] and vorinostat is known to induce p53 protein expression [60]. Panobinostat is a hydroxamic acid and blocks class I and II HDAC activity [58]. Panobinostat has recently gained FDA approval for relapsed/refractory MM in combination with bortezomib and dexamethasone, indicating that investigation of epigenetic regulation is indeed leading to new targets in this disease [61].

As mentioned previously, MMSET is a histone modifying enzyme that is known to be upregulated in all cases of t(4:14) translocated MM, which accounts for 15 % of all patients. Upregulation of MMSET results in global alterations in histone methylation patterns and constitutive activation of NF-KB. The NF-KB pathway is commonly disrupted in MM. Futhermore inhibition of MMSET in vitro results in reduced proliferation of MM cells [62, 63]. Several studies have shown the relevance of this interaction in MM and are likely to lead to promising targets in the future.

8   Epigenetic Regulation of Key Genes in MM

The most convincing evidence that miRNAs are indeed playing a critical role in MM development and progression, comes from studies demonstrating their role as potent regulators of key MM genes. One of the first studies to implicate deregulated miRNA expression with known MM prognostic genetic abnormalities was that by Gutierrez et al. in 2010 [64]. Amongst their findings was the concomitant expression of higher levels of miR-1 and miR-133a with the t(14;16) translocation in MM, which is known to be associated with a poor prognosis [64, 65].

Another important example is the t(4;14) translocation, which leads to overexpression of histone methyltransferase MMSET promoting the proliferation of MM cells via c-myc activation [36]. When found alone in MM patients the t(4;14) translocation is associated with a significantly reduced survival [66]. miRNA profiling of t(4;14) translocated MM cells identified miR-126 as being regulated by MMSET and predicted to target c-myc mRNA leading to translation inhibition and reduced proliferation [67]. Chi et al. stratified MM patients according to the common cytogenetic abnormalities in MM and identified specific miRNAs that are deregulated in each group. Comparison of MM cases harboring the IgH translocation to those that did not identified a number of deregulated miRNAs including upregulation of miR-590, 886, and 33b [28].

Correlation of miRNA deregulation to chromosomal locations known to be deregulated in MM was also studied by Lionetti et al. [68] and revealed that 16 deregulated miRNAs in MM mapped to chromosomal regions that are known to be altered in MM and implicated in disease pathobiology. This includes miR-22 at the critical location of 17p13.3. Deletion of 17p has been shown to negatively impact event-free and overall survival in MM and is critical target in MM [69]. Other deregulated miRNA's mapping to disease relevant locations included miR-106b and miR-25 at 17q22.1, miR-15a at 13q14.3, miR-21 at 17q23.1 and miR-92b at 1q22, all of which are regions that are found to be altered in MM patients.

Other interesting observations involve intronic miRNAs. Intronic miRNAs are usually orientated in the same direction as the pre-miRNA, which provides an opportunity to study their regulation alongside that of their host genes as they can expect to have coordinate expression and may be under the control of the same regulatory mechanisms. In MM such intronic miRNAs are deregulated in correlation with that of their host genes (miR-335-MEST, miR-342-3p-EVL) and putatively may play a role in plasma cell homing to the bone marrow given their predicted targets of genes responsible for actin polymerization and microtubule formation [70].

9 Epigenetic Regulation of the Bone Marrow Niche in MM

The bone marrow microenvironment in MM provides a supportive niche for MM cells, with growth and survival mediated through adhesion to BMSC's and cytokine-mediated mechanisms [71]. The complex interaction between BMSC's and MM cells has been a major focus of study in an attempt to gain a better understanding of this pro-survival relationship, which is pivotal in MM and a diversity of other neoplasias. In this supportive milieu growth, survival and drug resistance of MM cells is promoted in part through NF-kB, PI3 K/AKT and STAT-3 signaling [72]. The possible contribution of miRNAs to this pro-survival environment was investigated by Roccaro et al. Following pre-miRNA 15-a and 16-1 infection in MM1S cells, significant inhibition of adhesion to BMSC's and reduced migration to SDF-1 was demonstrated in vitro, while in vivo disruption of adhesion of MM cells to bone marrow niche was apparent resulting in reduced tumor burden in mice.

10 Conclusion

Epigentic regulation governs key genetic abberations in MGUS and MM and can be linked prognostically to disease progression. This gives epigenetics a strong footing in this disease as a reference point for target identification in the search for novel therapies in this currently incurable disease and indeed this is reflected in current literature [73].

Conflicts of interest: There are no conflicts of interest for any author.

References

1. Palumbo A, Anderson K (2011) Multiple myeloma. N Engl J Med 364(11):1046–1060
2. Rajkumar SV (2011) Treatment of multiple myeloma. Nat Rev Clin Oncol 8(8):479–491. PubMed PMID: 21522124. Pubmed Central PMCID: 3773461
3. American Cancer Society (2012) Cancer Facts and Figures 2012. Atlanta GACS, 2012
4. Kuehl WM, Bergsagel PL (2002) Multiple myeloma: evolving genetic events and host interactions. Nat Rev Cancer 2(3):175–187. PubMed PMID: 11990854. Epub 2002/05/07. eng
5. Fonseca R, Bergsagel PL, Drach J, Shaughnessy J, Gutierrez N, Stewart AK, et al (2009) International Myeloma Working Group molecular classification of multiple myeloma: spotlight review. Leukemia 23(12):2210–2221. PubMed PMID: 19798094. Pubmed Central PMCID: 2964268. Epub 2009/10/03. eng
6. Matsui W, Huff CA, Wang Q, Malehorn MT, Barber J, Tanhehco Y, et al (2004) Characterization of clonogenic multiple myeloma cells. Blood 103(6):2332–2336. PubMed PMID: 14630803. Pubmed Central PMCID: 3311914
7. Bergsagel PL, Mateos MV, Gutierrez NC, Rajkumar SV, San Miguel JF (2013) Improving overall survival and overcoming adverse prognosis in the treatment of cytogenetically high-risk multiple myeloma. Blood 121(6):884–892. PubMed PMID: 23165477. Pubmed Central PMCID: 3567336
8. Bird A (2002) DNA methylation patterns and epigenetic memory. Genes Dev 16(1):6–21
9. Esteller M (2008) Epigenetics in cancer. N Engl J Med 358(11):1148–1159
10. Jones PA, Baylin SB (2002) The fundamental role of epigenetic events in cancer. Nat Rev Genet 3(6):415–428
11. Zhang W, Wang YE, Zhang Y, Leleu X, Reagan M, Zhang Y, et al (2014) Global epigenetic regulation of microRNAs in multiple myeloma. PloS one 9(10):e110973. PubMed PMID: 25330074. Pubmed Central PMCID: 4201574
12. Walker BA, Wardell CP, Chiecchio L, Smith EM, Boyd KD, Neri A et al (2011) Aberrant global methylation patterns affect the molecular pathogenesis and prognosis of multiple myeloma. Blood 117(2):553–562
13. Heuck CJ, Mehta J, Bhagat T, Gundabolu K, Yu Y, Khan S et al (2013) Myeloma is characterized by stage-specific alterations in DNA methylation that occur early during myelomagenesis. J Immunol 190(6):2966–2975
14. Xie X, Lu J, Kulbokas EJ, Golub TR, Mootha V, Lindblad-Toh K, et al (2005) Systematic discovery of regulatory motifs in human promoters and 3' UTRs by comparison of several mammals. Nature 434(7031):338–345. PubMed PMID: 15735639. Pubmed Central PMCID: 2923337. Epub 2005/03/01. eng

15. Roldo C, Missiaglia E, Hagan JP, Falconi M, Capelli P, Bersani S, et al (2006) MicroRNA expression abnormalities in pancreatic endocrine and acinar tumors are associated with distinctive pathologic features and clinical behavior. J Clin Oncol 24(29):4677–4684. PubMed PMID: 16966691. Epub 2006/09/13. eng

16. He L, Hannon GJ (2004) MicroRNAs: small RNAs with a big role in gene regulation. Nat Rev Genet 5(7):522–531. PubMed PMID: 15211354. Epub 2004/06/24. eng

17. Volinia S, Calin GA, Liu CG, Ambs S, Cimmino A, Petrocca F, et al (2006) A microRNA expression signature of human solid tumors defines cancer gene targets. Proc Natl Acad Sci USA 103(7):2257–2261. PubMed PMID: 16461460. Pubmed Central PMCID: 1413718. Epub 2006/02/08. eng

18. Inui M, Martello G, Piccolo S (2010) MicroRNA control of signal transduction. Nat Rev Mol Cell Biol 11(4):252–263. PubMed PMID: 20216554. Epub 2010/03/11. eng

19. He L, Thomson JM, Hemann MT, Hernando-Monge E, Mu D, Goodson S, et al (2005) A microRNA polycistron as a potential human oncogene. Nature 435(7043):828–833. PubMed PMID: 15944707. Epub 2005/06/10. eng

20. Haidet AM, Rizo L, Handy C, Umapathi P, Eagle A, Shilling C, et al (2008) Long-term enhancement of skeletal muscle mass and strength by single gene administration of myostatin inhibitors. Proc Natl Acad Sci USA 105(11):4318–22. PubMed PMID: 18334646. Pubmed Central PMCID: 2393740. Epub 2008/03/13. eng

21. Cully M, You H, Levine AJ, Mak TW (2006) Beyond PTEN mutations: the PI3K pathway as an integrator of multiple inputs during tumorigenesis. Nat Rev Cancer 6(3):184–192. PubMed PMID: 16453012. Epub 2006/02/03. eng

22. Costinean S, Zanesi N, Pekarsky Y, Tili E, Volinia S, Heerema N, et al (2006) Pre-B cell proliferation and lymphoblastic leukemia/high-grade lymphoma in E(mu)-miR155 transgenic mice. Proc Natl Acad Sci USA 103(18):7024–7029. PubMed PMID: 16641092. Pubmed Central PMCID: 1459012. Epub 2006/04/28. eng

23. Calin GA, Dumitru CD, Shimizu M, Bichi R, Zupo S, Noch E, et al (2002) Frequent deletions and down-regulation of micro-RNA genes miR15 and miR16 at 13q14 in chronic lymphocytic leukemia. Proc Natl Acad Sci USA 99(24):15524–15529. PubMed PMID: 12434020. Pubmed Central PMCID: 137750. Epub 2002/11/16. eng

24. Lawrie CH (2008) MicroRNA expression in lymphoid malignancies: new hope for diagnosis and therapy? J Cell Mol Med 12(5A):1432–1444. PubMed PMID: 18624758. Epub 2008/07/16. eng

25. Lawrie CH, Chi J, Taylor S, Tramonti D, Ballabio E, Palazzo S, et al (2009) Expression of microRNAs in diffuse large B cell lymphoma is associated with immunophenotype, survival and transformation from follicular lymphoma. J Cell Mol Med 13(7):1248–1260. PubMed PMID: 19413891. Epub 2009/05/06. eng

26. Pichiorri F, Suh SS, Ladetto M, Kuehl M, Palumbo T, Drandi D, et al (2008) MicroRNAs regulate critical genes associated with multiple myeloma pathogenesis. Proc Natl Acad Sci USA 105(35):12885–12890. PubMed PMID: 18728182. Pubmed Central PMCID: 2529070

27. Pichiorri F, De Luca L, Aqeilan RI (2011) MicroRNAs: new players in multiple Myeloma. Front Genet 2:22. PubMed PMID: 22303318. Pubmed Central PMCID: 3268577. Epub 2012/02/04. eng

28. Chi J, Ballabio E, Chen XH, Kusec R, Taylor S, Hay D, et al (2011) MicroRNA expression in multiple myeloma is associated with genetic subtype, isotype and survival. Biol Direct 6:23. PubMed PMID: 21592325. Pubmed Central PMCID: 3120802. Epub 2011/05/20. eng

29. Fabbri M, Garzon R, Cimmino A, Liu Z, Zanesi N, Callegari E, et al (2007) MicroRNA-29 family reverts aberrant methylation in lung cancer by targeting DNA methyltransferases 3A and 3B. Proc Natl Acad Sci USA 104(40):15805–15810. PubMed PMID: 17890317. Pubmed Central PMCID: 2000384. Epub 2007/09/25. eng

30. Garzon R, Liu S, Fabbri M, Liu Z, Heaphy CE, Callegari E, et al (2009) MicroRNA-29b induces global DNA hypomethylation and tumor suppressor gene reexpression in acute

myeloid leukemia by targeting directly DNMT3A and 3B and indirectly DNMT1. Blood 113 (25):6411–6418. PubMed PMID: 19211935. Pubmed Central PMCID: 2710934. Epub 2009/02/13. eng

31. Galm O, Wilop S, Reichelt J, Jost E, Gehbauer G, Herman JG et al (2004) DNA methylation changes in multiple myeloma. Leukemia 18(10):1687–1692

32. Amodio N, Leotta M, Bellizzi D, Di Martino MT, D'Aquila P, Lionetti M et al (2012) DNA-demethylating and anti-tumor activity of synthetic miR-29b mimics in multiple myeloma. Oncotarget 3(10):1246–1258

33. Shaughnessy JD Jr, Zhan F, Burington BE, Huang Y, Colla S, Hanamura I, et al (2007) A validated gene expression model of high-risk multiple myeloma is defined by deregulated expression of genes mapping to chromosome 1. Blood 109(6):2276–2284. PubMed PMID: 17105813. Epub 2006/11/16. eng

34. Loffler D, Brocke-Heidrich K, Pfeifer G, Stocsits C, Hackermuller J, Kretzschmar AK et al (2007) Interleukin-6 dependent survival of multiple myeloma cells involves the Stat3-mediated induction of microRNA-21 through a highly conserved enhancer. Blood 110 (4):1330–1333

35. Roccaro AM, Sacco A, Thompson B, Leleu X, Azab AK, Azab F, et al (2009) MicroRNAs 15a and 16 regulate tumor proliferation in multiple myeloma. Blood 113(26):6669–6680. PubMed PMID: 19401561. Pubmed Central PMCID: 2710922

36. Fonseca R, Blood E, Rue M, Harrington D, Oken MM, Kyle RA, et al (2003) Clinical and biologic implications of recurrent genomic aberrations in myeloma. Blood 101(11):4569–4575. PubMed PMID: 12576322. Epub 2003/02/11. eng

37. Chen RW, Bemis LT, Amato CM, Myint H, Tran H, Birks DK, et al (2008) Truncation in CCND1 mRNA alters miR-16–1 regulation in mantle cell lymphoma. Blood 112(3):822–829. PubMed PMID: 18483394. Pubmed Central PMCID: 2481543. Epub 2008/05/17. eng

38. Annunziata CM, Davis RE, Demchenko Y, Bellamy W, Gabrea A, Zhan F, et al (2007) Frequent engagement of the classical and alternative NF-kappaB pathways by diverse genetic abnormalities in multiple myeloma. Cancer Cell 12(2):115–130. PubMed PMID: 17692804. Pubmed Central PMCID: 2730509. Epub 2007/08/19. eng

39. Hideshima T, Chauhan D, Richardson P, Mitsiades C, Mitsiades N, Hayashi T, et al (2002) NF-kappa B as a therapeutic target in multiple myeloma. J Biol Chem 277(19):16639–16647. PubMed PMID: 11872748. Epub 2002/03/02. eng

40. Leleu X, Eeckhoute J, Jia X, Roccaro AM, Moreau AS, Farag M, et al (2008) Targeting NF-kappaB in Waldenstrom macroglobulinemia. Blood 111(10):5068–5077. PubMed PMID: 18334673. Pubmed Central PMCID: 2384134. Epub 2008/03/13. eng

41. Keats JJ, Fonseca R, Chesi M, Schop R, Baker A, Chng WJ, et al (2007) Promiscuous mutations activate the noncanonical NF-kappaB pathway in multiple myeloma. Cancer Cell 12 (2):131–144. PubMed PMID: 17692805. Pubmed Central PMCID: 2083698. Epub 2007/08/19. eng

42. Zhou Y, Chen L, Barlogie B, Stephens O, Wu X, Williams DR, et al (2010) High-risk myeloma is associated with global elevation of miRNAs and overexpression of EIF2C2/AGO2. Proc Natl Acad Sci USA. 107(17):7904–7909. PubMed PMID: 20385818. Pubmed Central PMCID: 2867889. Epub 2010/04/14. eng

43. Ria R, Vacca A, Russo F, Cirulli T, Massaia M, Tosi P, et al (2004) A VEGF-dependent autocrine loop mediates proliferation and capillarogenesis in bone marrow endothelial cells of patients with multiple myeloma. Thromb Haemost 92(6):1438–1445. PubMed PMID: 15583754. Epub 2004/12/08. eng

44. Sun CY, She XM, Qin Y, Chu ZB, Chen L, Ai LS et al (2013) miR-15a and miR-16 affect the angiogenesis of multiple myeloma by targeting VEGF. Carcinogenesis 34(2):426–435

45. Ventura A, Young AG, Winslow MM, Lintault L, Meissner A, Erkeland SJ, et al (2008) Targeted deletion reveals essential and overlapping functions of the miR-17 through 92 family of miRNA clusters. Cell 132(5):875–886. PubMed PMID: 18329372. Pubmed Central PMCID: 2323338. Epub 2008/03/11. eng

46. Unno K, Zhou Y, Zimmerman T, Platanias LC, Wickrema A (2009) Identification of a novel microRNA cluster miR-193b-365 in multiple myeloma. Leuk Lymphoma 50(11):1865–1871. PubMed PMID: 19883314. Pubmed Central PMCID: 2774220. Epub 2009/11/04. eng

47. Yan LX, Huang XF, Shao Q, Huang MY, Deng L, Wu QL, et al (2008) MicroRNA miR-21 overexpression in human breast cancer is associated with advanced clinical stage, lymph node metastasis and patient poor prognosis. RNA 14(11):2348–2360. PubMed PMID: 18812439. Pubmed Central PMCID: 2578865

48. Wu W, Lin Z, Zhuang Z, Liang X (2009) Expression profile of mammalian microRNAs in endometrioid adenocarcinoma. Eur J Cancer Prev 18(1):50–55. PubMed PMID: 19077565. Epub 2008/12/17. eng

49. O'Carroll D, Mecklenbrauker I, Das PP, Santana A, Koenig U, Enright AJ, et al (2007) A Slicer-independent role for Argonaute 2 in hematopoiesis and the microRNA pathway. Genes Dev 21(16):1999–2004. PubMed PMID: 17626790. Pubmed Central PMCID: 1948855. Epub 2007/07/14. eng

50. Diederichs S, Haber DA (2007) Dual role for argonautes in microRNA processing and posttranscriptional regulation of microRNA expression. Cell 131(6):1097–1108. PubMed PMID: 18083100. Epub 2007/12/18. eng

51. Sarasquete ME, Gutierrez NC, Misiewicz-Krzeminska I, Paiva B, Chillon MC, Alcoceba M, et al (2011) Upregulation of Dicer is more frequent in monoclonal gammopathies of undetermined significance than in multiple myeloma patients and is associated with longer survival in symptomatic myeloma patients. Haematologica 96(3):468–471. PubMed PMID: 21160068. Pubmed Central PMCID: 3046281. Epub 2010/12/17. eng

52. Zhang XG, Klein B, Bataille R (1989) Interleukin-6 is a potent myeloma-cell growth factor in patients with aggressive multiple myeloma. Blood 74(1):11–13. PubMed PMID: 2787674. Epub 1989/07/01. eng

53. Linares LK, Kiernan R, Triboulet R, Chable-Bessia C, Latreille D, Cuvier O, et al (2007) Intrinsic ubiquitination activity of PCAF controls the stability of the oncoprotein Hdm2. Nat Cell Biol 9(3):331–338. PubMed PMID: 17293853. Epub 2007/02/13. eng

54. Pichiorri F, Suh SS, Rocci A, De Luca L, Taccioli C, Santhanam R, et al (2010) Downregulation of p53-inducible microRNAs 192, 194, and 215 impairs the p53/MDM2 autoregulatory loop in multiple myeloma development. Cancer Cell 18(4):367–381. PubMed PMID: 20951946. Pubmed Central PMCID: 3561766. Epub 2010/10/19. eng

55. Lavelle D, Chen YH, Hankewych M, DeSimone J (2001) Histone deacetylase inhibitors increase p21(WAF1) and induce apoptosis of human myeloma cell lines independent of decreased IL-6 receptor expression. Am J Hematol 68(3):170–178

56. Kouzarides T (2007) Chromatin modifications and their function. Cell 128(4):693–705

57. Lavrov SA, Kibanov MV (2007) Noncoding RNAs and chromatin structure. Biochem Biokhimiia 72(13):1422–1438

58. Hideshima T, Anderson KC (2013) Histone deacetylase inhibitors in the treatment for multiple myeloma. Int J Hematol 97(3):324–332

59. Mitsiades CS, Mitsiades NS, McMullan CJ, Poulaki V, Shringarpure R, Hideshima T, et al (2004) Transcriptional signature of histone deacetylase inhibition in multiple myeloma: biological and clinical implications. Proc Natl Acad Sci USA 101(2):540–545. PubMed PMID: 14695887. Pubmed Central PMCID: 327183

60. Mitsiades N, Mitsiades CS, Richardson PG, McMullan C, Poulaki V, Fanourakis G et al (2003) Molecular sequelae of histone deacetylase inhibition in human malignant B cells. Blood 101(10):4055–4062

61. (2015) Panobinostat approved for multiple myeloma. Cancer Discov 5(5):OF4. PubMed PMID: 25802326

62. Marango J, Shimoyama M, Nishio H, Meyer JA, Min DJ, Sirulnik A, et al (2008) The MMSET protein is a histone methyltransferase with characteristics of a transcriptional corepressor. Blood 111(6):3145–3154. PubMed PMID: 18156491. Pubmed Central PMCID: 2265454

63. Huang Z, Wu H, Chuai S, Xu F, Yan F, Englund N et al (2013) NSD2 is recruited through its PHD domain to oncogenic gene loci to drive multiple myeloma. Cancer Res 73(20):6277–6288

64. Gutierrez NC, Sarasquete ME, Misiewicz-Krzeminska I, Delgado M, De Las Rivas J, Ticona FV, et al (2010) Deregulation of microRNA expression in the different genetic subtypes of multiple myeloma and correlation with gene expression profiling. Leukemia 24 (3):629–37. PubMed PMID: 20054351. Epub 2010/01/08. eng

65. Munshi NC, Anderson KC, Bergsagel PL, Shaughnessy J, Palumbo A, Durie B, et al (2011) Consensus recommendations for risk stratification in multiple myeloma: report of the International Myeloma Workshop Consensus Panel 2. Blood 117(18):4696–4700. PubMed PMID: 21292777. Pubmed Central PMCID: 3293763. Epub 2011/02/05. eng

66. Gutierrez NC, Castellanos MV, Martin ML, Mateos MV, Hernandez JM, Fernandez M et al (2007) Prognostic and biological implications of genetic abnormalities in multiple myeloma undergoing autologous stem cell transplantation: t(4;14) is the most relevant adverse prognostic factor, whereas RB deletion as a unique abnormality is not associated with adverse prognosis. Leukemia 21(1):143–150

67. Min DJ, Ezponda T, Kim MK, Will CM, Martinez-Garcia E, Popovic R, et al (2012) MMSET stimulates myeloma cell growth through microRNA-mediated modulation of c-MYC. Leukemia. PubMed PMID: 22972034. Epub 2012/09/14. Eng

68. Lionetti M, Agnelli L, Mosca L, Fabris S, Andronache A, Todoerti K, et al (2009) Integrative high-resolution microarray analysis of human myeloma cell lines reveals deregulated miRNA expression associated with allelic imbalances and gene expression profiles. Genes Chromosomes Cancer 48(6):521–531. PubMed PMID: 19306352. Epub 2009/03/24. eng

69. Neben K, Jauch A, Bertsch U, Heiss C, Hielscher T, Seckinger A, et al (2010) Combining information regarding chromosomal aberrations t(4;14) and del(17p13) with the International Staging System classification allows stratification of myeloma patients undergoing autologous stem cell transplantation. Haematologica95(7):1150–1157. PubMed PMID: 20220069. Pubmed Central PMCID: 2895040. Epub 2010/03/12. eng

70. Ronchetti D, Lionetti M, Mosca L, Agnelli L, Andronache A, Fabris S, et al (2008) An integrative genomic approach reveals coordinated expression of intronic miR-335, miR-342, and miR-561 with deregulated host genes in multiple myeloma. BMC Med Genomics 1:37. PubMed PMID: 18700954. Pubmed Central PMCID: 2531129. Epub 2008/08/15. eng

71. Mitsiades CS, Mitsiades NS, Munshi NC, Richardson PG, Anderson KC (2006) The role of the bone microenvironment in the pathophysiology and therapeutic management of multiple myeloma: interplay of growth factors, their receptors and stromal interactions. Eur J Cancer 42 (11):1564–1573. PubMed PMID: 16765041. Epub 2006/06/13. eng

72. Katz BZ (2010) Adhesion molecules—the lifelines of multiple myeloma cells. Semin Cancer Biol 20(3):186–195 PubMed PMID: 20416379. Epub 2010/04/27. eng

73. Pawlyn C, Kaiser MF, Davies FE, Morgan GJ (2014) Current and potential epigenetic targets in multiple myeloma. Epigenomics 6(2):215–228

Role of Endothelial Cells and Fibroblasts in Multiple Myeloma Angiogenic Switch

Domenico Ribatti and Angelo Vacca

Abstract

Multiple myeloma (MM) mainly progresses in bone marrow (BM). Therefore, signals from the BM microenvironment are thought to play a critical role in maintaining plasma cell growth, migration, and survival. Reciprocal positive and negative interactions between plasma cells and microenvironmental cells, including endothelial cells (ECs) and fibroblasts may occur. The BM neovascularization is a constant hallmark of MM, and goes hand in hand with progression to leukemic phase. Microenvironmental factors induce MMECs and fibroblasts to become functionally different from monoclonal gammopathy of undetermined significance (MGUS) ECs (MGECs), i.e., to acquire an overangiogenic phenotype, and be similar to transformed cells. These alterations play an important role in MM progression and may represent new molecular markers for prognostic stratification of patients and prediction of response to antiangiogenic drugs, as well as new potential therapeutic targets.

D. Ribatti (✉)
Department of Basic Medical Sciences, Neurosciences and Sensory Organs, Section of Human Anatomy and Histology, University of Bari Medical School "Aldo Moro", Piazza G. Cesare, 11, 70124 Bari, Italy
e-mail: domenico.ribatti@uniba.it

D. Ribatti
National Cancer Institute, Giovanni Paolo II, Bari, Italy

A. Vacca (✉)
Department of Biomedical Sciences and Human Oncology (DIMO), Section of Internal Medicine "G. Baccelli", University of Bari Medical School "Aldo Moro", Piazza Giulio Cesare, 11, 70124 Bari, Italy
e-mail: angelo.vacca@uniba.it

© Springer International Publishing Switzerland 2016
A.M. Roccaro and I.M. Ghobrial (eds.), *Plasma Cell Dyscrasias*,
Cancer Treatment and Research 169, DOI 10.1007/978-3-319-40320-5_5

Keywords
Angiogenesis · Antiangiogenesis · Endothelial cells · Fibroblasts · Multiple myeloma

1 Tumor Microenvironment

Tumor microenvironment plays an important role in the initiation and progression of tumors [2]. Individuals affected by chronic inflammatory pathologies have increased risk of cancer development [1], and, accordingly, treatment with nonsteroidal antiinflammatory drugs reduces the incidence of several cancer [23].

The bone marrow (BM) is a primary lymphoid organ involved in B lymphocyte production as well as T cell precursor generation. In hematological malignancies, the BM represents the paradigmatic anatomical site in which tumor microenvironment expresses its morphofunctional features. The BM microenvironment includes hematopoietic stem cells (HSCs) and nonhematopoietic cells. HSCs give rise to all the blood cell types of the myeloid and lymphoid lineages [26]. The nonhematopoietic cells include endothelial cells, pericytes, fibroblasts, osteoblasts, osteoclasts, macrophages, mast cells, and mesenchymal stem cells (MSCs) [24]. All these cells constitute specialized niches, closed to the endosteum, named osteoblast or endosteal niche, or to the BM vasculature, named vascular niche [65].

Inflammatory cells in tumor microenvironment communicate via a complex network of intercellular signaling pathways, mediated by surface adhesion molecules, cytokines, and their receptors [46]. Immune cells cooperate and synergize with microenvironmental cells as well as malignant cells in stimulating tumor angiogenesis which is an important mechanism for tumor development and metastatic spread since it provides efficient vascular supply and easy pathway to escape.

Among inflammatory cells found in tumor microenvironment, tumor-associated macrophages and mast cells support tumor growth and neovascularization by production and secretion of a wide variety of angiogenic cytokines, including tumor necrosis factor alpha (TNF-α), transforming growth factor beta 1 (TGF-β1), fibroblast growth factor-2 (FGF-2), vascular endothelial growth factor (VEGF), platelet-derived growth factor (PDGF), interleukin-8 (IL-8), osteopontin, and nerve growth factor (NGF). On the contrary, macrophage- and mast cell-produced cytokines that may participate in antitumor response include interleukin (IL)-1, IL-2, IL-4, IL-10, and interferon gamma (IFN-γ) [44].

2 Angiogenesis in Multiple Myeloma

Under physiological conditions, angiogenesis depends on the balance of positive and negative angiogenic modulators within the vascular microenvironment. Tumor angiogenesis is linked to a switch in this balance, and mainly depends on the release by tumor cells of growth factors specific for endothelial cells and able to stimulate the growth of the host's blood vessels [45]. Numerous clinical studies have shown that the degree of angiogenesis or the levels of angiogenic factors are correlated with the extent of disease stage, prognosis, or response to therapy, suggesting that angiogenesis induction in solid and hematological tumors has a pathophysiologic relevance for disease progression.

Angiogenesis is a constant hallmark of multiple myeloma (MM) progression and has prognostic potential [54]. It is induced by plasma cells via angiogenic factors with the transition from monoclonal gammopathy of undetermined significance (MGUS) to MM, and probably with loss of angiostatic activity on the part of MGUS [30]. MGUS and nonactive MM (MM in complete or objective response) are the "avascular phase" of plasma cell tumors, while the active MM (MM at diagnosis, at relapse or in resistant phase) is the "vascular phase" which is associated with clonal expansion and the angiogenic switch [45]. The pathophysiology of MM-induced angiogenesis is complex and involves both direct production of angiogenic cytokines by plasma cells and their induction within the microenvironment.

BM stromal cells (BMSCs) increase the concentration of angiogenic factors and matrix degrading enzymes in the microenvironment by direct secretion or by stimulation of MM plasma cells or ECs through paracrine interactions [48, 46]. BMSCs, osteoclasts, osteoblasts, and ECs secrete several factors, including VEGF, FGF-2, TNF-α, IL-6, B-cell activating factor, stromal cell-derived factor-1α (SDF-1α, also known as CXCL12), and various Notch family members, which are further upregulated by the plasma cell adhesion to extracellular matrix proteins and/or BMSCs. Moreover, BMSCs and other cells supporting the plasma cell survival in the BM constitute potential therapeutic targets [48, 46]. Finally, circulating ECs and endothelial precursor cells (EPCs) contribute to the neovascularization, and the presence of EPCs suggests that vasculogenesis may also contribute to the full MM vascular tree [54].

3 Multiple Myeloma Endothelial Cells (MMECs)

Vacca et al. [56] for the first time isolated MMECs from BM of patients with active MM and compared them with human umbilical vein ECs (HUVECs). MMECs showed high expression of typical endothelial cell markers, including Tie2, vascular endothelial growth factor receptor-2 (VEGFR-2), FGF receptor-2 (FGFR-2), CD105-endoglin, vascular endothelial (VE)-cadherin, secretion of matrix metalloproteinases-2 and -9 (MMP-2 and MMP-9), and upregulation of angiogenic genes, including VEGF, FGF-2, Gro-α chemokine, TGFβ, hypoxia inducible factor 1 alpha (HIF-1α), ETS-1, and osteopontin. Moreover, MMECs expressed CD133, a marker of ECPs. MMECs showed intrinsic angiogenic ability in vitro and in vivo, they were ultrastructurally abnormal and metabolically activated.

Pellegrino et al. [36] demonstrated that MMECs secrete high amounts of the CXC chemokines CXCL8/IL-8, CXCL11/interferon-inducible T cell alpha chemoattractant (I-TAC), CXCL12/SDF-1α, and CCL2/monocyte chemotactic protein (MCP)-1 than HUVECs. Also, paired plasma cells and several MM cell lines expressed cognate receptors of each chemokine to a variable extent, suggesting that MMECs are able to recruit the plasma cells into the BM.

Hematopoietic stem and progenitor cells (HSPCs) of MM patients differentiate into cells with EC phenotype, losing CD133 expression and acquiring VEGFR-2, factor VIII-related antigen (FVIII-RA), and vascular endothelial (VE)-cadherin [42]. Platelet-derived growth factor (PDGF)-BB/PDGF receptor beta (PDGFRβ) promoted the transcription of MMEC-proangiogenic factors, such as VEGF, FGF-2, and IL-8 [7]. Moreover, a prolonged exposure of MMECs to dasatinib, a PDGFRβ/SrcTK inhibitor, prevented the expression of endogenous VEGF, and reduced the levels of secreted VEGF in the conditioned medium of MMECs.

Vacca et al. [56] demonstrated by means of a 96-gene cDNA array that MMECs [7] overexpressed angiogenesis-related genes, including FGF-2, VEGF-A, VEGF-C, thrombospondin-1 (TSP-1), fibronectin, osteopontin. Moreover, COL6A1 and COL6A3 (collagen isotypes), responsible for cell anchorage to the extracellular matrix, were downregulated in MMECs, which may account for their increased migratory activity. Vacca et al. [55] confirmed by means of DNA microarray and RT-PCR analysis the induction of VEGF, FGF-2, hepatocyte growth factor (HGF), insulin-like growth factor-1 (IGF-1), and insulin-like growth factor binding protein-3 (IGFBP-3) in active MMECs, nonactive MMECs, and MGUS ECs (MGECs) over HUVECs, and showed that exposure to thalidomide produced a significant downregulation of all these genes.

Ria et al. [43] showed that, among 36 genes, 8 genes were differentially expressed at high stringency in MMECs versus MGECs: the isoform 7 of the FGF, the VEGF isoforms VEGF-A and VEGF-C, fibronectin and TSP-2 were upregulated whereas the endothelial differentiating factor 1, CD105, and CD31 were downregulated in MMECs [43]. Moreover, the deregulated genes were involved in extracellular matrix formation and bone remodeling, cell adhesion, chemotaxis, angiogenesis, resistance to apoptosis, and cell cycle regulation. Validation was focused on BNIP3, IER3, SEPW1 CRYAB, SERPINF1, and SRPX genes, which were not previously found to be functionally correlated to the overangiogenic phenotype of MMECs. BNPI3 which belongs to the Bcl-2 family and is induced by HIF1-α [32], behaves as an antiapoptotic gene in MMECs, because BNIP3-small interfering (si)-RNA ECs increased apoptosis and decreased growth [43]. IER3, which acts as an antiapoptotic and a stress-inducible gene [66], is overexpressed in MM plasma cells [59] and si-RNA-silenced IER3 expression reduced cell proliferation and induced apoptosis in MMECs [43]. SERPIN1, a serine protease inhibitor of angiogenesis [20] through Fas/Fas ligand-mediated apoptosis [58], is downregulated in MMECs [43]. SEPW1, a gene with antioxidant function [27], is upregulated in MMECs, and si-RNA-silenced expression of this gene inhibited MMECs adhesion and angiogenic activity [43]. Finally, DIRAS3, which negatively regulates cell growth and is associated with disease progression in breast and ovary carcinoma [61], is downregulated in MMECs [43].

Berardi et al. [4] found that filamin A (FLNA), vimentin (VIM), a-crystallin B (CRYAB), and 14-3-3f/d protein (YWHAZ) were constantly overexpressed in MMECs versus MGECs and HUVECs, and enhanced by VEGF, FGF-2, HGF, and MM plasma cell conditioned medium.

Ferrucci et al. [13] demonstrated that MMECs expressed more HGF, cMET, and activated cMET (phospho [p]-cMET) at both mRNA and protein levels versus MGECs and healthy (control) ECs. MMECs maintained the HGF/cMET pathway activation in absence of external stimulation, while treatment with anti-HGF and anti-cMET neutralizing antibodies was able to inhibit the cMET activation. Moreover, the cMET pathway regulated several MMECs activities including chemotaxis, locomotion, adhesion, spreading, and angiogenesis. Its inhibition by SU11274 impaired these activities in a synergistic fashion when combined with bortezomib or lenalidomide, both in vitro and in vivo.

4 MM Associated Fibroblasts

In solid tumors, fibroblasts are referred as cancer-associated fibroblasts (CAFs) or tumor-associated fibroblasts (TAFs), and parallel higher malignancy grade, tumor progression, and poor prognosis [14, 21, 35, 51]. CAFs activation is accompanied by the acquisition or upregulation of the proangiogenic markers desmin-1, FGF-2, alpha smooth actin (α-SMA), VEGF, HGF, IL-6, IL-8, FGF-2, and angiopoietin-1 Ang-1 [5, 6, 41]. CAFs express MMP-1 and MMP-3 [24]. BM is a site that significantly contributes to CAFs generation [63]. In particular, cancer-derived soluble factors recruit BM-derived MSCs to tumor sites, where the latter cells acquire the expression of CAFs-specific markers such as α-SMA, fibroblast activation protein (FAP), tenascin-C, and TSP-1 [22, 53].

Primary BM fibroblasts have been isolated from MM patients and these cells presented multiple features of CAFs and promoted tumor growth [15]. CAFs expressing FSP1, aSMA, and FAP were identified in BM samples of patients with MM or MGUS [2] CAFs expressing FSP1, αSMA, and FAP in BM samples of patients with MM or MGUS. The highest proportions of CAFs were found in active MM patients. The CAFs population was heterogeneous since expressed cell markers are restricted to ECs, HSPCs, and MSCs, which implies their multiple cell derivation. Moreover, Frassanito et al. [15] demonstrated that MM plasma cells activate fibroblasts and recruit them via secretion of TGF-β. CAFs transformed the BM stroma by producing collagen and fibronectin, and by secreting TGF-β, HGF, IGF1, IL-1, IL-6 and SDF1α [21]. TGF-β and conditioned media from MM plasma cells and active MM CAFs converted patients' MMECs and HSPCs into CAFs-like cells. Finally, using the in vivo xenograft MM 5T33 mouse model, animals coinjected with active MM CAFs and MM cells showed faster tumor growth than those injected with MM cells alone, and inhibition of the SDF1α/CXCR4 axis affects the MM cell migration, adhesion, and proliferation indicating that MM CAFs recruit CXCR4$^+$ MM cells via SDF1α secretion [15].

5 Therapeutic Applications

VEGF and its receptors are expressed predominantly by clonal plasma cells in MM, and by both ECs and fibroblasts in the BM microenvironment. VEGFR complexes may be a specific target on tumor endothelium for antibodies in vivo. Targeting VEGF or its receptors with monoclonal antibodies (such as bevacizumab/ Avastin) or small molecule inhibitors of VEGFR tyrosine kinase has confirmed the anticancer activity of these agents. However, the results of MM patients treated with bevacizumab have been disappointing [52].

In MM treatment, thalidomide, lenalidomide, and bortezomib have changed clinical practice for both the newly presenting and the relapsed patients. Thalidomide inhibits angiogenesis in MM through inhibition of secretion of VEGF and IL-6 [12, 47, 55]. In addition to its antiangiogenic activity, thalidomide enhances T cell- and NK cell-mediated immunological responses, induces caspase-8 mediated apoptosis, and downregulates IL-6 production within the BM microenvironment in MM [8, 31].

Subsequently to thalidomide, a series of more potent immunomodulatory drugs (IMiDs) and lenalidomide are part of standard therapy regimens for patients with relapsed or refractory MM, as well as for patients with newly diagnosed MM. Lenalidomide reduces the expression of VEGF and FGF-2, exerts in vivo (CAM assay) a relevant antiangiogenic effect, whereas in vitro it inhibits MMECs proliferation and migration [29]. Moreover, MMECs treated with lenalidomide show changes in VEGF/VEGFR-2 signaling pathway and in several proteins controlling the MMECs motility, cytoskeleton remodeling, as well as energy metabolism pathways [29]. Lenalidomide inhibits VEGF-induced PI3K-Akt pathway signaling and HIF-1α expression [28], exerts an anti-TNF-α activity, modulates the immune response stimulating T cells and NK cells activities, induces apoptosis of tumor cells, and decreases the binding of MM cells to BM stromal cells [11, 16, 19, 31]. A retrospective analysis of clinical trials, with previously treated relapsed/refractory MM, demonstrated an improved response rate and increased median for patients treated with lenalidomide and dexamethasone, compared to those treated only with dexamethasone [9, 60, 62]. In a phase 2 study, lenalidomide/bortezomib/ dexamethasone gave responses in 84 % of relapsed/refractory patients, including complete response or near complete response in 21 % [10], and produced responses in 98–100 % of newly diagnosed patients [3].

Bortezomib induces EC apoptosis [64], and inhibits VEGF, IL-6, Ang-1 and Ang-2 and IGF-1 secretion in BM stromal cells and ECs derived from MM patients [18, 49]. The use of bortezomib in pretransplant induction therapy revealed a higher response rate, compared to other induction regimens [39]. Bortezomib and zoledronic acid inhibit macrophage proliferation, adhesion, migration, and expression of angiogenic cytokines and angiogenesis on Matrigel in MM patients. Moreover, VEGFR-2 and ERK1/2 phosphoactivation as well as NF-kB are also inhibited [34].

New small molecules with antiangiogenic properties are available, including pazopanib (GW 7866034), a multitargeted receptor tyrosine kinase inhibitor of VEGFRs, PDGFRs, and cKit, which exerts antiangiogenic activities on MMECs [37]. A phase II clinical trial of 21 refractory/relapsed MM patients showed no clinical responses [38]. The efficacy of vatalanib (PKT787/ZK222584), another VEGFRs inhibitor, has been tested in posttransplant maintenance therapy in MM patients without any significant decrease of microvascular density in BM biopsy and clinical benefit [57]. In a phase II clinical trial of vandetanib (ZD6474), a small tyrosine kinase inhibitor of VEGFRs and epidermal growth factor receptor (EGFR), no responses were found in 18 patients with relapsed MM [25]. SU5416, a small tyrosine kinase inhibitor of VEGFR-2, was tested in 27 patients with refractory MM, and no objective responses were observed [67]. Sorafenib targeting VEGFR-2, VEGFR-3, RAF, PBGFR-β, Flt-3, and c-Kit has shown in a preclinical study a significant anti-MM activity and synergistic activity with common anti-MM drugs [40].

The administration of inhibitors of osteoclasts activity, including bisphosphonates, not only prevents the MM-induced bone destruction, but also exerts an antiangiogenic activity. Therapeutic doses of zoledronic acid markedly inhibit in vitro proliferation, chemotaxis and angiogenesis of MMECs, and in vivo angiogenesis in the CAM assay [50]. These data suggest that the zoledronic acid antitumoral activity in MM is also sustained by antiangiogenesis, which would partly account for its therapeutic efficacy in MM [17, 33].

A very common side effect of antiangiogenic therapy is hypertension, which is associated with nitric oxide changes, pruning of normal vessels, as well as effects on renal salt homeostastis. Toxic peripheral neuropathy represents a dose-limiting debilitating side effect of the treatment of MM with thalidomide, bortezomib, and lenalidomide.

Although the introduction of antiangiogenic agents into clinical practice represented a milestone in cancer therapy (Table 1), their use alone either in early or refractory/progressive disease was disappointing due to the development of different mechanisms of resistance (Table 2). Moreover, survival benefits in patients with advanced tumors treated with antiangiogenic agents even combined with conventional chemotherapy was modest, because their activity was transient.

Both thalidomide and bortezomib showed response rates of 30–40 % when used as monotherapy in relapsed patients. However, when combined with steroids or alkylating agents, the response rates doubles.

Further, studies to increase our understanding of tumor angiogenesis and the development of resistance are required.

Table 1 FDA-approved angiogenesis inhibitors

Monoclonal antibodies
Bevacizumab
Cetuximab
Panitumumab
Small-molecule tyrosine kinase inhibitors
Sunitinib
Sorafenib
Erlotinib
Imatinib
Gefitinib
Pazopanib
Lapatinib
Other antiangiogenic agents
Thalidomide
TNP-470
Endostatin
Rapamycin

Table 2 Mechanisms of resistance

Upregulation of alternative proangiogenic signaling pathways
Recruitment of vascular progenitor cells and proangiogenic monocytes from the bone marrow
Increased pericyte coverage
Increased capabilities for invasion and metastasis
Hypovascularity
Mutational alterations of genes within endothelial cells

Acknowledgments The research leading to these results has received funding from the European Union Seventh Framework Programme (FP7/2007–2013) under grant agreement no. 278570 to DR and no. 278706 to AV.

References

1. Balkwill F, Charles KA, Mantovani A (2005) Smoldering and polarized inflammation in the initiation and promotion of malignant disease. Cancer Cell 7:211–217
2. Balkwill F, Mantovani A (2001) Inflammation and cancer: back to Virchow? Lancet 357:539–545
3. Barosi G, Merlini G, Billio A et al (2012) SIE, SIES, GIT MO evidence-based guidelines on novel agents (thalidomide, bortezomib, and lenalidomide) in the treatment of multiple myeloma. Ann Hematol 91:875–888
4. Berardi S, Caivano A, Ria R et al (2012) Four proteins governing overangiogenic endothelial cell phenotype in patients with multiple myeloma are plausible therapeutic targets. Oncogene 31:2258–2269
5. Chen L, Tredget EE, Wu PYG et al (2008) Paracrine factors of mesenchymal stem cells recruit macrophages and endothelial lineage cells and enhance wound healing. PLoS ONE 3(4):e1886

6. Cirri P, Chiarugi P (2012) Cancer-associated-fibroblasts and tumour cells: a diabolic liaison driving cancer progression. Cancer Metastasis Rev 31:195–208

7. Coluccia AM, Cirulli T, Neri T et al (2008) Validation of PDGFRβ and C-Src tyrosine kinases as tumor/vessel targets in patients with multiple myeloma: preclinical efficacy of the novel, orally available inihibitor dasatinib. Blood 112:1346–1356

8. Davies FE, Raje N, Hideshima T et al (2001) Thalidomide and immunomodulatory derivatives augment natural killer cell cytotoxicity in multiple myeloma. Blood 98:210–216

9. Dimopoulos S, Spencer A, Attal M et al (2007) Lenalidomide plus dexamethasone for relapsed or refractory multiple myeloma. N Engl J Med 357:2123–2132

10. Dimopoulos MA, Kastritis E, Christoulas D et al (2010) Treatment of patients with relapsed/refractory multiple myeloma with lenalidomide and dexametasone with or without bortezomib: prospective evaluation of the impact of cytogenetic abnormalities and of previous therapies. Leukemia 24:1769–1778

11. Dredge K, Horsfall R, Robinson SP et al (2005) Orally administered lenalidomide (CC-5013) is anti angiogenic in vivo and inhibits endothelial cell migration and Akt phosphorylation in vitro. Microvasc Res 69:56–63

12. Du W, Hattori Y, Hashiquuchi A et al (2004) Tumor angiogenesis in the bone marrow of multiple myeloma patients and its alterations by thalidomide treatment. Pathol Int 54:285–294

13. Ferrucci A, Moschetta A, Frassanito MA et al (2014) A HGF/cMET autocrine loop is operative in multiple myeloma bone marrow endothelial cells and may represent a novel therapeutic target. Clin Cancer Res 20(22):5796–5807

14. Franco OE, Shaw AK, Strand DW et al (2010) Cancer associated fibroblasts in cancer pathogenesis. Semin Cell Dev Biol 21:33–39

15. Frassanito MA, Rao L, Moschetta M et al (2014) Bone marrow fibroblasts parallel multiple myeloma progression in patients and mice: in vitro and in vivo studies. Leukemia 28:904–916

16. Görgün G, Calabrese E, Soydan E et al (2010) Immunomodulatory effects of lenalidomide and pomalidomide on interaction of tumor and bone marrow accessory cells in multiple myeloma. Blood 116:3227–3237

17. Henk HJ, Teitelbaum A, Perez JR et al (2012) Persistency with zoledronic acid is associated with clinical benefit in patients with multiple myeloma. Am J Hematol 87:490–495

18. Hideshima T, Chauhan D, Hayashi T et al (2003) Proteasome inhibitor PS-341 abrogates IL-6 triggered signaling cascades via caspase-dependent downregulation of gp130 in multiple myeloma. Oncogene 22:8386–8393

19. Hideshima T, Mitsiades C, Tonon G et al (2007) Understanding multiple myeloma pathogenesis in the bone marrow to identify new therapeutic targets. Nat Rev Cancer 8:585–598

20. Jian GR, Chunfa J, Conove T (2005) How PEDF prevents angiogenesis: a hypothesized pathway. Med Hypothesis 64:74–78

21. Kalluri R, Zeisberg M (2006) Fibroblasts in cancer. Nat Rev Cancer 6:392–3401

22. Kidd S, Spaeth E, Watson K et al (2012) Origins of the tumor microenvironment: quantitative assessment of adipose-derived and bone marrow-derived stroma. PLoS ONE 7(2):e30563

23. Koehne C-H, Dubois RN (2004) COX-2 inhibition and colorectal cancer. Semin Oncol 31(2 Suppl 7):12–21

24. Kopp H-G, Avecilla ST, Hooper AT, Rafii S (2005) The bone marrow vascular niche: home of HSC differentiation and mobilization. Physiology (Bethesda) 20:349–356

25. Kovacs MJ, Reece DE, Marcellus D et al (2006) A phase II study of ZD6474 (Zactima), a selective inhibitor of VEGFR and EGFR tyrosine kinase in patients with relapsed multiple myeloma. Invest New Durgs 24:529–535

26. Krause DS (2002) Regulation of hematopoietic stem cell fate. Oncogene 21:3262–3269

27. Loflin J, Lopez N, Whanger PD et al (2006) Selenoprotein W during development and oxidative stress. J Inorg Biochem 100:1679–1884

28. Lu L, Payvandi F, Wu L et al (2009) The anti-cancer drug lenalidomide inhibits angiogenesis and metastasis via multiple inhibitory effects on endothelial cell function in normoxic and hypoxic conditions. Microvasc Res 77:78–86
29. De Luisi A, Ferrucci A, Coluccia AM et al (2011) Lenalidomide restrains motility and overangiogenic potential of bone marrow endothelial cells in patients with active multiple myeloma. Clin Cancer Res 17(7):1935–1946
30. Mangieri D, Nico B, Benagiano V et al (2008) Angiogenic activity of multiple myeloma endothelial cells in vivo in the chick embryo chorioallantoic membrane assay is associated to a down-regulation in the expression of endogenous endostatin. J Cell Mol Med 12:1023–1028
31. Mitsiades N, Mitsiades CS, Poulaki V et al (2002) Apoptotic signaling induced by immunomodulatory thalidomide analogs in human multiple myeloma cells: therapeutic implications. Blood 99:4525–4530
32. Mizukami Y, Fujiki K, Duerr EM et al (2006) Hypoxic regulation of vascular endothelial growth factor through the induction of phosphatidylinositol3-kinase/Rho/ROCK and c-Myc. J Biol Chem 281:13957–13963
33. Morgan GJ, Davies FE, Gregory WM et al (2012) Effects of induction and maintenance plus long-term bisphosphonates on bone disease in patients with multiple myeloma: MRC Myeloma IX trial. Blood 119:5374–5383
34. Moschetta M, Di Pietro G, Ria R et al (2010) Bortezomib and zoledronic acid on angiogenic and vasculogenic activities of bone marrow macrophages in patients with multiple myeloma. Eur J Cancer 46:420–429
35. Orimo A, Gupta PB, Sgroi DC et al (2005) Stromal fibroblasts present in invasive human breast carcinomas promote tumor growth and angiogenesis through elevated SDF-1/CXCL12 secretion. Cell 121:335–348
36. Pellegrino A, Ria R, Di Pietro G et al (2005) Bone marrow endothelial cells in multiple myeloma secrete CXC chemokines that mediate interactions with plasma cells. Br J Haematol 129:248–256
37. Podar K, Tonon G, Sattler M et al (2006) The small molecule VEGF receptor inhibitor pazopanib (GW 786034B) targets both tumor and endothelial cells in multiple myeloma. Proc Natl Acad Sci USA 103:19478–19483
38. Prince HM, Hanemann D, Spencer A et al (2009) Vascular endothelial growth factor inhibition is not an effective therapeutic strategy for relapsed or refractory multiple myeloma: a phase 2 study of pazopanib (GW 786034). Blood 113:4819–4820
39. Rajkumar SV, Sonneveld P (2009) Front-line treatment in younger patients with multiple myeloma. Semin Hematol 46:118–126
40. Ramakrishnan V, Timm M, Haug JL et al (2010) Sorafenib, a dual rafkinase/vascular endothelial growth factor receptor inhibitor has significantly anti-myeloma activity and synergizes with common anti-myeloma drugs. Oncogene 29:1190–1202
41. Rasanen K, Vaheri A (2010) Activation of fibroblasts in cancer stroma. Exp Cell Res 316:2713–2722
42. Ria R, Piccoli C, Cirulli T et al (2008) Endothelial differentiation of hematopoietic stem cells and progenitor cells from patients with multiple myeloma. Clin Cancer Res 14:1678–1685
43. Ria R, Todoerti K, Berardi S et al (2009) Gene expression profiling of bone marrow endothelial cells in patients with multiple myeloma. Clin Cancer Res 15:5369–5378
44. Ribatti D (2013) Mast cells and macrophages exert beneficial and detrimental effects on tumor progression and angiogenesis. Immunol Lett 152:83–88
45. Ribatti D, Nico B, Crivellato E et al (2007) The history of the angiogenic switch concept. Leukemia 21:44–52
46. Ribatti D, Nico B, Vacca A (2006) Importance of the bone marrow microenvironment in inducing the angiogenic response in multiple myeloma. Oncogene 25:4257–4266
47. Ribatti D, Vacca A (2005) Therapeutic renaissance of thalidomide in the treatment of haematological malignancies. Leukemia 19:1525–1531

48. Ribatti D, Vacca A (2009) The role of monocytes-macrophages in vasculogenesis in multiple myeloma. Leukemia 23:1535–1536
49. Roccaro AM, Hideshima T, Raje N et al (2006) Bortezomib mediates antiangiogenesis in multiple myeloma via direct and indirect effects on endothelial cells. Cancer Res 66:184–191
50. Scavelli C, Di Pietro G, Cirulli T et al (2007) Zoledronic acid affects over-angiogenic phenotype of endothelial cells in patients with multiple myeloma. Mol Cancer Ther 6:3256–3262
51. Shimoda M, Mellody KT, Orimo A (2010) Carcinoma-associated fibroblasts are a rate-limiting determinant for tumour progression. Semin Cell Dev Biol 21:19–25
52. Somlo G, Lashkari A, Bellamy W et al (2011) Phase II randomized trial of bevacizumab versus bevacizumab and thalidomide for replasped/refractory multiple myeloma: a Californnia Cancer Consortium trial. Br J Haematol 154:533–535
53. Spaeth EL, Dembinski JL, Sasser AK et al (2009) Mesenchymal stem cell transition to tumor associated fibroblasts contributes to fibrovascular network expansion and tumor progression. PLoS ONE 4(4):e4992
54. Vacca A, Ribatti D (2006) Bone marrow angiogenesis in multiple myeloma. Leukemia 20:193–199
55. Vacca A, Scavelli C, Montefusco V et al (2005) Thalidomide downregulates angiogenic genes in bone marrow endothelial cells of patients with active multiple myeloma. J Clin Oncol 23:5534–5546
56. Vacca A, Semeraro F, Merchionne F et al (2003) Endothelial cells in the bone marrow of patients with multiple myeloma. Blood 102:3340–3348
57. Vij R, Ansstas G, Mosley JC et al (2010) Efficacy and tolerability of PTK787/ZK222584 in a phase II study of post-transplant maintenance therapy in patients with multiple myeloma following high-dose chemotherapy and autologous stem cell transplant. Leuk Lymphoma 51:1577–1579
58. Volpert OV, Zaichuk T, Zhow W et al (2002) Inducer-stimulated Fas targets activated endothelium for destruction by antiangiogenic thrombospondin-1 and pigment epithelium derived factor. Nat Med 8:349–357
59. De Vos J, Thykjaer T, Tarte K et al (2002) Comparison of gene expression profiling between malignant and normal plasma cells with oligonucleotide arrays. Oncogene 21:6848–6857
60. Wang M, Dimopoulos MA, Chen C et al (2008) Lenalidomide plus dexamethasone is more effective than dexamethasone alone in patients with relapsed or refractory multiple myeloma regardless of prior thalidomide exposure. Blood 112:4445–4451
61. Wang L, Hoque A, Luo RZ et al (2003) Loss of the expression of the tumor suppressor gene ARHI is associated with progression of breast cancer. Clin Cancer Res 9:3660–3666
62. Weber DM, Chen C, Niesvizky R et al (2007) Lenalidomide plus dexamethasone for relapsed multiple myeloma in North America. N Engl J Med 357:2133–2142
63. De Wever O, Van Bockstal M, Mareel M et al (2014) Carcinoma-associated fibroblasts provide operational flexibility in metastasis. Semin Cancer Biol 25:33–46
64. Williams S, Pettaway C, Song R et al (2003) Differential effects of the proteasome inhibitor bortezomib on apoptosis and angiogenesis in human prostate tumor xenografts. Mol Cancer Ther 2:835–843
65. Wilson A, Trumpp A (2006) Bone-marrow haematopoietic-stem-cell niches. Nat Rev Immunol 6:9093–9106
66. Wu MX, Ao Z, Prasad KV et al (1998) IEX-1L, an apoptosis inhibitor involved in NF kB-mediated cell survival. Science 281:998–1001
67. Zangari M, Anaissie E, Stopeck A et al (2004) Phase II study of SU5416, a small molecule vascular endothelial growth factor tyrosine kinase receptor inhibitor in patients with refractory multiple myeloma. Clin Cancer Res 10:88–95

Targeting the Bone Marrow Microenvironment

Michele Moschetta, Yawara Kawano and Klaus Podar

Abstract

Unprecedented advances in multiple myeloma (MM) therapy during the last 15 years are predominantly based on our increasing understanding of the pathophysiologic role of the bone marrow (BM) microenvironment. Indeed, new treatment paradigms, which incorporate thalidomide, immunomodulatory drugs (IMiDs), and proteasome inhibitors, target the tumor cell as well as its BM microenvironment. Ongoing translational research aims to understand in more detail how disordered BM-niche functions contribute to MM pathogenesis and to identify additional derived targeting agents. One of the most exciting advances in the field of MM treatment is the emergence of immune therapies including elotuzumab, daratumumab, the immune checkpoint inhibitors, Bispecific T-cell engagers (BiTes), and Chimeric antigen receptor (CAR)-T cells. This chapter will review our knowledge on the pathophysiology of the BM microenvironment and discuss derived novel agents that hold promise to further improve outcome in MM.

Keywords

Bone marrow microenvironment · Bone marrow · Immune checkpoint inhibition · CAR-T cells · BiTEs

M. Moschetta · Y. Kawano
Department of Medical Oncology, Dana-Farber Cancer Institute,
Harvard Medical School, Boston, MA, USA

K. Podar (✉)
Department of Medical Oncology, National Center for Tumor Diseases (NCT),
University of Heidelberg, Heidelberg, Germany
e-mail: klaus.podar@nct-heidelberg.de

© Springer International Publishing Switzerland 2016
A.M. Roccaro and I.M. Ghobrial (eds.), *Plasma Cell Dyscrasias*,
Cancer Treatment and Research 169, DOI 10.1007/978-3-319-40320-5_6

63

1 Introduction

The bone marrow (BM) environment consists of a cellular compartment with hematopoietic and nonhematopoietic cells and an extracellular compartment within a liquid *milieu* organized in a complex architecture of sub-microenvironments ("niches") within the protective coat of the vascularized and innervated bone. The *cellular BM compartment* is composed of hematopoietic cells including hematopoietic and mesenchymal stem cells (HSCs, MSCs); hematopoietic and mesenchymal progenitor and precursor cells; mesenchymal stroma cells; BM-derived circulating endothelial precursors (EPCs); immune cells (B lymphocytes, T lymphocytes, natural killer (NK) cells, cytotoxic T lymphocytes (CTLs), macrophages, monocytes, NKT cells, myeloid and plasmacytoid dendritic cells (mDCs, pDCs), regulatory T cells (Tregs), myeloid derived suppressor cells (MDSCs)); erythrocytes; megakaryocytes and platelets; and nonhematopoietic cells including adipocytes; endothelial progenitor cells (EPCs); endothelial cells (ECs); BM mesenchymal stroma cells (BM-MSCs); adipocytes; as well as cells involved in bone homeostasis including chondroclasts, osteoclasts (OCs), and osteoblasts (OBs). The *extracellular compartment* is composed of the extracellular matrix (ECM), an interlocking mesh of fibrous proteins and glycosaminoglycans. The *liquid milieu* contains a multitude of growth factors and cytokines; as well as matrix metalloproteinases. Moreover, the healthy BM, considered to be physiologically hypoxic [1, 2], contains a heterogeneous oxygen distribution. Low oxygen tension is present in the "endosteal" niche, which is located near trabecular bone, and high oxygen tension is present in the central "vascular" niche, which is associated with the sinusoidal endothelium and represents the anatomic barrier between the "hematopoietic" compartment within the BM and the peripheral circulation [3, 4]. Under physiologic conditions these components are highly organized and finely tuned by cell–cell and cell–matrix interactions within the *liquid milieu* to regulate the homing of mature cells to selective sites within the BM; to support normal hematopoiesis; and to mobilize blood and other cells into the blood stream. Moreover, the BM microenvironment exerts forces to keep occult tumors, which are present also in healthy individuals, check in [5].

In multiple myeloma (MM), this homeostasis is disrupted. Indeed, the development of MM is a complex multistep process not only involving early and late genetic changes in the tumor cells, but also selective supportive conditions of the BM and its niches. Outstanding questions concern the cellular complexity of the niche, the role of the endosteum and functional heterogeneity among perivascular microenvironments [6]. Ongoing studies aim to understand how disordered niche functions contribute to MM pathogenesis. It is suggested that nonactive MM and MGUS in which the tumor growth is arrested are "avascular phases" of plasma cell tumors located within the "endosteal niche." In contrast, active MM is the "vascular phase" of plasma cell tumors located within the "vascular niche," which is associated with clonal expansion and epigenetic modifications of the microenvironment as well as the "angiogenic switch." These findings correlate with disease progression and poor prognosis. Indeed, it was only the identification that the MM BM microenvironment, and BMSCs and ECs in particular, play a supportive role in MM pathogenesis that led to the clinical development of thalidomide, proteasome inhibitors, and the immunomodulatory drugs (IMiDs). Cell surface receptors, which mediate MM cell–stroma cell and MM cell–ECM binding include integrins, cadherins, selectins, syndecans, and the immunoglobulin superfamily of cell adhesion molecules including syndecan-1 (CD138), H-CAM (CD44), VLA-4 (CD49d/CD29), ICAM-1 (CD54), N-CAM (CD56), LFA-3 (CD58), αvβ3, CD56, CD74, HM1.24, VLA-5 (CD49e/CD29), VLA-6, and CD51 [7]; as well as the cell surface glycoprotein CD2 subset-1 (CS-1), a member of the immunoglobulin gene superfamily [8]. Signaling cascades activated by cytokines, growth factors and/or adhesion of MM cells to BM stroma cells and the ECM include the Ras/Raf/MEK/MAPK pathway, the phosphoinositide 3-kinase (PI3K)/Akt pathway, the Janus-activated kinase (JAK)/Stat3 pathway, the NF-kB pathway, the Notch-, and the Wnt pathway. Importantly, the complexity of signaling cascades is further enhanced by their co-simulation.

In addition to direct effects on MM cells, alterations within the BM induce immune suppression, lytic bone lesions, and enhance BM angiogenesis. Specifically, in MM the development of an effective anti-MM immune response is inhibited via induction of dysfunctional T regulatory cells; ineffective antigen presentation; and production of excessive proinflammatory cytokines. In turn, immune cells including pDCs and macrophages are able to trigger tumor cell proliferation, survival, and drug resistance. The usefulness of immunotherapies in MM patients has first been supported by the identification of the graft-versus-myeloma effect in the context of allogeneic BM transplantation. Moreover, the introduction of thalidomide and its derivatives, the IMiDs, as well as (immuno) proteasome inhibitors into MM therapies has radically improved patients' outcome. Ongoing research focuses on developing antibody- and peptide-based strategies (e.g., against CS-1 and CD38), as well as on targeting Btk, and immune checkpoints to enhance immune cell activity against MM cells. Bispecific T-cell engagers (BiTes) and Chimeric antigen receptor (CAR)-T cells represent yet another novel approach of immunotherapy in MM. Furthermore, up to 80 % of MM patients at diagnosis present with osteolytic lesions. Functionally, MM cells interfere with physiologic bone remodeling by releasing OC promoting cytokines as well as by inhibition of BM-MSC differentiation into OBs. In turn, MM-induced bone modifications support tumor growth and confer chemoresistance [9]. Indeed, bisphosphonates not only prevent skeletal-related events (SREs), but also inhibit MM activity. Additional approaches to treat MM-associated bone disease are ongoing.

Based on our increasing understanding of the pathophysiologic facets of the MM BM microenvironment and its interrelation with the MM cell, several novel agents have been identified. Novel biologically based treatment regimens not only target MM cells alone but also MM cell–stroma cell interactions and the *liquid* BM *milieu*. However, despite significant therapeutic advances during the last 15 years, MM remains as an incurable disease. Therefore, there is still an urgent need for more efficacious and tolerable drugs. Here, we will summarize current knowledge on the functional role of the cellular and extracellular compartments, as well as of hypoxia in MM pathogenesis and present derived novel microenvironment-targeting therapeutic approaches.

2 The Cellular Compartment

2.1 Accessory Cells

Normal BM cells are progressively replaced by clonal plasma cells in patients with MGUS, SMM, and MM [10]. Whether they contribute to MM pathogenesis by mediating transformation from premalignant monoclonal gammopathies to MM is still not entirely understood. Recent studies indicate a progressive increase in the incidence of copy number abnormalities (CNA) and chromosomal gains as well as a strong association between genetic lesions and fragile sites from MGUS to SMM and to MM [11]. In support of these findings, the MGUS disease stage is genetically less complex than MM, and high-risk smoldering MM (HR-SMM) is similar to MM [12]. Taken together, clonal progression seems to be a key feature in the transformation of HR-SMM to MM, and depends on accumulating changes in the BM microenvironment. Whether invasive subclones are amenable to therapeutic interventions that may prevent permissive changes in the microenvironment is currently under investigation.

Accessory BM cells, BM-MSCs, ECs, immune cells (e.g., pDCs), OCs, and OBs in particular, support MM cell proliferation, survival, migration, and drug resistance directly via cell–cell binding and indirectly via secretion of growth factors and cytokines. To critically understand the pathological basis of the interaction between MM cells and BM stromal cells, it is important to first define and understand the origin and differentiation of accessory BM cells. However to date, the development of accessory cells is still poorly understood, and their phenotypic and genotypic characteristics remain disputable [13]. Pathological conditions such as MM tumor growth in the BM significantly change the composition of the BM stroma compartment by acting on stroma cell progenitors/stroma cells and by modulating their functional and differentiating status [13]. This is in line with some evidences indicating that BM-MSCs derived from MM patients are inherently abnormal at genomic/transcriptional/functional [14] levels and remain abnormal after ex vivo isolation and MM cell removal [15]. Moreover, MM-induced changes in the cellular compartment are accompanied by changes in the noncellular compartment including the composition of the ECM [16, 17], and by changes in the liquid milieu [18], which in turn act on stroma cell differentiation thus creating a complex and self-sustaining vicious cycle. Ultimately, these changes lead to the creation of a BM niche more prone to support MM cell rather than hematopoietic stem cell growth [19]. Consequently, MM progression results in defective function of the hematopoietic cell compartment, with clinical consequences including anemia, and immune dysfunction development in MM patients [19]. BM-MSCs are the accessory BM cells predominantly utilized to study the pathophysiological relevance of interactions and cross talks with MM cells both in in vitro and in vivo MM models. BM-MSCs strongly adhere to MM cells via binding to surface molecules [13, 20]. They thereby promote MM cell proliferation, survival, and drug resistance via activation of several signaling pathways [20–22]. For example, the interaction between MM cells and BM-MSCs triggers NF-κB-dependent production and secretion of interleukin-6 (IL-6) in BM-MSCs [23]. In turn, IL-6 enhances the production and secretion of VEGF by MM cells [24, 25]. VEGF secretion then activates ECs and EPCs, which increase BM angiogenesis and thereby promote MM cell proliferation [26, 27]. Moreover, BM-MSCs suppress bortezomib-induced MM cell growth inhibition via cell–cell contact [28] and NF-kB-dependent IL-8 secretion [29]. Importantly, ex vivo isolated BM-MSCs have the capacity for mesoderm-like cell differentiation into osteogenic, chondrogenic, myogenic, and adipogenic lineages both in vitro and in vivo [30]. This finding is of particular interest because it suggests that MM cells may induce differentiation of BM-MSCs toward specific, terminally differentiated cell types that additionally support MM cell growth by direct binding. For example, MM cells induce differentiation of BM-MSCs toward the adipocyte lineage, which sustains MM growth at the expenses of osteoblastic lineage differentiation, which instead limits MM growth [31]. Moreover, it is likely that accumulating genetic changes in tumor cells, e.g., those that define high-risk disease, influence their interrelation with the cellular and noncellular BM microenvironment. For example, MM cells with a t(14;16) translocation overexpress c-Maf, and thereby induce β7-integrin upregulation and enhancement of MM cell adhesion to BM-MSCs, strongly indicating a therapeutic role for targeting c-Maf and β7-integrin in MM [32]. Although suggested by some authors, the existence of MM-specific abnormal BMSCs is still controversial. For example, Zdzisinska et al. show increased production of MMP-1, MMP-2, and TIMP-2 in BMSCs of MM patients *versus* healthy controls [18]. Importantly, accumulating evidence indicates that the BM microenvironment not only plays a supportive role in MM cell growth, survival, and drug resistance but may also act as a conduit of epigenetic information leading to behavioral changes in the tumor clone. For example, Cancer-Associated Fibroblasts (**CAFs**) comprise a heterogeneous population that resides within the BM microenvironment. They actively foster chemotaxis, adhesion, proliferation, and apoptosis resistance in MM cells through production of cytokines and chemokines, and the release of proinflammatory and proangiogenic factors, thereby creating a more supportive microenvironment [33, 34]. Moreover, Roccaro et al. recently demonstrated that BM-MSCs transfer exosomes, small nanometer-sized (50–100 nm) vesicles of endocytic origin, into MM cells. Exosomes contain microRNAs (miRs) as well as oncogenic proteins, cytokines, and protein kinases; they may therefore act as active vesicles responsible for molding the microenvironment surrounding MM cells, and thereby leading to MM growth, dissemination, and subsequent disease progression [35], dependent on heparanase activity [36].

Compared to healthy human umbilical vein EC (HUVEC), MM-associated ECs (**MMECs**) secrete higher amounts of the CXC chemokines (e.g., IL-8, SDF-1α, MCP-1), which act in a paracrine manner to mediate plasma cell proliferation and chemotaxis. In turn, MM cells and stromal cells prolong survival of ECs both by increased secretion of EC survival factors, such as VEGF, and by decreased secretion of anti-angiogenetic factors [37, 38]. Yet another facet to the complex multistep model of MM pathogenesis was added by studies, which indicated that MMECs (similar to ECs found in B-cell lymphomas) resemble transformed tumor cells. Specifically, MMECs were found to harbor 13q14 deletion, and genomic clonotypic IgH VDJ gene arrangements. In addition, they produced growth and invasive factors for MM cells including VEGF, FGF-2, MMP-2 as well as MMP-9 [39–41]. Four different mechanisms could explain this finding: (1) tumor cells as well as MMECs are derived from a common malignant precursor cell; (2) the EC carrying genetic alterations of the MM cell has arisen from a cell that was already committed to the myeloid lineage; (3) MM cell–EC fusion has occurred; or (4) apoptotic bodies from tumor cells have been taken up by ECs.

Moreover, by utilizing a niche-based screening technique, Chattopadhyay et al. identified BRD9876, an unusual ATP noncompetitive kinesin-5 (Eg5) inhibitor, which showed improved selectivity over hematopoietic progenitors [42].

Accumulating data also suggest the existence of a Hedgehog (Hh)-dependent MM cell subclone, the MM stem cell (**MMSC**), which has self-renewing capacities and is relatively chemoresistant [43–45]. It is hypothesized that MMSCs arise from aberrant signaling of the microenvironment (e.g., triggered by hypoxia, inflammation, and angiogenesis), which not only provides survival signals to MMSCs but also contributes to metastasis by induction of Epithelial–Mesenchymal Transition (EMT) [46]. Similar to HSCs, MMSCs may be maintained in an immature quiescent state in the endosteal niche, while the more oxygenated vascular niche promotes their maturation and proliferation, and facilitates their egress from the BM [47–49]. However, the phenotype of MM stem cells remains controversial, with respect to the expression of syndecan-1 (CD138) and CD20 in particular [50, 51]. Most recent data demonstrate that elevated expression of Bruton-Tyrosin kinase (BTK) in MM cells leads to AKT/WNT/β-catenin-dependent upregulation of key stemness genes (OCT4, SOX2, NANOG, and MYC) and enhanced self-renewal. Consequently, enforced transgenic expression of BTK in MM cells increases features of cancer stemness, including clonogenicity and resistance to widely used anti-MM drugs, whereas inducible knockdown of BTK abolished them [52]. Based on these data, clinical trials testing the small-drug Btk inhibitor ibrutinib alone or in combination with carfilzomib are ongoing (https://clinicaltrials.gov). In addition, also the Hh inhibitors cyclopamine and vismodegib are under clinical investigation [45, 53]. Moreover, current efforts aim to develop compounds that specifically modify the stem cell niche in order to block MM stem cell engraftment while still enabling HSC development.

MSCs, which differentiate in a context-specific manner into muscle, bone, fat, and other cell types, represent another potential therapeutic target in MM. BM-MSCs isolated from MM patients, as compared with normal MSCs, produce high levels of IL-6, DKK1, as well as factors associated with angiogenesis and osteogenic differentiation [15]. Moreover, they have decreased ability to inhibit T-cell proliferation [54]. Bortezomib induces MSCs to preferentially undergo OB differentiation in mice, in part by modulation of the bone-specifying transcription factor Runt-related transcription factor 2. Mice implanted with MSCs showed increased ectopic ossicle and bone formation after treatment with bortezomib. Bortezomib treatment increased bone formation and rescued bone loss in a mouse model of osteoporosis [55]. These results are consistent with the therapeutic benefits of bortezomib on MM bone disease [56].

Ongoing efforts aim to further enhance our understanding on the functional role of accessory stroma cells and their role in the formation of BM niches in MM, in order to develop improved targeted therapies.

2.2 The Immune Cell Microenvironment

An important step in tumor progression is the evasion and suppression of the host immune system [57, 58]. In the normal microenvironment the effector cells, mainly the natural killer (NK) cells and cytotoxic T lymphocytes (CTLs), are capable of driving potent antitumor responses. However, tumor cells often induce an immunosuppressive microenvironment in order to protect themselves from the host immune system. Like solid tumors, MM cells are capable of modifying the bone marrow (BM) microenvironment, which is rich of immune cell populations, in a suitable way for their own survival [59]. The two major immunosuppressive mechanisms in cancer are (1) expansion of regulatory immune cells (such as MDSCs and Tregs) and (2) activation of inhibitory T-cell pathways (especially Programmed cell Death-1 (PD-1)/PD-Ligand 1 (PD-L1) pathway).

Myeloid Derived Suppressor Cells (MDSCs) MDSCs are heterogeneous, immature, MPCs that differentiate into macrophages, granulocytes, or DCs under normal conditions. However, under pathological conditions such as cancer, differentiation of immature myeloid cells is inhibited resulting in accumulation of MDSCs [60]. In cancer patients and tumor models, MDSCs accumulate in the tumor microenvironment due to release of soluble factors by tumor cells or cells in the microenvironment [61, 62]. MDSCs can suppress T-cell proliferation through expression of immune suppressive factors such as arginase, reactive oxygen species (ROS), and nitric oxide (NO). In addition, MDSCs can induce the development of Tregs in vivo, which are anergic and suppressive [63]. Previous reports showed that cancer patients with higher MDSC levels have shorter survival compared to patients with lower MDSC levels [64, 65]. Depletion of MDSCs in tumor-bearing mice using anti-Gr-1 antibody [66, 67] or MDSC-specific peptides [68] suggest that MDSCs can be a good target of antitumor treatment. Two main subsets of MDSCs have been described, granulocytic MDSC (G-MDSC) or polymorphonuclear (PMN)-MDSCs and monocytic MDSC (Mo-MDSC). G-MDSCs have granulocyte-like morphology with increased levels of ROS and low levels of NO, whereas Mo-MDSCs have monocyte-like morphology with increased levels of NO, but low levels of ROS. Human G-MDSCs and Mo-MDSCs are usually defined as $CD11b^+ CD33^+ HLA-DR^{-/low}CD14^-$ and $CD11b^+ CD33^+ HLA-DR^{-/low} CD14^+$, respectively. In tumor-bearing mice, G-MDSCs are the main MDSC subsets to be expanded in peripheral lymphoid organs [69].

Previous reports have shown an increase in the number of MDSCs in the peripheral blood (PB) [70, 71] and BM [72] of MM patients compared to healthy donors. A recent report showed that increased frequency of Mo-MDSCs is associated with tumor progression and therapeutic response to bortezomib-based treatment in MM patients [73]. Similarly, the analysis of 5T2 and 5T33 murine MM model showed that the percentage of Ly6G^{low} MDSC (Mo-MDSC) within the CD11b$^+$ population was increased in the BM of tumor-bearing mice compared to control [74]. In addition, these CD11b^{high}Ly6G^{low} cells (Mo-MDSCs) were more suppressive than the CD11b^{high}Ly6G^{high} population (G-MDSCs). However, other reports show a significant increase in G-MDSCs in the BM [72] or PB [75] of MM patients. Further research is required to understand the differences and functions of MM-associated G-MDSCs and Mo-MDSCs.

MDSCs induce MM growth by suppressing T-cell-mediated immune responses, while MM cells induce the development of MDSCs from healthy donor PB mononuclear cells, confirming a bidirectional interaction between MDSCs and MM cells and immune effector cells [71]. Moreover, purified MDSCs from MM patients induce more Tregs than MDSCs from age-matched controls [75], leading to a more suppressive immune environment. Interestingly, MDSCs from mice injected with 5TGM1 murine MM cells display a significantly higher potential to differentiate into mature and functional OCs than MDSCs from nontumor controls. This finding indicates that tumor-induced MDSCs exacerbate cancer-associated bone destruction by directly serving as OC precursors [76].

Given that novel agents such as the IMiD lenalidomide and the proteasome inhibitor bortezomib target both MM cells and the BM microenvironment [20], the anti-MDSC activity of these drugs was studied. However, neither bortezomib nor lenalidomide were able to alter the suppressive activity of MDSCs [71]. This finding indicates that other strategies are needed to target MDSCs in the MM microenvironment. For example, phosphodiesterase-5 (PDE5) inhibitors reduced the suppressive machinery of tumor recruited MDSCs through downregulation of arginase 1 and NO synthase-2 expression in murine tumor models [66, 77, 78]. Noonan et al. recently reported that PDE5 inhibitor, tadalafil, reduced MDSC function in a relapsed/refractory MM patient [79]. Indeed, the strategy to target MDSCs in MM with PDE5 inhibitors may represent a novel approach that augments the efficacy of tumor-directed therapies.

Regulatory T Cells (Tregs) Tregs are a subset of CD4$^+$ T lymphocytes characterized by the expression of transcription factor FOXP3 [80]. Tregs suppress the function of antigen-presenting cells (APCs) and effector T cells by direct contact or by release of anti-inflammatory cytokines (IL-10 and TGF-beta). These cells accumulate in the tumor microenvironment and the peripheral blood of patients with cancer [81, 82]. The increased frequency of Tregs has been generally considered as a marker of poor prognosis due to Treg-mediated suppression of anti-tumor immunity [83, 84]. It has been shown using the diphtheria toxin inducible "depletion of regulatory T cell" (DEREG) mice [85] that Treg depletion induces regression of solid tumors and lymphomas, which was associated with an increased intratumoral accumulation of activated $CD8^+$ cytotoxic T cells [86, 87]. These data indicate that targeting Tregs in cancer represents a potential antitumor strategy.

Many groups have reported an increase of functional Tregs in MM patient's PB compared to healthy donors [70, 88–91]. In addition, MM patients with higher percentage of Tregs in the PB were shown to have shorter time to progression (TTP) (37) and shorter overall survival (OS) (36). A positive association of Treg frequency with international staging system (ISS) and paraprotein level was also reported [89]. Analysis of the 5T2 and 5T33 murine MM model showed that the increased numbers of functional Tregs in the myeloma-bearing mice was due to the increased Treg development in the thymus [92], leading to MM progression. Beyer et al. showed that Tregs from MM patients express increased levels of IL-10 and TGF-beta compared to healthy controls, indicating a higher suppressive function of MM patients derived Tregs [88]. However, there are some conflicting results showing decreased frequency and function of myeloma associated Tregs [93, 94]. These differences may be explained by different gating strategies of Tregs ($CD4^+$ $FOXP3^+$, $CD4^+$ $CD25^+$ $FOXP3^+$, $CD4^+$ $CD25^+$ $CD127^-$) and heterogeneous patient populations.

Tregs, in general, can be induced from naïve $CD4^+$ T cells in the presence of several cytokines, such as TGF-beta [95, 96], secreted in the microenvironment. However, there are few reports showing the mechanism of Treg induction by MM cells. Feyler et al. showed in an in vitro experimental model that MM cells can directly induce Tregs in an APC-independent manner mediated, at least in part, through MM expression of ICOS-L [97]. Frassanito et al. also reported that Treg induction by MM cells are mainly contact dependent and MM cells act as immature APCs [98]. Recent reports have shown the involvement of the PD-1/PD-L1 pathway in Treg induction, identifying this pathway as an attractive therapeutic target for controlling Treg cell plasticity [99, 100]. Since, MM cells express PD-L1 significantly higher than normal plasma cells [101, 102], the association of Treg induction by PD-L1 on MM cells should be further investigated.

Low-dose cyclophosphamide (CYC) has been shown to reduce the numbers and function of Tregs, and to induce antitumor, immune-mediated effects [103, 104]. In a MM mouse model, low-dose CYC showed a transient depletion of Tregs resulting in reduced occurrence of MM and improved survival rate [105]. The IMiDs lenalidomide and pomalidomide are reported to inhibit expansion and function of Tregs by decreasing FOXP3 mRNA expression [106]. However, contradictory results have been reported showing that newly diagnosed MM patients treated with IMiDs have increased number of Tregs [94, 107]. For more specific and effectve targeting of Tregs, it is nction are controlled at the molecular level.

Dendritic Cells (DCs) Dendritic cells (DCs) are BM-derived professional APCs which present self and nonself antigens to T cells, and promote immunity or tolerance [108]. Antigen presentation by DCs induces naive T cells to differentiate into effector and memory T cells, but it can also lead to different forms of T-cell tolerance, depending on the functional status of the DCs. mDCs and pDCs are the two major DC subsets that have been identified based on their origin, phenotype, and function [109]. Human mDCs are usually defined as Lin$^-$H-LADR$^+$CD11c$^+$CD123^{dim} cells, while pDCs are Lin$^-$CD11c$^-$CD4$^+$CD45RA$^+$CD123$^+$ILT3$^+$. Several studies have documented an increase of DCs in human tumor sites, which often correlated with adverse prognosis [110–112]. Indeed, loss of immune function of tumor-infiltrating DCs has been linked to the suppressive effects of the tumor microenvironment mediated by various cytokines [113]. Recent findings have demonstrated that tumor-infiltrating pDCs from solid tumors express high levels of ICOS-L, which explains their ability to induce Tregs [114, 115]. It was also shown that TGF-beta secreted by DCs from breast cancer patients was partially associated with induction of Tregs [116]. Similar findings of induction of Tregs by DCs were observed in MM patients [117].

DCs play an important role in normal plasma cell differentiation and survival [118, 119]. However, the frequency and function of DCs in MM patients compared to healthy individuals is still controversial [120, 121]. Chauhan et al. showed that pDCs are increased in MM patient's BM compared to healthy controls and pDCs confer growth, survival, chemotaxis, and drug resistance against MM cells [122]. Targeting Toll-like receptors (TLRs) with CpG oligodeoxynucleotides both restore pDC immune function and abrogates pDC-induced MM cell growth. TLR-9 agonist inhibited pDC-induced MM cell growth through interferon secretion and activation of TLR9/MyD88 signaling axis [123]. Kukreja et al. reported that DCs enhanced clonogenic growth of MM cell lines and primary tumor cells from MM patients [124]. This effect was inhibited by blockade of the RANK–RANK ligand and BAFF–APRIL-mediated interactions. Recently, Ray et al. showed that PD-L1 is highly expressed on pDCs and MM cells, implicating a two-pronged suppression of PD1-expressing T cell and NK cell immune function, and blockade of PD-L1/PD1 pathway generated robust MM-specific CD8$^+$ CTL activity, as well as enhances NK cell-mediated MM cell cytolytic activity [125]. These data suggest that MM–DC interactions may directly impact the biology of MM and may be a target for therapeutic intervention.

Macrophages Cells of the monocyte–macrophage lineage are an important component of the leukocyte infiltration in tumors, where they are able to promote tumor progression, tumor cell invasion, and metastasis [126].

Physical interaction between macrophages and MM cells activate signaling pathways that protect MM cells from apoptosis induced by drug treatment [127]. Interactions between P-selectin glycoprotein ligand 1 (PSGL-1) and intercellular adhesion molecule-1 (ICAM-1) on MM cells and E/P selectins and CD18 on macrophages, respectively, allow macrophages to protect MM cells from drug-induced apoptosis [128]. Macrophages are also able to protect MM cells from apoptosis through noncontact mediated mechanisms [129].

Human myeloma-associated monocytes/macrophages (MAM), but not MM cells, are the predominant source of interleukin-1b (IL-1b), IL-10, and tumor necrosis factor (TNF)-alpha, whereas IL-6 originates from both BM-MSCs and macrophages in line with previous results [130]. In this latter study, TPL2 (Cot/MAP3K8) pathway was found to ultimately activate MM-associated macrophages, and it may represent a new therapeutic target in MM, specifically acting on BM microenviroment and not on MM cells [130].

Tumor-associated macrophages are also a rich source of potent proangiogenic cytokines and growth factors, such as VEGF, interleukin-8 and FGF-2 and express a broad array of angiogenesis modulating enzymes, including matrix metalloproteinases, cycloxygenase-2, and colony-stimulating factor-1 (CSF-1) [131]; they may have a crucial role in promoting MM-associated neovessel formation and angiogenesis and represent targets for development of new anti-angiogenic drugs in MM.

Natural Killer Cells (NK Cells) NK cells represent a heterogeneous lymphocyte population with cytotoxic antitumor capacity and multiple immunoregulatory properties. One of the NK cell activating receptors is Natural Killer Group 2D (NKG2D), which recognizes various proteins expressed on the surface of target cells in response to several forms of cellular stress. MHC class I polypeptide-related sequence A (MICA) is one of the ligands for NKG2D. Target tumor cells ectopically expressing MICA are efficiently killed via NKG2D despite the expression of MHC class I molecules [132].

NK cells in MM patients are increased in the PB [133, 134] and BM [135, 136] compared to healthy individuals. However, the expansion of NK cells in MM patients is not associated with their activation. Importantly, NKG2D expression on the surface of NK cells isolated from MM patients is decreased [137, 138], which may lead to the escape of MM from immunosurveillance. Indeed, elevated levels of soluble MICA in the circulation of MM patients may trigger downregulation of NKG2D and impaired lymphocyte cytotoxicity [137]. The functional defect of NK cells in MM patients can also be explained by the expression of PD-1 on NK cells of MM patients [139]. Engagement of PD-1 with their ligand PD-L1, which is expressed on MM cells, can downmodulate the NK cell versus MM effect.

In MM, the therapeutic efficacy of IMiDs is known to originate, at least in part, from the activation of NK cells. IMiDs are able to stimulate T cells to produce IFN-γ and IL-2 leading to NK cell activation [140, 141]. Lenalidomide upregulates CD16, CD40L, and LFA1 on NK cells, thereby facilitating antibody-dependent cell cytotoxicity (ADCC) against MM cells [142]. Salvage therapy with lenalidomide after allogenic stem cell transplantation for MM leads to an increase of activated NKp44$^+$ NK cells [143]. Also the proteasome inhibitor bortezomib has been shown to promote NK cell activation by increasing the levels of MICA on the surface of MM cells [137]. These results show that, at least in part, the efficacy of novel anti-MM agents is associated with NK cell activation.

The Immune Checkpoint Pathway PD-1 is a type I transmembrane protein which belongs to the CD28 family [144]. PD-1 is expressed on activated and exhausted T and B cells and has two ligands PD-L1 and PD-L2. PD-L1 is not expressed on normal epithelial tissues but it is aberrantly expressed on a variety of solid tumors [145], while PD-L2 is more broadly expressed on normal healthy tissues. Binding of PD-L1 to PD-1 reduces cytokine production and activation of the target T cells, leading to an immunosuppressive microenvironment.

Importantly PD-L1 is only expressed on primary MM cells but not on normal plasma cells [101, 102]. In vitro analysis has shown that cytokines [101] and BM-MSCs [102] increase PD-L1 expression on MM cells, indicating that the BM microenvironment plays a role in the activation of the PD-1/PD-L1 pathway. It has been demonstrated that PD-1 expression is upregulated on T cells [146] and NK cells [139] isolated from patients with MM compared to healthy donors, likely leading to an inhibition of antitumor immunity through the expression of PD-L1.

Clinical trials targeting PD-1/PD-L1 pathway to overcome tumor-associated immune suppression have shown unprecedented results in a variety of heavily pretreated patients with solid tumors, melanoma, and lung cancer in particular. Most recently, significant activity of nivolumab as well as pembrolizumab, PD-1 blocking antibodies, has also been observed in hematologic malignancies. Specifically, substantial therapeutic activity and an acceptable safety profile were observed in patients with previously heavily pretreated relapsed/refractory Hodgkin's lymphoma [147]. Moreover, the efficacy of inhibiting the PD-1/PD-L1 pathway has also been demonstrated in preclinical studies of MM. Rosenblatt et al. [146] showed that pidilizumab/CT-011, an anti-PD1 antibody, enhanced activated T-cell responses after DC/tumor fusion stimulation in MM. Furthermore, Hallet et al. [148] showed that PD-L1 blockade combined with stem cell transplant and whole-cell vaccination increased the survival of myeloma bearing mice. Kearl et al. [149] showed that PD-L1 antibody improves survival of murine MM when combined with whole body irradiation. Similarly, Jing et al. demonstrated synergistic or additive increases of survival in a 5T33 murine MM model upon combining low dose of whole body irradiation and combinations of blocking antibodies to PD-L1 LAG-3, TIM-3, CD48 and CTLA4 [150].

Considering the elevation of PD-1 and its ligand in the MM microenvironment, inhibition of the PD-1/PD-L1 pathway has the potential to substantially change microenvironment-targeted therapy in MM. However, in contrast to solid tumors, monotherapy with immune checkpoint inhibitors in MM is not sufficient. Further research is therefore required to investigate their therapeutic potential when combined with other novel agents or a series of immune checkpoint inhibitors.

Bispecific Antibodies and Bispecific T- Cell Engagers (BiTEs) Bispecific antibodies are two monoclonal antibodies incorporated into a single molecular species. One of the effective formats is the bispecific T-cell engagers (BiTEs), in which a tumor-reactive single-chain variable antibody fragment (scFv) is translated in tandem with a second scFv that binds CD3 [151]. BiTEs promote the formation of immunologic synapses and mediate serial triggering of tumor cell cytotoxicity. In hematological malignancies, blinatumomab, which simultaneously engages CD3 and the pan B-cell antigen CD19, showed clinical efficacy in refractory B-ALL at an early clinical trial [152]. In MM, several bispecific antibodies and BiTEs have been tested in preclinical models. Von Strandmann et al. developed a bispecific protein targeting CD138 on MM cells and the NKG2D receptor on NK cells, which had potent antitumor activity against human MM in vivo [153]. Rossi et al. reported that IFN-alpha2b immunocytokine targeting CD20 and HLA-DR was effective to human MM cell line KMS-12BM, which is CD20$^+$ HLA-DR$^+$ [154]. Recently, Zou et al. successfully developed a ScFv combination of anti-CD3 ScFv and anti-CD138 ScFv with the hIgG1 Fc (hIgFc) sequence, which is able to target T cells, NK cells, and MM cell lines (RPMI-8226 or U266) [155]. The antibodies showed potent antitumor activity both in vitro and in vivo. In summary, BiTEs have the potential to increase the efficacy of preclinically used monoclonal antibodies in MM treatment (i.e., CD38, CD138, and CS1). Additional antibody combinations should be considered for more efficient treatment response of BiTEs in MM.

Chimeric Antigen Receptor Modified T Cells (CAR-T Cells) Chimeric antigen receptors (CARs) are recombinant receptors that can target native cell surface molecules. First-generation CARs comprise an antigen recognition domain from the single-chain variable fragments (scFv) of a monoclonal antibody, and an intracellular T-cell signaling domain (usually CD3ζ), whereas second- and third-generation CARs additionally incorporate one or two costimulatory domains (such as CD28, 4-1BB and ICOS), respectively [156]. Unlike T-cell receptors (TCRs), CARs engage molecules that do not require peptide processing or HLA expression to be recognized. Adoptive transfer of CAR modified T cells (CAR-T cells) is a promising anticancer therapeutic, which induces immune responses against tumor-associated antigens. The most investigated target for CAR-T cell therapies in hematological malignancies is CD19 for B-cell malignancies. For instance, Davila et al. reported the first large cohort of B-ALL patients in a phase I trial treated with CD19-targeted CAR-T cells with an 88 % overall complete response rate [157]. Multiple preclinical studies for CARs have been done in MM, targeting different surface molecules. Similar to the case of monoclonal antibodies used in clinical trials, CD38 [158] and CS1 [159] have been studied as potential target antigens for CAR-T cell therapy in MM. Additionally, CAR-T therapy targeting CD138 has entered into a phase I/II clinical trial in China (NCT01886976). Other potential targets in MM have also been identified such as BCMA [160], Lewis Y antigen [161] and CD44v6 [162]. However, multiple factors such as CAR design, off target effects, and disease burden still require consideration when adapting the therapy to individuals.

2.3 Focus on MM Bone Disease

The balance between bone resorption and new bone formation is fundamental for preserving the functional integrity of bone tissue throughout the adult life [163]. This balance is lost in most of MM cases, resulting in bone destruction and the development of osteolytic lesions, which represent paradigmatic features of MM [164]. Overall data suggest that bone degradation is an early event in MM; patients diagnosed with MGUS few months to one year before development of MM have an increased bone degradation compared with MGUS patients who did not progress to MM [165].

OCs are the cells responsible for bone resorption; they originate from hematopoietic precursors and are part of the monocyte–macrophage cell lineage [166]. OBs are responsible for the formation of new bone following OC-mediated bone resorption. OBs originate from Runx2- and wingless type (Wnt)-dependent differentiation of MSCs [166]. Overall it is now clear whether MM cells are able to both increase the bone resorption by stimulating OCs, and to reduce bone formation by inhibiting OBs or MSC-to-OB differentiation [167]. There are several factors that have been implicated in activation and proliferation of OCs, including receptor activator of NF-κB ligand (RANKL), stromal-derived factor 1-alpha (SDF-1 alpha), vascular endothelial growth factor (VEGF), macrophage colony-stimulating factor (M-CSF), macrophage inflammatory protein-1a (MIP-1a), interleukin-3 (IL-3) and IL-6 [168]. RANKL is a member of the tumor necrosis factor (TNF) family and plays a pivotal role in the increased osteoclastogenesis implicated in MM bone disease [169]. **RANK** is a transmembrane receptor expressed by OCs, which binds to RANKL expressed by both MM cells and BMSCs within the BM; activation of RANK receptor by its interaction with RANKL leads to differentiation of OC precursors, and activation, inhibition of apoptosis, and proliferation of mature OCs via NF-κB and JunN-terminal kinase pathways [170]. On the other hand, osteoprotegerin (OPG) is a soluble receptor, secreted by OBs and BM-MSCs, that exerts the exact opposite biological activity to RANKL; in fact, OPG is able to antagonize RANKL by direct binding [171].

Tightly regulated under physiological conditions, the equilibrium between RANKL and OPG expression in patients with MM is markedly disrupted, with an increase in the expression of RANKL and a decrease in OPG expression, leading to increased bone resorption [172]. Conversely, blockade of RANKL with a soluble form of RANK inhibits not only bone loss but also decreases tumor burden in MM in vivo models [173, 174]. Bone-targeting strategies based on the use of the potent bisphosphonate zoledronic acid have demonstrated the ability to significantly increase survival of MM patients in a phase III clinical trial [175]. Consequently, research on new therapeutic tools able to prevent and halt progression of MM bone disease is now becoming critical. Denosumab is a humanized antibody with high affinity for RANKL, mimicking the activity of OPG; it has been tested in phase II and phase III clinical trials showing activity as an antiresorptive agent in MM patients [176]. In a phase III trial MM patients were randomized to treatment with either the gold standard treatment zoledronic acid or denosumab. Denosumab was found to be equivalent to zoledronic acid in delaying time to first on-study skeletal-related event with a subanalysis demonstrating an increase in survival in MM denosumab treated patients [177]. Besides MM cell migration and differentiation, the **SDF-1 alpha**/CXCR4 complex plays an important role in OC activity and bone resorption [178]. Indeed, anti-CXCR4 antibodies have demonstrated therapeutic activity in preclinical MM models indicating a direct effect on OCs [179, 180]. In addition to its implication in BM angiogenesis [181], **VEGF** has been also associated with the promotion of OC-mediated MM bone resorption [182, 183]. VEGF therefore represents a promising therapeutic target in MM. Clinical trials using VEGF and VEGFR inhibitors are ongoing. **MIP-1α**, a chemokine produced by MM cells, promotes proliferation and differentiation of OCs and thereby bone resorption [168]. Increased serum levels of MIP-1α in MM patients correlate with the severity of bone destruction [184]. Additional liquid factors known to stimulate OCs and thereby contribute to MM bone disease include M-CSF, IL-6, TNF-α, IL-3, and IL-11 [167, 185]. Finally, direct as well as indirect interactions between MM cells and OCs increase viability of MM cells and OC proliferation and activation [186, 187]. Similarly, OBs contribute to MM pathogenesis by supporting MM cell growth, proliferation and survival [188]. Moreover, reduced recruitment of OBs into the bone causes reduced mineral deposition [168, 189]. For example, MM-OB cocultures stimulate IL-6 production and secretion by MM cells thereby triggering autocrine MM cell proliferation [188]. Moreover, OBs secrete OPG, which in turn blocks TRAIL-mediated MM cell apoptosis [190]. Several liquid factors are responsible for suppression of osteoblast activity in MM [191]. DKK1, a Wnt signaling antagonist secreted by MM cells inhibits osteoblast differentiation. Indeed, in patients with MM bone disease DKK1 blood and BM serum levels are increased [192]. Therefore, we and others hypothesized that blocking DKK1 or activating Wnt signaling pathway prevents MM bone disease and reduces tumor burden [193]. The anti-DKK1 human antibody BHQ880 increases OBs differentiation, the number of OBs and trabecular thickness in murine MM models [194]. Clinical trials with BHQ880 and other DKK1 inhibitors are currently ongoing in MM and smoldering MM patients [195] (https://clinicaltrials.gov). Sclerostin, sFRP-2, and sFRP-3, which are expressed by MM cells, are other inhibitors of Wnt signaling that have been implicated in MM bone disease. They may therefore represent additional therapeutic targets for MM bone disease [191]. Moreover, TGF-β, which is secreted by bone matrix during OC-mediated bone destruction, inhibits OB differentiation [196]. Inhibition of TGF-β signaling pathways results in the reversion of the inhibitory action of MM cells on OB differentiation [197]. Thus TGF-β may be implicated in sustaining progression of MM disease via promotion of bone remodeling. Interestingly, IL-3 inhibits differentiation of primary BM-MSCs into OBs [198]; and IL-3 levels in the BM serum of MM patients are increased compared to healthy individuals [199]. Importantly, IL-3 also promotes activation of OCs [199]. Finally, hepatocyte growth factor (HGF) is another factor expressed by MM cells, which inhibits osteoblastogenesis [200]. Implicated also in MM BM angiogenesis [201], and MM cell proliferation [202] HGF may therefore represent a promising therapeutic target.

Taken together, these studies show the complexity of the pathogenesis of MM bone disease, and indicate new therapeutic approaches that may be used in the near future to implement currently available bisphosphonate based therapy for the prevention and treatment of bone destruction in MM patients.

2.4 Bone Marrow Adipose Tissues

The set of accepted MM risk factors includes increasing age, male gender, black race, positive family history, and the MGUS predisposing condition [203]. Several studies have now identified obesity as an additional risk factor associated with MM development and aggressiveness [204–206]. Similarly, an increased risk of MM development is associated with type 2 diabetes (T2D) [207, 208], a condition closely linked to obesity. MGUS incidence seems higher in obese people, supporting the hypothesis that myelomagenesis is linked with obesity [209]. The circulating levels of adiponectin are negatively correlated with obesity and it exists an inverse relationship between circulating adipokines and risk of MM development [210]; in this context adiponectin may play an important role in obesity-related myelomagenesis [210]. Obesity may also have a role as a prognostic factor in MM. Although a significant shorter OS has been linked to obese MM patients, the relationship between BMI and MM prognosis is more complex [211]. The effects of systemic obesity and T2D on hematopoiesis are currently under intense investigation [212]. Overall, data shows that obesity impairs immunity both in humans and mice by deregulating BM hematopoiesis. Many studies in mice have demonstrated an effect of adiposity on reducing lymphocyte populations and increasing numbers of myeloid progenitors [212]. Interestingly, diet-induced obesity (DIO) induced significant trabecular bone loss probably due to OB dysfuntion and B-cell depletion in mice suggesting that obesity affects the BM hematopoietic niche [213]; accordingly, increase in BM adiposity slows haematopoietic recovery following high dose chemotherapy in mice and possibly in humans [214]. DIO induces BM lymphoid depletion, thymic adiposity and defective T-cell production that may explain immune deregulation; DIO impairs the function and maintenance of memory T cells, Treg cells, and it inhibits cytotoxic T cells as well as NK activity [212]. Taken together these changes induced by obesity on hematopoiesis could partially explain evidences linking obesity to MM. In addition, adipocytes accumulating in BM may also directly promote MM cell growth; thus it is important to investigate putative BM adipocytes–MM cell interactions in the MM BM microenvironment. BM adipocytes are derived from stroma cell progenitor differentiation and their number progressively increases with advancing age, resulting in adipocytic deposits occupying up to 70 % of the BM cavity in elderly persons [215]. Considering that MM is typically a disease of the elderly people and that its incidence increases with age [203], a positive association between obesity and MM development is likely. To test this hypothesis, Caers et al. [216] assessed the effects of both an adipocyte cell line and primary adipocytes on MM cells. The authors found that adipocytes positively promote MM growth, survival and migration. Of note, these effects were partially mediated by leptin, which is secreted by adipocytes and acts via binding to the leptin receptor, which is expressed on MM cell line and primary cells. Importantly, during MM progression, the invasion of MM cells into the BM stroma is progressively accompanied by a decrease in BM adipocytes. The importance of adipocytes may therefore be mainly restricted to the initial disease stages before a remodeling of the BM microenvironment occurs, the MGUS and SMM transition to active MM in particular [216]. In line with these observations a recent study by Lwin et al. [217] showed that 5-week high-fat diet was not able to further promote MM growth in the myeloma-permissive KaLwRij mice after tail vein injection of syngenic 5TGM1 MM cells. Importantly, DIO created a permissive environment for MM in nonpermissive C57Bl6 mice enabling the engraftment with 5TGM1 cells. Taken together, obesity may create a permissive environment promoting development of an MGUS-like condition that eventually progresses to overt MM. Consequently, targeting of adipocytes and obesity treatment may be effective in the early stages of myelomagenesis or MM prevention, in particular.

3 The Extracellular Compartment and the Liquid Milieu

3.1 The Extracellular Matrix (ECM)

The ECM consists of proteoglycans, nonproteoglycans, and fibers (collagen, elastin) as well as fibronectin and laminin. These components are produced by various cell types, including fibroblasts, and OBs. Although the composition of the ECM varies dependent on the tissue context, cell adhesion, cell-to-cell communication and differentiation are common functions of the ECM [218]. In addition, it acts as a local store by sequestering growth factors and cytokines. Physiologic or pathophysiologic changes trigger protease or metalloproteinase activities thereby causing the immediate release of factors from these stores and allowing rapid and local growth factor-mediated activation of cellular functions. Cell adhesion to the ECM is either mediated via focal adhesions connecting the ECM to actin filaments of the cell, or via hemidesmosomes connecting the ECM to intermediate filaments such as keratin. Integrins are specific cell surface cellular adhesion molecules (CAM) that bind cells to ECM structures, such as fibronectin and laminin, but also to integrin proteins on the surface of other cells. The attachment of fibronectin to the extracellular domain initiates intracellular signaling pathways as well as association with the cellular cytoskeleton via a set of adaptor molecules such as actin. Unlike growth factor receptors, integrins have no intrinsic enzymatic activity but trigger signaling pathways by clustering with other kinases (receptor tyrosine kinases or cytoplasmic kinases) or proteins of focal/adhesion/cytoskeleton complexes. Key integrins mediating MM cell–ECM adhesion are $\alpha4\beta1$ (CD49d/CD29 or VLA-4) and $\alpha v\beta3$-integrin. MM cell adhesion to fibronectin is predominantly mediated through VLA-4 and directly protects tumor cells from DNA damaging drugs (i.e., anthracyclines and alkylating agents) by induction of CAM drug resistance (CAM-DR), a reversible G1 arrest associated with increased p27kip1 (encoded by CDKN1B) levels [7, 219]. MM cell adhesion to vitronectin and fibronectin is predominantly mediated through $\alpha v\beta3$-integrin-binding and triggers production and release of urokinase-type plasminogen activator, MMP-2 and MMP-9, thereby promoting tumor cell invasion and spreading [220, 221]. Interestingly, a recent study indicates that ECM remodeling by BM-MSCs may play an important role in the progression of MGUS to MM [222]. Since integrins are easily accessible and readily targeted by antibodies they may provide excellent drug targets. Another potential target is CD147 also known as ECM metalloproteinase (MMP) inducer (EMMPRIN), which has been implicated in the evolution from MGUS to MM progression [223].

Finally, changes in glycosylation of cell surface adhesion molecules such as selectin ligands, integrins and mucins have been implicated in the pathogenesis of several solid and hematological malignancies, often with prognostic implications [224]. Most recent studies demonstrated high expression of β-galactoside α-2,3-sialyltransferase, ST3GAL6, in MM cell lines and patients. This gene plays a key role in selectin ligand synthesis, which is involved in the mediation of adhesion to MM BM stromal cells and fibronectin, and is significantly associated with inferior overall survival [225]. Therefore, targeting glycosylation of selectin ligands represents a potential therapeutic target. Moreover, recent advances to introduce anti-adhesion strategies as a novel therapeutic concept in oncology in general, and MM in particular, hold great promise. Importantly, thalidomide, bortezomib, and lenalidomide exert their anti-MM activity, at least in part, by inhibition of MM cell binding to ECM proteins. Our own data demonstrate anti-MM activity of the humanized anti-α4 antibody natalizumab in MM [226]. However, a clinical trial using natalizumab in relapsed/refractory MM was terminated in late 2014 due to low enrollment. A clinical trial evaluating the humanized anti-vitronectin receptor (anti-αvβ3) antibody etaracizumab (Abegrin™ previously known as Vitaxin® or MEDI-522) is ongoing.

3.2 The Liquid Milieu

Initially considered to be the sole contributor of maintenance and expansion of MM cells within the BM, the liquid compartment consists of cytokines and growth factors, most prominently including IL-6, VEGF, IGF-1, and SDF-1. They are produced and secreted by MM cells as well as other BM stroma cells both via autocrine and paracrine loops and cell–cell adhesion.

IL-6. Predominantly produced and secreted by BMSCs and osteoblasts, IL-6 is a key growth and survival factor in MM. IL-6 levels correlate with MM tumor cell mass, disease stage and prognosis [227, 228]. IL-6 triggers caveolin-1/Hck/Gab1/2-dependent activation of MEK/MAPK-, JAK/STAT3-, and PI3K/Akt signaling pathways [229]. Moreover, it triggers JAK/STAT3-dependent upregulation/activation of antiapoptotic proteins Mcl-1 and Bcl-xL, Pim1 as well as c-Myc. Besides MM cell growth and survival, IL-6 confers drug resistance, to dexamethasone in particular, via activation of PI3K- Akt- and SHP2-related adhesion focal tyrosine kinase (RAFTK) and mitochondrial release of second activator of apoptosis (Smac) [230, 231]. Compounds targeting IL-6 signaling pathways include antibodies against IL-6 and IL-6 receptor, for example, siltuximab/CNTO 328, IL-6 antisense oligonucleotides and IL-6 super antagonist Sant7 [232]. A Japanese phase 1 study of siltuximab in relapsed/refractory MM showed no dose-limiting toxicities at a recommended dose of 11 mg/kg once every 3 weeks [233]. Additional clinical trials evaluating the safety and efficacy of siltuximab alone or in combination with other agents including bortezomib, lenalidomide are ongoing in patients with high-risk SMM, relapsed or refractory MM (https://clinicaltrials.gov). However, many MM cell lines grow independently of IL-6. Moreover, binding of MM cells to

BMSCs trigger survival even after inhibition of the IL-6/gp130/STAT3 pathway, suggesting MM growth mechanisms other than IL-6. These findings may also explain why therapeutic approaches targeting IL-6 have not induced responses in phase I clinical trials. Taken together, these data show that IL-6 is a crucial, but not a sole factor in MM pathogenesis.

TNFα superfamily-induced signaling pathways in MM. The TNFα superfamily includes SDF-1α, CD40, BAFF, and APRIL. In MM, SDF-1α and its G-protein-linked cognate receptor CXCR4 (CD184) are expressed in the BM of MM patients. SDF-1α is primarily produced by BMSCs, but also by MM cells. Functionally, SDF-1α rapidly and transiently upregulates LFA-1-, VLA-4-, and VLA5-mediated MM cell adhesion and migration [234, 235]; promotes proliferation and protects against dexamethasone-induced apoptosis in MM cells; and stimulates secretion of IL-6 and VEGF in BMSCs [236]. In addition, SDF-1α activates the CXCR7 receptor [237], which modulates trafficking and adhesion of human malignant hematopoietic cells. Most importantly SDF-1α is a critical regulator of MM cell homing [236]. Indeed, a recent study demonstrates that treatment with the high-affinity anti-SDF-1 PEGylated mirror-image l-oligonucleotide (olaptesed pegol) renders the BM microenvironment less receptive for MM cells and reduces MM cell homing and growth, thereby inhibiting MM disease progression [179]. Moreover, current clinical trials investigate the role of the CXCR4 inhibitor AMD3100 (Genzyme, Cambridge, MA, USA) in the inhibition of MM cell homing [238]. *CD40* is expressed by antigen-presenting cells, T cells, as well as B-cell malignancies including MM. Functionally, CD40 mediates p53-dependent increases in MM cell growth, PI3K/Akt/NF-kB-dependent MM cell migration, triggers VEGF secretion and induces membrane translocation of Ku86 and Ku70 proteins involved in IgH class switching. Moreover, CD40-activated MM cells adhere to fibronectin and are protected against apoptosis triggered by irradiation and doxorubicin [239]. A clinical phase I trial using the anti-CD40 antibody dacetuzumab (SGN-40) showed good tolerance, with the best clinical response of stable disease in 20 % of patients. Based on preclinical studies [142] two trials evaluating the therapeutic potential of dacetuzumab in combination with lenalidomide/dexamethasone, or bortezomib, respectively, have now been completed. Results are pending. TNFα is mainly secreted by macrophages, and triggers only modest MM cell proliferation, survival and drug resistance. However, it markedly upregulates (fivefold) secretion of IL-6 in BMSCs and induces NF-kB-dependent expression of CD11a/LFA-1, CD54/ICAM-1, CD106/VCAM-1, CD49d/VLA-4 and/or MUC-1 on MM cell lines; as well as CD106/VCAM-1 and CD54/ICAM-1 expression on BMSCs. Expression of these molecules results in increased (two to fourfold) specific binding of MM cells to BM-MSCs, with related induction of IL-6 transcription and secretion, as well as CAM-DR. Agents that target TNFα including bortezomib, thalidomide and IMiDs, at least in part, abrogate the paracrine growth and survival advantage conferred by MM cell adhesion in the BM microenvironment [240]. B lymphocyte stimulator (BAFF) is normally expressed by monocytes, macrophages, DCs, T cells, OCs and BM-MSCs, and exists both as a membrane-bound and a cleaved soluble protein. In MM, both tumor cells and BM-MSCs express high levels of BAFF and APRIL and their receptors [241]. BAFF secretion by BM-MSCs is further augmented upon adhesion to MM cells [231]. Serum BAFF levels are related to angiogenesis and prognosis in MM patients [242]. Functionally, BAFF and APRIL protect MM cells from apoptosis induced by IL-6 deprivation and dexamethasone and promote MM cell growth as well as adhesion to BM-MSCs through activation of NF-kB-, PI3K/Akt-, and MAPK pathways. Furthermore, both BAFF and APRIL induce strong upregulation of Mcl-1 and Bcl-2, and regulate TACI- and c-Maf-dependent expression of both cyclin D2 and integrin β7 [231, 241]. Importantly, high TACI expression TACI (hi)) displays mature plasma cell gene signature indicating dependence on the BM environment, while low TACI expression (TACI (lo)) displays a gene signature of plasma blasts, suggesting an attenuated dependence on the BM microenvironment. Taken together, these data strongly suggest the therapeutic value of antibodies or small-molecule inhibitors, which target BAFF/APRIL-induced signaling pathways, in MM patients with TACI (hi) in particular [243].

Insulin-like growth factor-1-induced signaling pathways in MM. In MM, IGF-1 promotes proliferation and drug resistance in MM cells through activation of MAPK and PI3K/Akt signaling cascades and MM cell migration and invasion through a PI3K-dependent Akt-independent protein kinase D/PKCm/RhoA/β1-integrin-associated pathway [232]. Moreover, IGF-1 regulates the expression of Bcl-2 proteins; and the IGF-1 receptor inhibitor picropodophyllin potentiates the anti-MM activity of BH3-mimetics ABT737, 263 and 199 [244]. Importantly, inhibition of the IGF-1R overcomes bortezomib resistance [245], and sensitizes MM cells to bortezomib via therapeutic enhancement of ER stress [246]. As for IL-6 and VEGF-signaling pathways, caveolae are also required for IGF-1-signaling sequelae [247]; and cross-activation of IGF-1 and IL-6 receptors is facilitated by the close proximity of these two receptors at lipid rafts on the plasma membrane [248]. Consequently, inhibition of IGF-1 receptor using NVP-ADW742 also blocks the IL-6-triggered response in MM cells [249]. A clinical trial investigating the IGF-1R inhibitor ASP7487 (OSI-906) in combination with bortezomib for the treatment of relapsed MM is ongoing (https://clinicaltrials.gov).

4   Recent New Insights on Signaling Molecules

Binding of MM cells to stroma cells and the ECM as well as changes in the secretion of cytokine- and growth factor levels lead to tumor cell proliferation, survival, migration, and drug resistance via activation of numerous signaling cascades. Several approaches to target surface receptors or to neutralize cytokines, growth factors and their respective receptors as well as downstream signaling molecules are under investigation. For example, Raf is a key regulator of cellular proliferation and survival within the MAPK pathway. BAY43-9006/sorafenib/ Nexavar (Bayer Pharmaceuticals, West Haven, CT, USA) is the first oral multikinase inhibitor (PDGFR, VEGFR-1,-2,-3 and c-Kit) that targets c-Raf. Single agent use of sorafenib in MM patients with relapsing and resistant MM did not exhibit anti-MM activity (SWOG S0434 trial [250]). Based on preclinical studies, which demonstrated significant anti-MM activity and synergism when given in combination with common anti-MM drugs [251, 252], ongoing clinical trials investigate the activity of sorafenib when combined with bortezomib, or lenalidomide in relapsed or refractory MM (https://clinicaltrials.gov). Moreover, in an initial genome sequencing analysis of MM B-Raf mutations were observed in 4 % of patients [253]. Indeed, treatment of a MM patient with extensive extramedullary disease, who was refractory to all approved therapeutic options and who carried the B-Raf V600E mutation, with vemurafenib induced rapid and durable responses [254]. A clinical phase I study in patients with B-Raf V600E-positive cancers including MM is ongoing. An additional novel target is ERK5 [255]. Clinical trials using the ERK5 inhibitor TG02-101 in MM are ongoing.

5 Hypoxia within the Bone Marrow Microenvironment

In MM, the hypoxic BM microenvironment of the endosteal niche supports the selection of aggressive MM cell clones and their survival and growth [256]. These effects are predominantly mediated via activation of HIF-1 and HIF-2. In addition HIFs increase the production of angiogenic but also osteoclastogenic factors within the BM and thereby stimulate, at least in part, BM angiogenesis and osteoclastogenesis. Importantly, when deregulated HIF collaborates with oncogenic c-Myc in inducing the expression of VEGF, PDK1, and hexokinase 2 [257]. Constitutive expression of HIF-1α has been observed in about 35 % of MM patients. Interestingly, recent studies demonstrate that hypoxia also activates EMT-related machinery in MM cells and stroma cells, including activation of HIFs, activation of SNAIL, and decreased expression of E-cadherin leading to decreased adhesion of MM cells to stroma cells, decreased SDF-1α secretion from stroma, and enhanced egress of MM cells to the circulation [46]. Moreover hypoxia reduces CD138 expression and induces an immature and stem cell-like transcription program in MM cells [258]. HIF-1α is therefore a promising therapeutic target. EZN-2968, a small 3rd generation antisense oligonucleotide against HIF-1α induced a permanent cell cycle arrest and mild apoptotic cell death [259]. Another approach to target hypoxia in MM is the use of hypoxia-activated prodrug TH-302, which selectively targets hypoxic MM cells triggers apoptosis and decreases paracodein secretion [256]. In addition synergistic induction of apoptosis in MM cells by bortezomib together with TH-302 was observed in preclinical in vitro and in vivo studies [260].

6 Concluding Remarks

It is now well established that the BM microenvironment plays a key role in MM pathogenesis. However, despite unprecedented advances in derived MM therapy it remains an incurable disease with a median survival of 7–8 years. One of the most exciting advances in the field of MM treatment is the emergence of immune therapies. Another striking finding of recently completed next-generation sequencing studies has been the high degree of heterogeneity in MM cells [12, 253, 261–264]. These data confirm analogous reports based on copy number variations [265, 266]; and flow cytometry analysis [267, 268]. Ongoing studies investigate whether disease progression depends on heterogeneity-driven modifications of the microenvironment; which in turn confer selective advantage of more aggressive MM subclones. New insights into these processes will lead to the identification of additional therapeutic targets and the development of derived novel agents. The foremost challenge in the clinical development of novel agents is the selection of the most promising compounds. Another challenge is the safety of novel agents. Moreover, given the profound heterogeneity of MM further improvements are likely only reachable by personalized treatment approaches, which simultaneously target both MM subclones as well as tumor-supportive constituents of the BM MM microenvironment. Well-designed clinical trials will be needed to identify those combination regimens with maximal activity and minimal toxicity. We are confident that continuing efforts in preclinical and clinical MM research will help to turn MM into a chronic disease with sustained complete response in many of our patients in near future.

Conflict of Interests

The Authors declare no competing interests

References

1. Danet GH, Pan Y, Luongo JL, Bonnet DA, Simon MC (2003) Expansion of human SCID-repopulating cells under hypoxic conditions. J Clin Investig 112:126–135
2. Pennathur-Das R, Levitt L (1987) Augmentation of in vitro human marrow erythropoiesis under physiological oxygen tensions is mediated by monocytes and T lymphocytes. Blood 69:899–907
3. Levesque JP, Winkler IG, Hendy J, Williams B, Helwani F, Barbier V, Nowlan B, Nilsson SK (2007) Hematopoietic progenitor cell mobilization results in hypoxia with increased hypoxia-inducible transcription factor-1 alpha and vascular endothelial growth factor A in bone marrow. Stem Cells 25:1954–1965
4. Podar K, Anderson KC (2005) The pathophysiologic role of VEGF in hematologic malignancies: therapeutic implications. Blood 105:1383–1395
5. Bissell MJ, Hines WC (2011) Why don't we get more cancer? A proposed role of the microenvironment in restraining cancer progression. Nat Med 17:320–329
6. Morrison SJ, Scadden DT (2014) The bone marrow niche for haematopoietic stem cells. Nature 505:327–334
7. Hazlehurst LA, Damiano JS, Buyuksal I, Pledger WJ, Dalton WS (2000) Adhesion to fibronectin via beta1 integrins regulates p27kip1 levels and contributes to cell adhesion mediated drug resistance (CAM-DR). Oncogene 19:4319–4327
8. Tai YT, Dillon M, Song W, Leiba M, Li XF, Burger P, Lee AI, Podar K, Hideshima T, Rice AG, van Abbema A, Jesaitis L, Caras I, Law D, Weller E, Xie W, Richardson P, Munshi NC, Mathiot C, Avet-Loiseau H, Afar DE, Anderson KC (2008) Anti-CS1 humanized monoclonal antibody HuLuc63 inhibits myeloma cell adhesion and induces antibody-dependent cellular cytotoxicity in the bone marrow milieu. Blood 112:1329–1337

9. Raje N, Roodman GD (2011) Advances in the biology and treatment of bone disease in multiple myeloma. Clin Cancer Res: Official J Am Assoc Cancer Res 17:1278–1286

10. Paiva B, Perez-Andres M, Vidriales MB, Almeida J, de las Heras N, Mateos MV, Lopez-Corral L, Gutierrez NC, Blanco J, Oriol A, Hernandez MT, de Arriba F, de Coca AG, Terol MJ, de la Rubia J, Gonzalez Y, Martin A, Sureda A, Schmidt-Hieber M, Schmitz A, Johnsen HE, Lahuerta JJ, Blade J, San-Miguel JF, Orfao A, Gem P (2011) N. Myeloma Stem Cell, Competition between clonal plasma cells and normal cells for potentially overlapping bone marrow niches is associated with a progressively altered cellular distribution in MGUS vs myeloma Leukemia 25:697–706

11. Lopez-Corral L, Corchete LA, Sarasquete ME, Mateos MV, Garcia-Sanz R, Ferminan E, Lahuerta JJ, Blade J, Oriol A, Teruel AI, Martino ML, Hernandez J, Hernandez-Rivas JM, Burguillo FJ, San Miguel JF, Gutierrez NC (2014) Transcriptome analysis reveals molecular profiles associated with evolving steps of monoclonal gammopathies. Haematologica 99:1365–1372

12. Walker BA, Wardell CP, Melchor L, Brioli A, Johnson DC, Kaiser MF, Mirabella F, Lopez-Corral L, Humphray S, Murray L, Ross M, Bentley D, Gutierrez NC, Garcia-Sanz R, San Miguel J, Davies FE, Gonzalez D, Morgan GJ (2014) Intraclonal heterogeneity is a critical early event in the development of myeloma and precedes the development of clinical symptoms. Leukemia 28:384–390

13. Reagan MR, Ghobrial IM (2012) Multiple myeloma mesenchymal stem cells: characterization, origin, and tumor-promoting effects. Clin Cancer Res: Official J Am Assoc Cancer Res 18:342–349

14. Garayoa M, Garcia JL, Santamaria C, Garcia-Gomez A, Blanco JF, Pandiella A, Hernandez JM, Sanchez-Guijo FM, del Canizo MC, Gutierrez NC, San Miguel JF (2009) Mesenchymal stem cells from multiple myeloma patients display distinct genomic profile as compared with those from normal donors. Leukemia 23:1515–1527

15. Corre J, Mahtouk K, Attal M, Gadelorge M, Huynh A, Fleury-Cappellesso S, Danho C, Laharrague P, Klein B, Reme T, Bourin P (2007) Bone marrow mesenchymal stem cells are abnormal in multiple myeloma. Leukemia 21:1079–1088

16. Harvey A, Yen TY, Aizman I, Tate C, Case C (2013) Proteomic analysis of the extracellular matrix produced by mesenchymal stromal cells: implications for cell therapy mechanism. PLoS ONE 8:e79283

17. Tancred TM, Belch AR, Reiman T, Pilarski LM, Kirshner J (2009) Altered expression of fibronectin and collagens I and IV in multiple myeloma and monoclonal gammopathy of undetermined significance. J Histochem Cytochem: Official J Histochem Soc 57:239–247

18. Zdzisinska B, Bojarska-Junak A, Dmoszynska A, Kandefer-Szerszen M (2008) Abnormal cytokine production by bone marrow stromal cells of multiple myeloma patients in response to RPMI8226 myeloma cells. Archivum immunologiae et therapiae experimentalis 56:207–221

19. Basak GW, Srivastava AS, Malhotra R, Carrier E (2009) Multiple myeloma bone marrow niche. Curr Pharm Biotechnol 10:345–346

20. Hideshima T, Mitsiades C, Tonon G, Richardson PG, Anderson KC (2007) Understanding multiple myeloma pathogenesis in the bone marrow to identify new therapeutic targets. Nat Rev Cancer 7:585–598

21. Mitsiades CS, Mitsiades NS, Munshi NC, Richardson PG, Anderson KC (2006) The role of the bone microenvironment in the pathophysiology and therapeutic management of multiple myeloma: interplay of growth factors, their receptors and stromal interactions. Eur J Cancer 42:1564–1573

22. Nefedova Y, Cheng P, Alsina M, Dalton WS, Gabrilovich DI (2004) Involvement of Notch-1 signaling in bone marrow stroma-mediated de novo drug resistance of myeloma and other malignant lymphoid cell lines. Blood 103:3503–3510

23. Kumar S, Witzig TE, Timm M, Haug J, Wellik L, Fonseca R, Greipp PR, Rajkumar SV (2003) Expression of VEGF and its receptors by myeloma cells. Leukemia 17:2025–2031

24. Dankbar B, Padro T, Leo R, Feldmann B, Kropff M, Mesters RM, Serve H, Berdel WE, Kienast J (2000) Vascular endothelial growth factor and interleukin-6 in paracrine tumor-stromal cell interactions in multiple myeloma. Blood 95:2630–2636

25. Podar K, Tai YT, Davies FE, Lentzsch S, Sattler M, Hideshima T, Lin BK, Gupta D, Shima Y, Chauhan D, Mitsiades C, Raje N, Richardson P, Anderson KC (2001) Vascular endothelial growth factor triggers signaling cascades mediating multiple myeloma cell growth and migration. Blood 98:428–435

26. Ribatti D, Moschetta M, Vacca A (2014) Microenvironment and multiple myeloma spread. Thromb Res 133(Suppl 2):S102–106

27. Moschetta M, Mishima Y, Sahin I, Manier S, Glavey S, Vacca A, Roccaro AM, Ghobrial IM (1846) Role of endothelial progenitor cells in cancer progression. Biochim Biophys Acta 2014:26–39

28. Hao M, Zhang L, An G, Meng H, Han Y, Xie Z, Xu Y, Li C, Yu Z, Chang H, Qiu L (2011) Bone marrow stromal cells protect myeloma cells from bortezomib induced apoptosis by suppressing microRNA-15a expression. Leuk lymphoma 52:1787–1794

29. Markovina S, Callander NS, O'Connor SL, Xu G, Shi Y, Leith CP, Kim K, Trivedi P, Kim J, Hematti P, Miyamoto S (2010) Bone marrow stromal cells from multiple myeloma patients uniquely induce bortezomib resistant NF-kappaB activity in myeloma cells. Molecular cancer 9:176

30. Ohishi M, Schipani E (2010) Bone marrow mesenchymal stem cells. J Cell Biochem 109:277–282

31. Savopoulos C, Dokos C, Kaiafa G, Hatzitolios A (2011) Adipogenesis and osteoblastogenesis: trans-differentiation in the pathophysiology of bone disorders. Hippokratia 15:18–21

32. Morito N, Yoh K, Fujioka Y, Nakano T, Shimohata H, Hashimoto Y, Yamada A, Maeda A, Matsuno F, Hata H, Suzuki A, Imagawa S, Mitsuya H, Esumi H, Koyama A, Yamamoto M, Mori N, Takahashi S (2006) Overexpression of c-Maf contributes to T-cell lymphoma in both mice and human. Cancer Res 66:812–819

33. De Veirman K, Rao L, De Bruyne E, Menu E, Van Valckenborgh E, Van Riet I, Frassanito MA, Di Marzo L, Vacca A, Vanderkerken K (2014) Cancer associated fibroblasts and tumor growth: focus on multiple myeloma. Cancers 6:1363–1381

34. Frassanito MA, Rao L, Moschetta M, Ria R, Di Marzo L, De Luisi A, Racanelli V, Catacchio I, Berardi S, Basile A, Menu E, Ruggieri S, Nico B, Ribatti D, Fumarulo R, Dammacco F, Vanderkerken K, Vacca A (2014) Bone marrow fibroblasts parallel multiple myeloma progression in patients and mice: in vitro and in vivo studies. Leukemia 28:904–916

35. Roccaro AM, Sacco A, Maiso P, Azab AK, Tai YT, Reagan M, Azab F, Flores LM, Campigotto F, Weller E, Anderson KC, Scadden DT, Ghobrial IM (2013) BM mesenchymal stromal cell-derived exosomes facilitate multiple myeloma progression. J Clin Investig 123:1542–1555

36. Thompson CA, Purushothaman A, Ramani VC, Vlodavsky I, Sanderson RD (2013) Heparanase regulates secretion, composition, and function of tumor cell-derived exosomes. J Biol Chem 288:10093–10099

37. Heissig B, Ohki Y, Sato Y, Rafii S, Werb Z, Hattori K (2005) A role for niches in hematopoietic cell development. Hematology 10:247–253

38. Vacca A, Ribatti D (2011) Angiogenesis and vasculogenesis in multiple myeloma: role of inflammatory cells. Recent Results Cancer Res 183:87–95

39. Braunstein M, Ozcelik T, Bagislar S, Vakil V, Smith EL, Dai K, Akyerli CB, Batuman OA (2006) Endothelial progenitor cells display clonal restriction in multiple myeloma. BMC Cancer 6:161

40. Ria R, Todoerti K, Berardi S, Coluccia AM, De Luisi A, Mattioli M, Ronchetti D, Morabito F, Guarini A, Petrucci MT, Dammacco F, Ribatti D, Neri A, Vacca A (2009) Gene expression profiling of bone marrow endothelial cells in patients with multiple myeloma. Clin Cancer Res: Official J Am Assoc Cancer Res 15:5369–5378

41. Streubel B, Chott A, Huber D, Exner M, Jager U, Wagner O, Schwarzinger I (2004) Lymphoma-specific genetic aberrations in microvascular endothelial cells in B-cell lymphomas. N Engl J Med 351:250–259

42. Chattopadhyay S, Stewart AL, Mukherjee S, Huang C, Hartwell KA, Miller PG, Subramanian R, Carmody LC, Yusuf RZ, Sykes DB, Paulk J, Vetere A, Vallet S, Santo L, Cirstea DD, Hideshima T, Dancik V, Majireck MM, Hussain MM, Singh S, Quiroz R, Iaconelli J, Karmacharya R, Tolliday NJ, Clemons PA, Moore MA, Stern AM, Shamji AF, Ebert BL, Golub TR, Raje NS, Scadden DT, Schreiber SL (2015) Niche-based screening in multiple myeloma identifies a kinesin-5 inhibitor with improved selectivity over hematopoietic progenitors. Cell Reports

43. Matsui W, Huff CA, Wang Q, Malehorn MT, Barber J, Tanhehco Y, Smith BD, Civin CI, Jones RJ (2004) Characterization of clonogenic multiple myeloma cells. Blood 103:2332–2336

44. Matsui W, Wang Q, Barber JP, Brennan S, Smith BD, Borrello I, McNiece I, Lin L, Ambinder RF, Peacock C, Watkins DN, Huff CA, Jones RJ (2008) Clonogenic multiple myeloma progenitors, stem cell properties, and drug resistance. Cancer Res 68:190–197

45. Peacock CD, Wang Q, Gesell GS, Corcoran-Schwartz IM, Jones E, Kim J, Devereux WL, Rhodes JT, Huff CA, Beachy PA, Watkins DN, Matsui W (2007) Hedgehog signaling maintains a tumor stem cell compartment in multiple myeloma. Proc Natl Acad Sci USA 104:4048–4053

46. Azab AK, Hu J, Quang P, Azab F, Pitsillides C, Awwad R, Thompson B, Maiso P, Sun JD, Hart CP, Roccaro AM, Sacco A, Ngo HT, Lin CP, Kung AL, Carrasco RD, Vanderkerken K, Ghobrial IM (2012) Hypoxia promotes dissemination of multiple myeloma through acquisition of epithelial to mesenchymal transition-like features. Blood 119:5782–5794

47. Scadden DT (2006) The stem-cell niche as an entity of action. Nature 441:1075–1079

48. Saltarella I, Lamanuzzi A, Reale A, Vacca A, Ria R (2015) Identify multiple myeloma stem cells: Utopia? World J stem cells 7:84–95

49. Wilson A, Laurenti E, Trumpp A (2009) Balancing dormant and self-renewing hematopoietic stem cells. Curr Opin Genet Dev 19:461–468

50. Paino T, Ocio EM, Paiva B, San-Segundo L, Garayoa M, Gutierrez NC, Sarasquete ME, Pandiella A, Orfao A, San JF (2012) Miguel, CD20 positive cells are undetectable in the majority of multiple myeloma cell lines and are not associated with a cancer stem cell phenotype. Haematologica 97:1110–1114

51. Paiva B, Paino T, Sayagues JM, Garayoa M, San-Segundo L, Martin M, Mota I, Sanchez ML, Barcena P, Aires-Mejia I, Corchete L, Jimenez C, Garcia-Sanz R, Gutierrez NC, Ocio EM, Mateos MV, Vidriales MB, Orfao A, San Miguel JF (2013) Detailed characterization of multiple myeloma circulating tumor cells shows unique phenotypic, cytogenetic, functional, and circadian distribution profile. Blood 122:3591–3598

52. Yang Y, Shi J, Gu Z, Salama ME, Das S, Wendlandt E, Xu H, Huang J, Tao Y, Hao M, Franqui R, Levasseur D, Janz S, Tricot G, Zhan F (2015) Bruton tyrosine kinase is a therapeutic target in stem-like cells from multiple myeloma. Cancer Res 75:594–604

53. Blotta S, Jakubikova J, Calimeri T, Roccaro AM, Amodio N, Azab AK, Foresta U, Mitsiades CS, Rossi M, Todoerti K, Molica S, Morabito F, Neri A, Tagliaferri P, Tassone P, Anderson KC, Munshi NC (2012) Canonical and noncanonical Hedgehog pathway in the pathogenesis of multiple myeloma. Blood 120:5002–5013

54. Arnulf B, Lecourt S, Soulier J, Ternaux B, Lacassagne MN, Crinquette A, Dessoly J, Sciaini AK, Benbunan M, Chomienne C, Fermand JP, Marolleau JP, Larghero J (2007) Phenotypic and functional characterization of bone marrow mesenchymal stem cells derived from patients with multiple myeloma. Leukemia 21:158–163

55. Mukherjee S, Raje N, Schoonmaker JA, Liu JC, Hideshima T, Wein MN, Jones DC, Vallet S, Bouxsein ML, Pozzi S, Chhetri S, Seo YD, Aronson JP, Patel C, Fulciniti M, Purton LE, Glimcher LH, Lian JB, Stein G, Anderson KC, Scadden DT (2008)

Pharmacologic targeting of a stem/progenitor population in vivo is associated with enhanced bone regeneration in mice. J Clin Investig 118:491–504

56. Giuliani N, Morandi F, Tagliaferri S, Lazzaretti M, Bonomini S, Crugnola M, Mancini C, Martella E, Ferrari L, Tabilio A, Rizzoli V (2007) The proteasome inhibitor bortezomib affects osteoblast differentiation in vitro and in vivo in multiple myeloma patients. Blood 110:334–338

57. Quail DF, Joyce JA (2013) Microenvironmental regulation of tumor progression and metastasis. Nat Med 19:1423–1437

58. Swann JB, Smyth MJ (2007) Immune surveillance of tumors. J Clin Investig 117:1137–1146

59. Kawano Y, Moschetta M, Manier S, Glavey S, Gorgun GT, Roccaro AM, Anderson KC, Ghobrial IM (2015) Targeting the bone marrow microenvironment in multiple myeloma. Immunol Rev 263:160–172

60. Gabrilovich DI, Nagaraj S (2009) Myeloid-derived suppressor cells as regulators of the immune system. Nat Rev Immunol 9:162–174

61. Almand B, Clark JI, Nikitina E, van Beynen J, English NR, Knight SC, Carbone DP, Gabrilovich DI (2001) Increased production of immature myeloid cells in cancer patients: a mechanism of immunosuppression in cancer. J Immunol 166:678–689

62. Diaz-Montero CM, Salem ML, Nishimura MI, Garrett-Mayer E, Cole DJ, Montero AJ (2009) Increased circulating myeloid-derived suppressor cells correlate with clinical cancer stage, metastatic tumor burden, and doxorubicin-cyclophosphamide chemotherapy. Cancer Immunol immunother: CII 58:49–59

63. Huang B, Pan PY, Li Q, Sato AI, Levy DE, Bromberg J, Divino CM, Chen SH (2006) Gr-1 +CD115+immature myeloid suppressor cells mediate the development of tumor-induced T regulatory cells and T-cell anergy in tumor-bearing host. Cancer Res 66:1123–1131

64. Walter S, Weinschenk T, Stenzl A, Zdrojowy R, Pluzanska A, Szczylik C, Staehler M, Brugger W, Dietrich PY, Mendrzyk R, Hilf N, Schoor O, Fritsche J, Mahr A, Maurer D, Vass V, Trautwein C, Lewandrowski P, Flohr C, Pohla H, Stanczak JJ, Bronte V, Mandruzzato S, Biedermann T, Pawelec G, Derhovanessian E, Yamagishi H, Miki T, Hongo F, Takaha N, Hirakawa K, Tanaka H, Stevanovic S, Frisch J, Mayer-Mokler A, Kirner A, Rammensee HG, Reinhardt C, Singh-Jasuja H (2012) Multipeptide immune response to cancer vaccine IMA901 after single-dose cyclophosphamide associates with longer patient survival. Nat Med 18:1254–1261

65. Solito S, Falisi E, Diaz-Montero CM, Doni A, Pinton L, Rosato A, Francescato S, Basso G, Zanovello P, Onicescu G, Garrett-Mayer E, Montero AJ, Bronte V, Mandruzzato S (2011) A human promyelocytic-like population is responsible for the immune suppression mediated by myeloid-derived suppressor cells. Blood 118:2254–2265

66. Serafini P, Meckel K, Kelso M, Noonan K, Califano J, Koch W, Dolcetti L, Bronte V, Borrello I (2006) Phosphodiesterase-5 inhibition augments endogenous antitumor immunity by reducing myeloid-derived suppressor cell function. J Exp Med 203:2691–2702

67. Li H, Han Y, Guo Q, Zhang M, Cao X (2009) Cancer-expanded myeloid-derived suppressor cells induce anergy of NK cells through membrane-bound TGF-beta 1. J Immunol 182:240–249

68. Qin H, Lerman B, Sakamaki I, Wei G, Cha SC, Rao SS, Qian J, Hailemichael Y, Nurieva R, Dwyer KC, Roth J, Yi Q, Overwijk WW, Kwak LW (2014) Generation of a new therapeutic peptide that depletes myeloid-derived suppressor cells in tumor-bearing mice. Nat Med 20:676–681

69. Youn JI, Nagaraj S, Collazo M, Gabrilovich DI (2008) Subsets of myeloid-derived suppressor cells in tumor-bearing mice. J Immunol 181:5791–5802

70. Brimnes MK, Vangsted AJ, Knudsen LM, Gimsing P, Gang AO, Johnsen HE, Svane IM (2010) Increased level of both CD4+FOXP3+regulatory T cells and CD14+HLA-DR(-)/low myeloid-derived suppressor cells and decreased level of dendritic cells in patients with multiple myeloma. Scand J Immunol 72:540–547

71. Gorgun GT, Whitehill G, Anderson JL, Hideshima T, Maguire C, Laubach J, Raje N, Munshi NC, Richardson PG, Anderson KC (2013) Tumor-promoting immune-suppressive myeloid-derived suppressor cells in the multiple myeloma microenvironment in humans. Blood 121:2975–2987

72. Ramachandran IR, Martner A, Pisklakova A, Condamine T, Chase T, Vogl T, Roth J, Gabrilovich D, Nefedova Y (2013) Myeloid-derived suppressor cells regulate growth of multiple myeloma by inhibiting T cells in bone marrow. J Immunol 190:3815–3823

73. Wang Z, Zhang L, Wang H, Xiong S, Li Y, Tao Q, Xiao W, Qin H, Wang Y, Zhai Z (2015) Tumor-induced CD14(+)HLA-DR (-/low) myeloid-derived suppressor cells correlate with tumor progression and outcome of therapy in multiple myeloma patients. Cancer Immunol immunother: CII 64:389–399

74. Van Valckenborgh E, Schouppe E, Movahedi K, De Bruyne E, Menu E, De Baetselier P, Vanderkerken K, Van Ginderachter JA (2012) Multiple myeloma induces the immunosuppressive capacity of distinct myeloid-derived suppressor cell subpopulations in the bone marrow. Leukemia 26:2424–2428

75. Favaloro J, Liyadipitiya T, Brown R, Yang S, Suen H, Woodland N, Nassif N, Hart D, Fromm P, Weatherburn C, Gibson J, Ho PJ, Joshua D (2014) Myeloid derived suppressor cells are numerically, functionally and phenotypically different in patients with multiple myeloma. Leuk lymphoma 1–8

76. Zhuang J, Zhang J, Lwin ST, Edwards JR, Edwards CM, Mundy GR, Yang X (2012) Osteoclasts in multiple myeloma are derived from Gr-1+CD11b+myeloid-derived suppressor cells. PLoS ONE 7:e48871

77. Serafini P, Mgebroff S, Noonan K, Borrello I (2008) Myeloid-derived suppressor cells promote cross-tolerance in B-cell lymphoma by expanding regulatory T cells. Cancer Res 68:5439–5449

78. Meyer C, Sevko A, Ramacher M, Bazhin AV, Falk CS, Osen W, Borrello I, Kato M, Schadendorf D, Baniyash M, Umansky V (2011) Chronic inflammation promotes myeloid-derived suppressor cell activation blocking antitumor immunity in transgenic mouse melanoma model. Proc Natl Acad Sci USA 108:17111–17116

79. Noonan KA, Ghosh N, L. Rudraraju, M. Bui, I. Borrello, Targeting immune suppression with PDE5 inhibition in end-stage multiple myeloma. Cancer Immunol Res

80. Fontenot JD, Gavin MA, Rudensky AY (2003) Foxp3 programs the development and function of CD4+CD25+regulatory T cells. Nat Immunol 4:330–336

81. Nishikawa H, Sakaguchi S (2010) Regulatory T cells in tumor immunity. Int J Cancer 127:759–767

82. Mougiakakos D, Choudhury A, Lladser A, Kiessling R, Johansson CC (2010) Regulatory T cells in cancer. Adv Cancer Res 107:57–117

83. Curiel TJ, Coukos G, Zou L, Alvarez X, Cheng P, Mottram P, Evdemon-Hogan M, Conejo-Garcia JR, Zhang L, Burow M, Zhu Y, Wei S, Kryczek I, Daniel B, Gordon A, Myers L, Lackner A, Disis ML, Knutson KL, Chen L, Zou W (2004) Specific recruitment of regulatory T cells in ovarian carcinoma fosters immune privilege and predicts reduced survival. Nat Med 10:942–949

84. Bates GJ, Fox SB, Han C, Leek RD, Garcia JF, Harris AL, Banham AH (2006) Quantification of regulatory T cells enables the identification of high-risk breast cancer patients and those at risk of late relapse. J Clin. Oncol: Official J Am Soc Clin Oncol 24:5373–5380

85. Lahl K, Loddenkemper C, Drouin C, Freyer J, Arnason J, Eberl G, Hamann A, Wagner H, Huehn J, Sparwasser T (2007) Selective depletion of Foxp3+regulatory T cells induces a scurfy-like disease. J Exp Med 204:57–63

86. Klages K, Mayer CT, Lahl K, Loddenkemper C, Teng MW, Ngiow SF, Smyth MJ, Hamann A, Huehn J, Sparwasser T (2010) Selective depletion of Foxp3 + regulatory T cells improves effective therapeutic vaccination against established melanoma. Cancer Res 70:7788–7799

87. Teng MW, Ngiow SF, von Scheidt B, McLaughlin N, Sparwasser T, Smyth MJ (2010) Conditional regulatory T-cell depletion releases adaptive immunity preventing carcinogenesis and suppressing established tumor growth. Cancer Res 70:7800–7809

88. Beyer M, Kochanek M, Giese T, Endl E, Weihrauch MR, Knolle PA, Classen S, Schultze JL (2006) In vivo peripheral expansion of naive CD4+CD25high FoxP3+regulatory T cells in patients with multiple myeloma. Blood 107:3940–3949

89. Feyler S, von Lilienfeld-Toal M, Jarmin S, Marles L, Rawstron A, Ashcroft AJ, Owen RG, Selby PJ, Cook G (2009) CD4(+)CD25(+)FoxP3(+) regulatory T cells are increased whilst CD3(+)CD4(-)CD8(-)alphabetaTCR(+) double negative T cells are decreased in the peripheral blood of patients with multiple myeloma which correlates with disease burden. Br J Haematol 144:686–695

90. Giannopoulos K, Kaminska W, Hus I, Dmoszynska A (2012) The frequency of T regulatory cells modulates the survival of multiple myeloma patients: detailed characterisation of immune status in multiple myeloma. Br J Cancer 106:546–552

91. Muthu Raja KR, Rihova L, Zahradova L, Klincova M, Penka M, Hajek R (2012) Increased T regulatory cells are associated with adverse clinical features and predict progression in multiple myeloma. PLoS ONE 7:e47077

92. Laronne-Bar-On A, Zipori D, Haran-Ghera N (2008) Increased regulatory versus effector T cell development is associated with thymus atrophy in mouse models of multiple myeloma. J Immunol 181:3714–3724

93. Prabhala RH, Neri P, Bae JE, Tassone P, Shammas MA, Allam CK, Daley JF, Chauhan D, Blanchard E, Thatte HS, Anderson KC, Munshi NC (2006) Dysfunctional T regulatory cells in multiple myeloma. Blood 107:301–304

94. Gupta R, Ganeshan P, Hakim M, Verma R, Sharma A, Kumar L (2011) Significantly reduced regulatory T cell population in patients with untreated multiple myeloma. Leuk Res 35:874–878

95. Chen W, Jin W, Hardegen N, Lei KJ, Li L, Marinos N, McGrady G, Wahl SM (2003) Conversion of peripheral CD4+CD25- naive T cells to CD4+CD25+regulatory T cells by TGF-beta induction of transcription factor Foxp3. J Exp Med 198:1875–1886

96. Coombes JL, Siddiqui KR, Arancibia-Carcamo CV, Hall J, Sun CM, Belkaid Y, Powrie F (2007) A functionally specialized population of mucosal CD103+DCs induces Foxp3 +regulatory T cells via a TGF-beta and retinoic acid-dependent mechanism. J Exp Med 204:1757–1764

97. Feyler S, Scott GB, Parrish C, Jarmin S, Evans P, Short M, McKinley K, Selby PJ, Cook G (2012) Tumour cell generation of inducible regulatory T-cells in multiple myeloma is contact-dependent and antigen-presenting cell-independent. PLoS ONE 7:e35981

98. Frassanito MA, Ruggieri S, Desantis V, Di Marzo L, Leone P, Racanelli V, Fumarulo R, Dammacco F, Vacca A (2014) Myeloma cells act as tolerogenic antigen-presenting cells and induce regulatory T cells in vitro. Eur J Haematol

99. Francisco LM, Salinas VH, Brown KE, Vanguri VK, Freeman GJ, Kuchroo VK, Sharpe AH (2009) PD-L1 regulates the development, maintenance, and function of induced regulatory T cells. J Exp Med 206:3015–3029

100. Amarnath S, Mangus CW, Wang JC, Wei F, He A, Kapoor V, Foley JE, Massey PR, Felizardo TC, Riley JL, Levine BL, June CH, Medin JA, Fowler DH (2011) The PDL1-PD1 axis converts human TH1 cells into regulatory T cells. Sci Transl Med 3:111ra120

101. Liu J, Hamrouni A, Wolowiec D, Coiteux V, Kuliczkowski K, Hetuin D, Saudemont A, Quesnel B (2007) Plasma cells from multiple myeloma patients express B7-H1 (PD-L1) and increase expression after stimulation with IFN-{gamma} and TLR ligands via a MyD88-, TRAF6-, and MEK-dependent pathway. Blood 110:296–304

102. Tamura H, Ishibashi M, Yamashita T, Tanosaki S, Okuyama N, Kondo A, Hyodo H, Shinya E, Takahashi H, Dong H, Tamada K, Chen L, Dan K, Ogata K (2013) Marrow stromal cells induce B7-H1 expression on myeloma cells, generating aggressive characteristics in multiple myeloma. Leukemia 27:464–472

103. Lutsiak ME, Semnani RT, De Pascalis R, Kashmiri SV, Schlom J, Sabzevari H (2005) Inhibition of CD4(+)25+T regulatory cell function implicated in enhanced immune response by low-dose cyclophosphamide. Blood 105:2862–2868

104. Ghiringhelli F, Larmonier N, Schmitt E, Parcellier A, Cathelin D, Garrido C, Chauffert B, Solary E, Bonnotte B, Martin F (2004) CD4+CD25+regulatory T cells suppress tumor immunity but are sensitive to cyclophosphamide which allows immunotherapy of established tumors to be curative. Eur J Immunol 34:336–344

105. Sharabi A, Laronne-Bar-On A, Meshorer A, Haran-Ghera N (2010) Chemoimmunotherapy reduces the progression of multiple myeloma in a mouse model. Cancer Prev Res (Phila) 3:1265–1276

106. Galustian C, Meyer B, Labarthe MC, Dredge K, Klaschka D, Henry J, Todryk S, Chen R, Muller G, Stirling D, Schafer P, Bartlett JB, Dalgleish AG (2009) The anti-cancer agents lenalidomide and pomalidomide inhibit the proliferation and function of T regulatory cells. Cancer Immunol Immunother: CII 58:1033–1045

107. Muthu KR, Raja L, Kovarova R (2012) Hajek, Induction by lenalidomide and dexamethasone combination increases regulatory cells of patients with previously untreated multiple myeloma. Leuk lymphoma 53:1406–1408

108. Banchereau J, Steinman RM (1998) Dendritic cells and the control of immunity. Nature 392:245–252

109. O'Doherty U, Peng M, Gezelter S, Swiggard WJ, Betjes M, Bhardwaj N, Steinman RM (1994) Human blood contains two subsets of dendritic cells, one immunologically mature and the other immature. Immunology 82:487–493

110. Bell D, Chomarat P, Broyles D, Netto G, Harb GM, Lebecque S, Valladeau J, Davoust J, Palucka KA, Banchereau J (1999) In breast carcinoma tissue, immature dendritic cells reside within the tumor, whereas mature dendritic cells are located in peritumoral areas. J Exp Med 190:1417–1426

111. Treilleux I, Blay JY, Bendriss-Vermare N, Ray-Coquard I, Bachelot T, Guastalla JP, Bremond A, Goddard S, Pin JJ, Barthelemy-Dubois C, Lebecque S (2004) Dendritic cell infiltration and prognosis of early stage breast cancer. Clin Cancer Res: Official J Am Assoc Cancer Res 10:7466–7474

112. Sandel MH, Dadabayev AR, Menon AG, Morreau H, Melief CJ, Offringa R, van der Burg SH, Janssen-van Rhijn CM, Ensink NG, Tollenaar RA, van de Velde CJ, Kuppen PJ (2005) Prognostic value of tumor-infiltrating dendritic cells in colorectal cancer: role of maturation status and intratumoral localization. Clin Cancer Res: Official J Am Assoc Cancer Res 11:2576–2582

113. Zou W (2005) Immunosuppressive networks in the tumour environment and their therapeutic relevance. Nat Rev Cancer 5:263–274

114. Conrad C, Gregorio J, Wang YH, Ito T, Meller S, Hanabuchi S, Anderson S, Atkinson N, Ramirez PT, Liu YJ, Freedman R, Gilliet M (2012) Plasmacytoid dendritic cells promote immunosuppression in ovarian cancer via ICOS costimulation of Foxp3(+) T-regulatory cells. Cancer Res 72:5240–5249

115. Faget J, Bendriss-Vermare N, Gobert M, Durand I, Olive D, Biota C, Bachelot T, Treilleux I, Goddard-Leon S, Lavergne E, Chabaud S, Blay JY, Caux C, Menetrier-Caux C (2012) ICOS-ligand expression on plasmacytoid dendritic cells supports breast cancer progression by promoting the accumulation of immunosuppressive CD4 + T cells. Cancer Res 72:6130–6141

116. Ramos RN, Chin LS, Dos Santos AP, Bergami-Santos PC, Laginha F, Barbuto JA (2012) Monocyte-derived dendritic cells from breast cancer patients are biased to induce CD4 + CD25 + Foxp3 + regulatory T cells. J Leukoc Biol 92:673–682

117. Banerjee DK, Dhodapkar MV, Matayeva E, Steinman RM, Dhodapkar KM (2006) Expansion of FOXP3high regulatory T cells by human dendritic cells (DCs) in vitro and after injection of cytokine-matured DCs in myeloma patients. Blood 108:2655–2661

118. Garcia De Vinuesa C, Gulbranson-Judge A, Khan M, O'Leary P, Cascalho M, Wabl M, Klaus GG, Owen MJ, MacLennan IC (1999) Dendritic cells associated with plasmablast survival. Eur J Immunol 29:3712–3721

119. Jego G, Palucka AK, Blanck JP, Chalouni C, Pascual V, Banchereau J (2003) Plasmacytoid dendritic cells induce plasma cell differentiation through type I interferon and interleukin 6. Immunity 19:225–234

120. Brown RD, Pope B, Murray A, Esdale W, Sze DM, Gibson J, Ho PJ, Hart D, Joshua D (2001) Dendritic cells from patients with myeloma are numerically normal but functionally defective as they fail to up-regulate CD80 (B7-1) expression after huCD40LT stimulation because of inhibition by transforming growth factor-beta1 and interleukin-10. Blood 98:2992–2998

121. Brimnes MK, Svane IM, Johnsen HE (2006) Impaired functionality and phenotypic profile of dendritic cells from patients with multiple myeloma. Clin Exp Immunol 144:76–84

122. Chauhan D, Singh AV, Brahmandam M, Carrasco R, Bandi M, Hideshima T, Bianchi G, Podar K, Tai YT, Mitsiades C, Raje N, Jaye DL, Kumar SK, Richardson P, Munshi N, Anderson KC (2009) Functional interaction of plasmacytoid dendritic cells with multiple myeloma cells: a therapeutic target. Cancer Cell 16:309–323

123. Ray A, Tian Z, Das DS, Coffman RL, Richardson P, Chauhan D, Anderson KC (2014) A novel TLR-9 agonist C792 inhibits plasmacytoid dendritic cell-induced myeloma cell growth and enhance cytotoxicity of bortezomib. Leukemia

124. Kukreja A, Hutchinson A, Dhodapkar K, Mazumder A, Vesole D, Angitapalli R, Jagannath S, Dhodapkar MV (2006) Enhancement of clonogenicity of human multiple myeloma by dendritic cells. J Exp Med 203:1859–1865

125. Ray A, Das DS, Song Y, Richardson P, Munshi NC, Chauhan D, Anderson KC (2015) Targeting PD1-PDL1 immune checkpoint in plasmacytoid dendritic cell interactions with T cells, natural killer cells and multiple myeloma cells. Leukemia

126. Cook J, Hagemann T (2013) Tumour-associated macrophages and cancer. Curr Opin Pharmacol 13:595–601

127. Zheng Y, Cai Z, Wang S, Zhang X, Qian J, Hong S, Li H, Wang M, Yang J, Yi Q (2009) Macrophages are an abundant component of myeloma microenvironment and protect myeloma cells from chemotherapy drug-induced apoptosis. Blood 114:3625–3628

128. Zheng Y, Yang J, Qian J, Qiu P, Hanabuchi S, Lu Y, Wang Z, Liu Z, Li H, He J, Lin P, Weber D, Davis RE, Kwak L, Cai Z, Yi Q (2013) PSGL-1/selectin and ICAM-1/CD18 interactions are involved in macrophage-induced drug resistance in myeloma. Leukemia 27:702–710

129. Kim J, Denu RA, Dollar BA, Escalante LE, Kuether JP, Callander NS, Asimakopoulos F, Hematti P (2012) Macrophages and mesenchymal stromal cells support survival and proliferation of multiple myeloma cells. Br J Haematol 158:336–346

130. Hope C, Ollar SJ, Heninger E, Hebron E, Jensen JL, Kim J, Maroulakou I, Miyamoto S, Leith C, Yang DT, Callander N, Hematti P, Chesi M, Bergsagel PL, Asimakopoulos F (2014) TPL2 kinase regulates the inflammatory milieu of the myeloma niche. Blood 123:3305–3315

131. Berardi S, Ria R, Reale A, De Luisi A, Catacchio I, Moschetta M, Vacca A (2013) Multiple myeloma macrophages: pivotal players in the tumor microenvironment. J Oncol 2013:183602

132. Groh V, Rhinehart R, Secrist H, Bauer S, Grabstein KH, Spies T (1999) Broad tumor-associated expression and recognition by tumor-derived gamma delta T cells of MICA and MICB. Proc Natl Acad Sci USA 96:6879–6884

133. Famularo G, D'Ambrosio A, Quintieri F, Di Giovanni S, Parzanese I, Pizzuto F, Giacomelli R, Pugliese O, Tonietti G (1992) Natural killer cell frequency and function in patients with monoclonal gammopathies. J Clin Lab Immunol 37:99–109

134. Frassanito MA, Silvestris F, Cafforio P, Silvestris N, Dammacco F (1997) IgG M-components in active myeloma patients induce a down-regulation of natural killer cell activity. Int J Clin Lab Res 27:48–54

135. Sawanobori M, Suzuki K, Nakagawa Y, Inoue Y, Utsuyama M, Hirokawa K (1997) Natural killer cell frequency and serum cytokine levels in monoclonal gammopathies: correlation of bone marrow granular lymphocytes to prognosis. Acta Haematol 98:150–154

136. Pessoa de Magalhaes RJ, Vidriales MB, Paiva B, Fernandez-Gimenez C, Garcia-Sanz R, Mateos MV, Gutierrez NC, Lecrevisse Q, Blanco JF, Hernandez J, de las Heras N, Martinez-Lopez J, Roig M, Costa ES, Ocio EM, Perez-Andres M, Maiolino A, Nucci M, De La Rubia J, Lahuerta JJ, San-Miguel JF, Orfao A (2013) Analysis of the immune system of multiple myeloma patients achieving long-term disease control by multidimensional flow cytometry. Haematologica 98:79–86

137. Jinushi M, Vanneman M, Munshi NC, Tai YT, Prabhala RH, Ritz J, Neuberg D, Anderson KC, Carrasco DR, Dranoff G (2008) MHC class I chain-related protein A antibodies and shedding are associated with the progression of multiple myeloma. Proc Natl Acad Sci USA 105:1285–1290

138. von Lilienfeld-Toal M, Frank S, Leyendecker C, Feyler S, Jarmin S, Morgan R, Glasmacher A, Marten A, Schmidt-Wolf IG, Brossart P, Cook G (2010) Reduced immune effector cell NKG2D expression and increased levels of soluble NKG2D ligands in multiple myeloma may not be causally linked. Cancer Immunol Immunother: CII 59:829–839

139. Benson DM Jr, Bakan CE, Mishra A, Hofmeister CC, Efebera Y, Becknell B, Baiocchi RA, Zhang J, Yu J, Smith MK, Greenfield CN, Porcu P, Devine SM, Rotem-Yehudar R, Lozanski G, Byrd JC, Caligiuri MA (2010) The PD-1/PD-L1 axis modulates the natural killer cell versus multiple myeloma effect: a therapeutic target for CT-011, a novel monoclonal anti-PD-1 antibody. Blood 116:2286–2294

140. Davies FE, Raje N, Hideshima T, Lentzsch S, Young G, Tai YT, Lin B, Podar K, Gupta D, Chauhan D, Treon SP, Richardson PG, Schlossman RL, Morgan GJ, Muller GW, Stirling DI, Anderson KC (2001) Thalidomide and immunomodulatory derivatives augment natural killer cell cytotoxicity in multiple myeloma. Blood 98:210–216

141. Hayashi T, Hideshima T, Akiyama M, Podar K, Yasui H, Raje N, Kumar S, Chauhan D, Treon SP, Richardson P, Anderson KC (2005) Molecular mechanisms whereby immunomodulatory drugs activate natural killer cells: clinical application. Br J Haematol 128:192–203

142. Tai YT, Li XF, Catley L, Coffey R, Breitkreutz I, Bae J, Song W, Podar K, Hideshima T, Chauhan D, Schlossman R, Richardson P, Treon SP, Grewal IS, Munshi NC, Anderson KC (2005) Immunomodulatory drug lenalidomide (CC-5013, IMiD3) augments anti-CD40 SGN-40-induced cytotoxicity in human multiple myeloma: clinical implications. Cancer Res 65:11712–11720

143. Lioznov M, El-Cheikh J Jr, Hoffmann F, Hildebrandt Y, Ayuk F, Wolschke C, Atanackovic D, Schilling G, Badbaran A, Bacher U, Fehse B, Zander AR, Blaise D, Mohty M, Kroger N (2010) Lenalidomide as salvage therapy after allo-SCT for multiple myeloma is effective and leads to an increase of activated NK (NKp44(+)) and T (HLA-DR (+)) cells. Bone Marrow Transplant 45:349–353

144. Ishida Y, Agata Y, Shibahara K, Honjo T (1992) Induced expression of PD-1, a novel member of the immunoglobulin gene superfamily, upon programmed cell death. EMBO J 11:3887–3895

145. Dong H, Strome SE, Salomao DR, Tamura H, Hirano F, Flies DB, Roche PC, Lu J, Zhu G, Tamada K, Lennon VA, Celis E, Chen L (2002) Tumor-associated B7-H1 promotes T-cell apoptosis: a potential mechanism of immune evasion. Nat Med 8:793–800

146. Rosenblatt J, Glotzbecker B, Mills H, Vasir B, Tzachanis D, Levine JD, Joyce RM, Wellenstein K, Keefe W, Schickler M, Rotem-Yehudar R, Kufe D, Avigan D (2011) PD-1 blockade by CT-011, anti-PD-1 antibody, enhances ex vivo T-cell responses to autologous dendritic cell/myeloma fusion vaccine. J Immunother 34:409–418

147. Ansell SM, Lesokhin AM, Borrello I, Halwani A, Scott EC, Gutierrez M, Schuster SJ, Millenson MM, Cattry D, Freeman GJ, Rodig SJ, Chapuy B, Ligon AH, Zhu L, Grosso JF, Kim SY, Timmerman JM, Shipp MA, Armand P (2015) PD-1 blockade with nivolumab in relapsed or refractory Hodgkin's lymphoma. N Engl J Med 372:311–319

148. Hallett WH, Jing W, Drobyski WR, Johnson BD (2011) Immunosuppressive effects of multiple myeloma are overcome by PD-L1 blockade. Biol Blood Marrow Transplant: J Am Soc Blood Marrow Transplant 17:1133–1145

149. Kearl TJ, Jing W, Gershan JA, Johnson BD (2013) Programmed death receptor-1/programmed death receptor ligand-1 blockade after transient lymphodepletion to treat myeloma. J Immunol 190:5620–5628

150. Jing W, Gershan JA, Weber J, Tlomak D, McOlash L, Sabatos-Peyton C, Johnson BD (2015) Combined immune checkpoint protein blockade and low dose whole body irradiation as immunotherapy for myeloma. J Immunol Cancer 3:2

151. Maher J, Adami AA (2013) Antitumor immunity: Easy as 1, 2, 3 with monoclonal bispecific trifunctional antibodies? Cancer Res 73:5613–5617

152. Topp MS, Kufer P, Gokbuget N, Goebeler M, Klinger M, Neumann S, Horst HA, Raff T, Viardot A, Schmid M, Stelljes M, Schaich M, Degenhard E, Kohne-Volland R, Bruggemann M, Ottmann O, Pfeifer H, Burmeister T, Nagorsen D, Schmidt M, Lutterbuese R, Reinhardt C, Baeuerle PA, Kneba M, Einsele H, Riethmuller G, Hoelzer D, Zugmaier G, Bargou RC (2011) Targeted therapy with the T-cell-engaging antibody blinatumomab of chemotherapy-refractory minimal residual disease in B-lineage acute lymphoblastic leukemia patients results in high response rate and prolonged leukemia-free survival. J Clin Oncol: Official J Am Soc Clin Oncol 29:2493–2498

153. von Strandmann EP, Hansen HP, Reiners KS, Schnell R, Borchmann P, Merkert S, Simhadri VR, Draube A, Reiser M, Purr I, Hallek M, Engert A (2006) A novel bispecific protein (ULBP2-BB4) targeting the NKG2D receptor on natural killer (NK) cells and CD138 activates NK cells and has potent antitumor activity against human multiple myeloma in vitro and in vivo. Blood 107:1955–1962

154. Rossi EA, Rossi DL, Stein R, Goldenberg DM, Chang CH (2010) A bispecific antibody-IFNalpha2b immunocytokine targeting CD20 and HLA-DR is highly toxic to human lymphoma and multiple myeloma cells. Cancer Res 70:7600–7609

155. Zou J, Chen D, Zong Y, Ye S, Tang J, Meng H, An G, Zhang X, Yang L (2015) BiTE-hIgFc-based immunotherapy as a new therapeutic strategy in multiple myeloma. Cancer Sci

156. Sadelain M, Brentjens R, Riviere I (2013) The basic principles of chimeric antigen receptor design. Cancer discovery 3:388–398

157. Davila ML, Riviere I, Wang X, Bartido S, Park J, Curran K, Chung SS, Stefanski J, Borquez-Ojeda O, Olszewska M, Qu J, Wasielewska T, He Q, Fink M, Shinglot H, Youssif M, Satter M, Wang Y, Hosey J, Quintanilla H, Halton E, Bernal Y, Bouhassira DC, Arcila ME, Gonen M, Roboz GJ, Maslak P, Douer D, Frattini MG, Giralt S, Sadelain M, Brentjens R (2014) Efficacy and toxicity management of 19-28z CAR T cell therapy in B cell acute lymphoblastic leukemia. Sci Transl Med 6:224–225

158. Mihara K, Bhattacharyya J, Kitanaka A, Yanagihara K, Kubo T, Takei Y, Asaoku H, Takihara Y, Kimura A (2012) T-cell immunotherapy with a chimeric receptor against CD38 is effective in eliminating myeloma cells. Leukemia 26:365–367

159. Chu J, He S, Deng Y, Zhang J, Peng Y, Hughes T, Yi L, Kwon CH, Wang QE, Devine SM, He X, Bai XF, Hofmeister CC, Yu J (2014) Genetic modification of T cells redirected toward CS1 enhances eradication of myeloma cells. Clin Cancer Res: Official J Am Assoc Cancer Res 20:3989–4000

160. Carpenter RO, Evbuomwan MO, Pittaluga S, Rose JJ, Raffeld M, Yang S, Gress RE, Hakim FT, Kochenderfer JN (2013) B-cell maturation antigen is a promising target for adoptive T-cell therapy of multiple myeloma. Clin Cancer Res: Official J Am Assoc Cancer Res 19:2048–2060

161. Peinert S, Prince HM, Guru PM, Kershaw MH, Smyth MJ, Trapani JA, Gambell P, Harrison S, Scott AM, Smyth FE, Darcy PK, Tainton K, Neeson P, Ritchie DS, Honemann D (2010) Gene-modified T cells as immunotherapy for multiple myeloma and acute myeloid leukemia expressing the Lewis Y antigen. Gene Ther 17:678–686

162. Casucci M, Nicolis di Robilant B, Falcone L, Camisa B, Norelli M, Genovese P, Gentner B, Gullotta F, Ponzoni M, Bernardi M, Marcatti M, Saudemont A, Bordignon C, Savoldo B, Ciceri F, Naldini L, Dotti G, Bonini C, Bondanza A (2013) CD44v6-targeted T cells mediate potent antitumor effects against acute myeloid leukemia and multiple myeloma. Blood 122:3461–3472

163. Raggatt LJ, Partridge NC (2010) Cellular and molecular mechanisms of bone remodeling. J Biol Chem 285:25103–25108

164. Bataille R, Chappard D, Marcelli C, Dessauw P, Sany J, Baldet P, Alexandre C (1989) Mechanisms of bone destruction in multiple myeloma: the importance of an unbalanced process in determining the severity of lytic bone disease. J Clin Oncol: Official J Am Soc Clin Oncol 7:1909–1914

165. Bataille R, Chappard D, Marcelli C, Rossi JF, Dessauw P, Baldet P, Sany J, Alexandre C (1990) Osteoblast stimulation in multiple myeloma lacking lytic bone lesions. Br J Haematol 76:484–487

166. Oranger A, Carbone C, Izzo M, Grano M (2013) Cellular mechanisms of multiple myeloma bone disease. Clin Dev Immunol 2013:289458

167. Hameed A, Brady JJ, Dowling P, Clynes M, O'Gorman P (2014) Bone disease in multiple myeloma: pathophysiology and management. Cancer Growth Metastasis 7:33–42

168. Roodman GD (2010) Pathogenesis of myeloma bone disease. J Cell Biochem 109:283–291

169. Ehrlich LA, Roodman GD (2005) The role of immune cells and inflammatory cytokines in Paget's disease and multiple myeloma. Immunol Rev 208:252–266

170. Terpos E, Szydlo R, Apperley JF, Hatjiharissi E, Politou M, Meletis J, Viniou N, Yataganas X, Goldman JM, Rahemtulla A (2003) Soluble receptor activator of nuclear factor kappaB ligand-osteoprotegerin ratio predicts survival in multiple myeloma: proposal for a novel prognostic index. Blood 102:1064–1069

171. Pearse RN, Sordillo EM, Yaccoby S, Wong BR, Liau DF, Colman N, Michaeli J, Epstein J, Choi Y (2001) Multiple myeloma disrupts the TRANCE/osteoprotegerin cytokine axis to trigger bone destruction and promote tumor progression. Proc Natl Acad Sci USA 98:11581–11586

172. Sezer O, Heider U, Zavrski I, Kuhne CA, Hofbauer LC (2003) RANK ligand and osteoprotegerin in myeloma bone disease. Blood 101:2094–2098

173. Kostenuik PJ, Nguyen HQ, McCabe J, Warmington KS, Kurahara C, Sun N, Chen C, Li L, Cattley RC, Van G, Scully S, Elliott R, Grisanti M, Morony S, Tan HL, Asuncion F, Li X, Ominsky MS, Stolina M, Dwyer D, Dougall WC, Hawkins N, Boyle WJ, Simonet WS, Sullivan JK (2009) Denosumab, a fully human monoclonal antibody to RANKL, inhibits bone resorption and increases BMD in knock-in mice that express chimeric (murine/human) RANKL. J Bone Miner Res: Official J Am Soc Bone Miner Res 24:182–195

174. Yaccoby S, Pearse RN, Johnson CL, Barlogie B, Choi Y, Epstein J (2002) Myeloma interacts with the bone marrow microenvironment to induce osteoclastogenesis and is dependent on osteoclast activity. Br J Haematol 116:278–290

175. Morgan GJ, Davies FE, Gregory WM, Cocks K, Bell SE, Szubert AJ, Navarro-Coy N, Drayson MT, Owen RG, Feyler S, Ashcroft AJ, Ross F, Byrne J, Roddie H, Rudin C, Cook G, Jackson GH, Child JA, National G (2010) Cancer research institute haematological oncology clinical study, first-line treatment with zoledronic acid as compared with clodronic acid in multiple myeloma (MRC Myeloma IX): a randomised controlled trial. Lancet 376:1989–1999

176. Henry DH, Costa L, Goldwasser F, Hirsh V, Hungria V, Prausova J, Scagliotti GV, Sleeboom H, Spencer A, Vadhan-Raj S, von Moos R, Willenbacher W, Woll PJ, Wang J, Jiang Q, Jun S, Dansey R, Yeh H (2011) Randomized, double-blind study of denosumab

versus zoledronic acid in the treatment of bone metastases in patients with advanced cancer (excluding breast and prostate cancer) or multiple myeloma. J Clin Oncol: Official J Am Soc Clin Oncol 29:1125–1132

177. Vadhan-Raj S, von Moos R, Fallowfield LJ, Patrick DL, Goldwasser F, Cleeland CS, Henry DH, Novello S, Hungria V, Qian Y, Feng A, Yeh H, Chung K (2012) Clinical benefit in patients with metastatic bone disease: results of a phase 3 study of denosumab versus zoledronic acid. Ann Oncol: Official J Eur Soc Med Oncol/ESMO 23:3045–3051

178. Zannettino AC, Farrugia AN, Kortesidis A, Manavis J, To LB, Martin SK, Diamond P, Tamamura H, Lapidot T, Fujii N, Gronthos S (2005) Elevated serum levels of stromal-derived factor-1alpha are associated with increased osteoclast activity and osteolytic bone disease in multiple myeloma patients. Cancer Res 65:1700–1709

179. Roccaro AM, Sacco A, Purschke WG, Moschetta M, Buchner K, Maasch C, Zboralski D, Zollner S, Vonhoff S, Mishima Y, Maiso P, Reagan MR, Lonardi S, Ungari M, Facchetti F, Eulberg D, Kruschinski A, Vater A, Rossi G, Klussmann S, Ghobrial IM (2014) SDF-1 inhibition targets the bone marrow niche for cancer therapy. Cell Rep 9:118–128

180. Azab AK, Runnels JM, Pitsillides C, Moreau AS, Azab F, Leleu X, Jia X, Wright R, Ospina B, Carlson AL, Alt C, Burwick N, Roccaro AM, Ngo HT, Farag M, Melhem MR, Sacco A, Munshi NC, Hideshima T, Rollins BJ, Anderson KC, Kung AL, Lin CP, Ghobrial IM (2009) CXCR4 inhibitor AMD3100 disrupts the interaction of multiple myeloma cells with the bone marrow microenvironment and enhances their sensitivity to therapy. Blood 113:4341–4351

181. Ria R, Reale A, De Luisi A, Ferrucci A, Moschetta M, Vacca A (2011) Bone marrow angiogenesis and progression in multiple myeloma. Am J Blood Res 1:76–89

182. Niida S, Kaku M, Amano H, Yoshida H, Kataoka H, Nishikawa S, Tanne K, Maeda N, Nishikawa S, Kodama H (1999) Vascular endothelial growth factor can substitute for macrophage colony-stimulating factor in the support of osteoclastic bone resorption. J Exp Med 190:293–298

183. Tanaka Y, Abe M, Hiasa M, Oda A, Amou H, Nakano A, Takeuchi K, Kitazoe K, Kido S, Inoue D, Moriyama K, Hashimoto T, Ozaki S, Matsumoto T (2007) Myeloma cell-osteoclast interaction enhances angiogenesis together with bone resorption: a role for vascular endothelial cell growth factor and osteopontin. Clin Cancer Res: Official J Am Assoc Cancer Res 13:816–823

184. Terpos E, Politou M, Szydlo R, Goldman JM, Apperley JF, Rahemtulla A (2003) Serum levels of macrophage inflammatory protein-1 alpha (MIP-1alpha) correlate with the extent of bone disease and survival in patients with multiple myeloma. Br J Haematol 123:106–109

185. Papamerkouriou YM, Kenanidis E, Gamie Z, Papavasiliou K, Kostakos T, Potoupnis M, Sarris I, Tsiridis E, Kyrkos J (2015) Treatment of multiple myeloma bone disease: experimental and clinical data. Expert Opin Biol Ther 15:213–230

186. Yaccoby S, Wezeman MJ, Henderson A, Cottler-Fox M, Yi Q, Barlogie B, Epstein J (2004) Cancer and the microenvironment: myeloma-osteoclast interactions as a model. Cancer Res 64:2016–2023

187. Abe M, Hiura K, Wilde J, Shioyasono A, Moriyama K, Hashimoto T, Kido S, Oshima T, Shibata H, Ozaki S, Inoue D, Matsumoto T (2004) Osteoclasts enhance myeloma cell growth and survival via cell-cell contact: a vicious cycle between bone destruction and myeloma expansion. Blood 104:2484–2491

188. Karadag A, Oyajobi BO, Apperley JF, Russell RG, Croucher PI (2000) Human myeloma cells promote the production of interleukin 6 by primary human osteoblasts. Br J Haematol 108:383–390

189. Taube T, Beneton MN, McCloskey EV, Rogers S, Greaves M, Kanis JA (1992) Abnormal bone remodelling in patients with myelomatosis and normal biochemical indices of bone resorption. Eur J Haematol 49:192–198

190. Shipman CM, Croucher PI (2003) Osteoprotegerin is a soluble decoy receptor for tumor necrosis factor-related apoptosis-inducing ligand/Apo2 ligand and can function as a paracrine survival factor for human myeloma cells. Cancer Res 63:912–916
191. Reagan MR, Liaw L, Rosen CJ, Ghobrial IM (2015) Dynamic interplay between bone and multiple myeloma: emerging roles of the osteoblast. Bone
192. Tian E, Zhan F, Walker R, Rasmussen E, Ma Y, Barlogie B, Shaughnessy JD Jr (2003) The role of the Wnt-signaling antagonist DKK1 in the development of osteolytic lesions in multiple myeloma. N Engl J Med 349:2483–2494
193. Yaccoby S, Ling W, Zhan F, Walker R, Barlogie B, Shaughnessy JD Jr (2007) Antibody-based inhibition of DKK1 suppresses tumor-induced bone resorption and multiple myeloma growth in vivo. Blood 109:2106–2111
194. Fulciniti M, Tassone P, Hideshima T, Vallet S, Nanjappa P, Ettenberg SA, Shen Z, Patel N, Tai YT, Chauhan D, Mitsiades C, Prabhala R, Raje N, Anderson KC, Stover DR, Munshi NC (2009) Anti-DKK1 mAb (BHQ880) as a potential therapeutic agent for multiple myeloma. Blood 114:371–379
195. Danylesko I, Beider K, Shimoni A, Nagler A (2012) Monoclonal antibody-based immunotherapy for multiple myeloma. Immunotherapy 4:919–938
196. Papadopoulou EC, Batzios SP, Dimitriadou M, Perifanis V, Garipidou V (2010) Multiple myeloma and bone disease: pathogenesis and current therapeutic approaches. Hippokratia 14:76–81
197. Vallet S, Mukherjee S, Vaghela N, Hideshima T, Fulciniti M, Pozzi S, Santo L, Cirstea D, Patel K, Sohani AR, Guimaraes A, Xie W, Chauhan D, Schoonmaker JA, Attar E, Churchill M, Weller E, Munshi N, Seehra JS, Weissleder R, Anderson KC, Scadden DT, Raje N (2010) Activin A promotes multiple myeloma-induced osteolysis and is a promising target for myeloma bone disease. Proc Natl Acad Sci USA 107:5124–5129
198. Barhanpurkar AP, Gupta N, Srivastava RK, Tomar GB, Naik SP, Joshi SR, Pote ST, Mishra GC, Wani MR (2012) IL-3 promotes osteoblast differentiation and bone formation in human mesenchymal stem cells. Biochemical and biophysical research communications 418:669–675
199. Lee JW, Chung HY, Ehrlich LA, Jelinek DF, Callander NS, Roodman GD, Choi SJ (2004) IL-3 expression by myeloma cells increases both osteoclast formation and growth of myeloma cells. Blood 103:2308–2315
200. Standal T, Abildgaard N, Fagerli UM, Stordal B, Hjertner O, Borset M, Sundan A (2007) HGF inhibits BMP-induced osteoblastogenesis: possible implications for the bone disease of multiple myeloma. Blood 109:3024–3030
201. Ferrucci A, Moschetta M, Frassanito MA, Berardi S, Catacchio I, Ria R, Racanelli V, Caivano A, Solimando AG, Vergara D, Maffia M, Latorre D, Rizzello A, Zito A, Ditonno P, Maiorano E, Ribatti D, Vacca A (2014) A HGF/cMET autocrine loop is operative in multiple myeloma bone marrow endothelial cells and may represent a novel therapeutic target. Clin Cancer Res: Official J Am Assoc Cancer Res 20:5796–5807
202. Moschetta M, Basile A, Ferrucci A, Frassanito MA, Rao L, Ria R, Solimando AG, Giuliani N, Boccarelli A, Fumarola F, Coluccia M, Rossini B, Ruggieri S, Nico B, Maiorano E, Ribatti D, Roccaro AM, Vacca A (2013) Novel targeting of phospho-cMET overcomes drug resistance and induces antitumor activity in multiple myeloma. Clin Cancer Res: Official J Am Assoc Cancer Res 19:4371–4382
203. Alexander DD, Mink PJ, Adami HO, Cole P, Mandel JS, Oken MM, Trichopoulos D (2007) Multiple myeloma: a review of the epidemiologic literature. Int J Cancer 120(Suppl 12): 40–61
204. Larsson SC, Wolk A (2007) Body mass index and risk of multiple myeloma: a meta-analysis, International journal of cancer. Int J Cancer 121:2512–2516
205. Renehan AG, Tyson M, Egger M, Heller RF, Zwahlen M (2008) Body-mass index and incidence of cancer: a systematic review and meta-analysis of prospective observational studies. Lancet 371:569–578

206. Wallin A, Larsson SC (2011) Body mass index and risk of multiple myeloma: a meta-analysis of prospective studies. Eur J Cancer 47:1606–1615
207. Castillo JJ, Mull N, Reagan JL, Nemr S, Mitri J (2012) Increased incidence of non-Hodgkin lymphoma, leukemia, and myeloma in patients with diabetes mellitus type 2: a meta-analysis of observational studies. Blood 119:4845–4850
208. Chou YS, Yang CF, Chen HS, Yang SH, Yu YB, Hong YC, Liu CY, Gau JP, Liu JH, Chen PM, Chiou TJ, Tzeng CH, Hsiao LT (2012) Pre-existing diabetes mellitus in patients with multiple myeloma. Eur J Haematol 89:320–327
209. Landgren O, Rajkumar SV, Pfeiffer RM, Kyle RA, Katzmann JA, Dispenzieri A, Cai Q, Goldin LR, Caporaso NE, Fraumeni JF, Blot WJ, Signorello LB (2010) Obesity is associated with an increased risk of monoclonal gammopathy of undetermined significance among black and white women. Blood 116:1056–1059
210. Hofmann JN, Liao LM, Pollak MN, Wang Y, Pfeiffer RM, Baris D, Andreotti G, Lan Q, Landgren O, Rothman N, Purdue MP (2012) A prospective study of circulating adipokine levels and risk of multiple myeloma. Blood 120:4418–4420
211. Beason TS, Chang SH, Sanfilippo KM, Luo S, Colditz GA, Vij R, Tomasson MH, Dipersio JF, Stockerl-Goldstein K, Ganti A, Wildes T, Carson KR (2013) Influence of body mass index on survival in veterans with multiple myeloma. Oncologist 18:1074–1079
212. Adler BJ, Kaushansky K, Rubin CT (2014) Obesity-driven disruption of haematopoiesis and the bone marrow niche, Nature reviews. Endocrinology 10:737–748
213. Chan ME, Adler BJ, Green DE, Rubin CT (2012) Bone structure and B-cell populations, crippled by obesity, are partially rescued by brief daily exposure to low-magnitude mechanical signals. FASEB J: Official Publ Fed Am Soc Exp Biol 26:4855–4863
214. Zhu RJ, Wu MQ, Li ZJ, Zhang Y, Liu KY (2013) Hematopoietic recovery following chemotherapy is improved by BADGE-induced inhibition of adipogenesis. Int J Hematol 97:58–72
215. Justesen J, Stenderup K, Ebbesen EN, Mosekilde L, Steiniche T, Kassem M (2001) Adipocyte tissue volume in bone marrow is increased with aging and in patients with osteoporosis. Biogerontology 2:165–171
216. Caers J, Deleu S, Belaid Z, De Raeve H, Van Valckenborgh E, De Bruyne E, Defresne MP, Van Riet I, Van Camp B, Vanderkerken K (2007) Neighboring adipocytes participate in the bone marrow microenvironment of multiple myeloma cells. Leukemia 21:1580–1584
217. Lwin ST, Olechnowicz SW, Fowler JA, Edwards CM (2015) Diet-induced obesity promotes a myeloma-like condition in vivo. Leukemia 29:507–510
218. Abedin M, King N (2010) Diverse evolutionary paths to cell adhesion. Trends Cell Biol 20:734–742
219. Damiano JS, Cress AE, Hazlehurst LA, Shtil AA, Dalton WS (1999) Cell adhesion mediated drug resistance (CAM-DR): role of integrins and resistance to apoptosis in human myeloma cell lines. Blood 93:1658–1667
220. Vacca A, Ria R, Presta M, Ribatti D, Iurlaro M, Merchionne F, Tanghetti E, Dammacco F (2001) alpha(v)beta(3) integrin engagement modulates cell adhesion, proliferation, and protease secretion in human lymphoid tumor cells. Exp Hematol 29:993–1003
221. Ria R, Vacca A, Ribatti D, Di Raimondo F, Merchionne F, Dammacco F (2002) Alpha (v)beta(3) integrin engagement enhances cell invasiveness in human multiple myeloma. Haematologica 87:836–845
222. Slany A, Haudek-Prinz V, Meshcheryakova A, Bileck A, Lamm W, Zielinski C, Gerner C, Drach J (2014) Extracellular matrix remodeling by bone marrow fibroblast-like cells correlates with disease progression in multiple myeloma. J Proteome Res 13:844–854
223. Arendt BK, Walters DK, Wu X, Tschumper RC, Huddleston PM, Henderson KJ, Dispenzieri A, Jelinek DF (2012) Increased expression of extracellular matrix metalloproteinase inducer (CD147) in multiple myeloma: role in regulation of myeloma cell proliferation. Leukemia 26:2286–2296

224. Glavey SV, Huynh D, Reagan MR, Manier S, Moschetta M, Kawano Y, Roccaro AM, Ghobrial IM, Joshi L, O'Dwyer ME (2015) The cancer glycome: carbohydrates as mediators of metastasis. Blood Rev

225. Glavey SV, Manier S, Natoni A, Sacco A, Moschetta M, Reagan MR, Murillo LS, Sahin I, Wu P, Mishima Y, Zhang Y, Zhang W, Zhang Y, Morgan G, Joshi L, Roccaro AM, Ghobrial IM, O'Dwyer ME (2014) The sialyltransferase ST3GAL6 influences homing and survival in multiple myeloma. Blood 124:1765–1776

226. Podar K, Zimmerhackl A, Fulciniti M, Tonon G, Hainz U, Tai YT, Vallet S, Halama N, Jager D, Olson DL, Sattler M, Chauhan D, Anderson KC (2011) The selective adhesion molecule inhibitor Natalizumab decreases multiple myeloma cell growth in the bone marrow microenvironment: therapeutic implications. Br J Haematol 155:438–448

227. Kawano M, Hirano T, Matsuda T, Taga T, Horii Y, Iwato K, Asaoku H, Tang B, Tanabe O, Tanaka H et al (1988) Autocrine generation and requirement of BSF-2/IL-6 for human multiple myelomas. Nature 332:83–85

228. Klein B, Zhang XG, Lu ZY, Bataille R (1995) Interleukin-6 in human multiple myeloma. Blood 85:863–872

229. Podar K, Chauhan D, Anderson KC (2009) Bone marrow microenvironment and the identification of new targets for myeloma therapy. Leukemia 23:10–24

230. Le Gouill S, Podar K, Harousseau JL, Anderson KC (2004) Mcl-1 regulation and its role in multiple myeloma. Cell Cycle 3:1259–1262

231. Tai YT, Li XF, Breitkreutz I, Song W, Neri P, Catley L, Podar K, Hideshima T, Chauhan D, Raje N, Schlossman R, Richardson P, Munshi NC, Anderson KC (2006) Role of B-cell-activating factor in adhesion and growth of human multiple myeloma cells in the bone marrow microenvironment. Cancer Res 66:6675–6682

232. Podar K (2012) Novel targets and derived small molecule inhibitors in multiple myeloma. Curr Cancer Drug Targets 12:797–813

233. Suzuki K, Ogura M, Abe Y, Suzuki T, Tobinai K, Ando K, Taniwaki M, Maruyama D, Kojima M, Kuroda J, Achira M, Iizuka K (2015) Phase 1 study in Japan of siltuximab, an anti-IL-6 monoclonal antibody, in relapsed/refractory multiple myeloma. Int J Hematol

234. Dar A, Kollet O, Lapidot T (2006) Mutual, reciprocal SDF-1/CXCR4 interactions between hematopoietic and bone marrow stromal cells regulate human stem cell migration and development in NOD/SCID chimeric mice. Exp Hematol 34:967–975

235. Kucia M, Reca R, Miekus K, Wanzeck J, Wojakowski W, Janowska-Wieczorek A, Ratajczak J, Ratajczak MZ (2005) Trafficking of normal stem cells and metastasis of cancer stem cells involve similar mechanisms: pivotal role of the SDF-1-CXCR4 axis. Stem Cells 23:879–894

236. Alsayed Y, Ngo H, Runnels J, Leleu X, Singha UK, Pitsillides CM, Spencer JA, Kimlinger T, Ghobrial JM, Jia X, Lu G, Timm M, Kumar A, Cote D, Veilleux I, Hedin KE, Roodman GD, Witzig TE, Kung AL, Hideshima T, Anderson KC, Lin CP, Ghobrial IM (2007) Mechanisms of regulation of CXCR4/SDF-1 (CXCL12)-dependent migration and homing in multiple myeloma. Blood 109:2708–2717

237. Tarnowski M, Liu R, Wysoczynski M, Ratajczak J, Kucia M, Ratajczak MZ (2010) CXCR7: a new SDF-1-binding receptor in contrast to normal CD34(+) progenitors is functional and is expressed at higher level in human malignant hematopoietic cells. Eur J Haematol 85:472–483

238. De Clercq E (2003) The bicyclam AMD3100 story. Nat Rev Drug Discov 2:581–587

239. Tai YT, Catley LP, Mitsiades CS, Burger R, Podar K, Shringpaure R, Hideshima T, Chauhan D, Hamasaki M, Ishitsuka K, Richardson P, Treon SP, Munshi NC, Anderson KC (2004) Mechanisms by which SGN-40, a humanized anti-CD40 antibody, induces cytotoxicity in human multiple myeloma cells: clinical implications. Cancer Res 64:2846–2852

240. Hideshima T, Chauhan D, Schlossman R, Richardson P, Anderson KC (2001) The role of tumor necrosis factor alpha in the pathophysiology of human multiple myeloma: therapeutic applications. Oncogene 20:4519–4527
241. Moreaux J, Legouffe E, Jourdan E, Quittet P, Reme T, Lugagne C, Moine P, Rossi JF, Klein B, Tarte K (2004) BAFF and APRIL protect myeloma cells from apoptosis induced by interleukin 6 deprivation and dexamethasone. Blood 103:3148–3157
242. Fragioudaki M, Tsirakis G, Pappa CA, Aristeidou I, Tsioutis C, Alegakis A, Kyriakou DS, Stathopoulos EN, Alexandrakis MG (2012) Serum BAFF levels are related to angiogenesis and prognosis in patients with multiple myeloma. Leuk Res 36:1004–1008
243. Moreaux J, Cremer FW, Reme T, Raab M, Mahtouk K, Kaukel P, Pantesco V, De Vos J, Jourdan E, Jauch A, Legouffe E, Moos M, Fiol G, Goldschmidt H, Rossi JF, Hose D, Klein B (2005) The level of TACI gene expression in myeloma cells is associated with a signature of microenvironment dependence versus a plasmablastic signature. Blood 106:1021–1030
244. Bieghs L, Lub S, Fostier K, Maes K, Van Valckenborgh E, Menu E, Johnsen HE, Overgaard MT, Larsson O, Axelson M, Nyegaard M, Schots R, Jernberg-Wiklund H, Vanderkerken K, De Bruyne E (2014) The IGF-1 receptor inhibitor picropodophyllin potentiates the anti-myeloma activity of a BH3-mimetic. Oncotarget 5:11193–11208
245. Kuhn DJ, Berkova Z, Jones RJ, Woessner R, Bjorklund CC, Ma W, Davis RE, Lin P, Wang H, Madden TL, Wei C, Baladandayuthapani V, Wang M, Thomas SK, Shah JJ, Weber DM, Orlowski RZ (2012) Targeting the insulin-like growth factor-1 receptor to overcome bortezomib resistance in preclinical models of multiple myeloma. Blood 120:3260–3270
246. Tagoug I, Jordheim LP, Herveau S, Matera EL, Huber AL, Chettab K, Manie S, Dumontet C (2013) Therapeutic enhancement of ER stress by insulin-like growth factor I sensitizes myeloma cells to proteasomal inhibitors. Clin Cancer Res: Official J Am Assoc Cancer Res 19:3556–3566
247. Podar K, Anderson KC (2006) Caveolin-1 as a potential new therapeutic target in multiple myeloma. Cancer Lett 233:10–15
248. Abroun S, Ishikawa H, Tsuyama N, Liu S, Li FJ, Otsuyama K, Zheng X, Obata M, Kawano MM (2004) Receptor synergy of interleukin-6 (IL-6) and insulin-like growth factor-I in myeloma cells that highly express IL-6 receptor alpha [corrected]. Blood 103:2291–2298
249. Mitsiades CS, Mitsiades NS, McMullan CJ, Poulaki V, Shringarpure R, Akiyama M, Hideshima T, Chauhan D, Joseph M, Libermann TA, Garcia-Echeverria C, Pearson MA, Hofmann F, Anderson KC, Kung AL (2004) Inhibition of the insulin-like growth factor receptor-1 tyrosine kinase activity as a therapeutic strategy for multiple myeloma, other hematologic malignancies, and solid tumors. Cancer Cell 5:221–230
250. Srkalovic G, Hussein MA, Hoering A, Zonder JA, Popplewell LL, Trivedi H, Mazzoni S, Sexton R, Orlowski RZ, Barlogie B (2014) A phase II trial of BAY 43-9006 (sorafenib) (NSC-724772) in patients with relapsing and resistant multiple myeloma: SWOG S0434. Cancer Med 3:1275–1283
251. Kharaziha P, De Raeve H, Fristedt C, Li Q, Gruber A, Johnsson P, Kokaraki G, Panzar M, Laane E, Osterborg A, Zhivotovsky B, Jernberg-Wiklund H, Grander D, Celsing F, Bjorkholm M, Vanderkerken K, Panaretakis T (2012) Sorafenib has potent antitumor activity against multiple myeloma in vitro, ex vivo, and in vivo in the 5T33MM mouse model. Cancer Res 72:5348–5362
252. Ramakrishnan V, Timm M, Haug JL, Kimlinger TK, Wellik LE, Witzig TE, Rajkumar SV, Adjei AA, Kumar S (2010) Sorafenib, a dual Raf kinase/vascular endothelial growth factor receptor inhibitor has significant anti-myeloma activity and synergizes with common anti-myeloma drugs. Oncogene 29:1190–1202
253. Chapman MA, Lawrence MS, Keats JJ, Cibulskis K, Sougnez C, Schinzel AC, Harview CL, Brunet JP, Ahmann GJ, Adli M, Anderson KC, Ardlie KG, Auclair D, Baker A, Bergsagel PL, Bernstein BE, Drier Y, Fonseca R, Gabriel SB, Hofmeister CC, Jagannath S,

Jakubowiak AJ, Krishnan A, Levy J, Liefeld T, Lonial S, Mahan S, Mfuko B, Monti S, Perkins LM, Onofrio R, Pugh TJ, Rajkumar SV, Ramos AH, Siegel DS, Sivachenko A, Stewart AK, Trudel S, Vij R, Voet D, Winckler W, Zimmerman T, Carpten J, Trent J, Hahn WC, Garraway LA, Meyerson M, Lander ES, Getz G, Golub TR (2011) Initial genome sequencing and analysis of multiple myeloma. Nature 471:467–472

254. Andrulis M, Lehners N, Capper D, Penzel R, Heining C, Huellein J, Zenz T, von Deimling A, Schirmacher P, Ho AD, Goldschmidt H, Neben K, Raab MS (2013) Targeting the BRAF V600E mutation in multiple myeloma. Cancer Discov 3:862–869

255. Alvarez-Fernandez S, Ortiz-Ruiz MJ, Parrott T, Zaknoen S, Ocio EM, San Miguel J, Burrows FJ, Esparis-Ogando A, Pandiella A (2013) Potent antimyeloma activity of a novel ERK5/CDK inhibitor. Clin Cancer Res: Official J Am Assoc Cancer Res 19:2677–2687

256. Hu J, Handisides DR, Van Valckenborgh E, De Raeve H, Menu E, Vande Broek I, Liu Q, Sun JD, Van Camp B, Hart CP, Vanderkerken K (2010) Targeting the multiple myeloma hypoxic niche with TH-302, a hypoxia-activated prodrug. Blood 116:1524–1527

257. Podar K, Anderson KC (2010) A therapeutic role for targeting c-Myc/Hif-1-dependent signaling pathways. Cell Cycle 9:1722–1728

258. Kawano Y, Kikukawa Y, Fujiwara S, Wada N, Okuno Y, Mitsuya H, Hata H (2013) Hypoxia reduces CD138 expression and induces an immature and stem cell-like transcriptional program in myeloma cells. Int J Oncol 43:1809–1816

259. Borsi E, Perrone G, Terragna C, Martello M, Dico AF, Solaini G, Baracca A, Sgarbi G, Pasquinelli G, Valente S, Zamagni E, Tacchetti P, Martinelli G, Cavo M (2014) Hypoxia inducible factor-1 alpha as a therapeutic target in multiple myeloma. Oncotarget 5:1779–1792

260. Hu J, Van Valckenborgh E, Xu D, Menu E, De Raeve H, De Bryune E, Xu S, Van Camp B, Handisides D, Hart CP, Vanderkerken K (2013) Synergistic induction of apoptosis in multiple myeloma cells by bortezomib and hypoxia-activated prodrug TH-302, in vivo and in vitro. Mol Cancer Ther 12:1763–1773

261. Lohr JG, Stojanov P, Carter SL, Cruz-Gordillo P, Lawrence MS, Auclair D, Sougnez C, Knoechel B, Gould J, Saksena G, Cibulskis K, McKenna A, Chapman MA, Straussman R, Levy J, Perkins LM, Keats JJ, Schumacher SE, Rosenberg M, Multiple Myeloma Research C, Getz G, Golub TR (2014) Widespread genetic heterogeneity in multiple myeloma: implications for targeted therapy. Cancer Cell 25:91–101

262. Bolli N, Avet-Loiseau H, Wedge DC, Van Loo P, Alexandrov LB, Martincorena I, Dawson KJ, Iorio F, Nik-Zainal S, Bignell GR, Hinton JW, Li Y, Tubio JM, McLaren S, O' Meara S, Butler AP, Teague JW, Mudie L, Anderson E, Rashid N, Tai YT, Shammas MA, Sperling AS, Fulciniti M, Richardson PG, Parmigiani G, Magrangeas F, Minvielle S, Moreau P, Attal M, Facon T, Futreal PA, Anderson KC, Campbell PJ, Munshi NC (2014) Heterogeneity of genomic evolution and mutational profiles in multiple myeloma. Nat Commun 5:2997

263. Melchor L, Brioli A, Wardell CP, Murison A, Potter NE, Kaiser MF, Fryer RA, Johnson DC, Begum DB, Hulkki Wilson S, Vijayaraghavan G, Titley I, Cavo M, Davies FE, Walker BA, Morgan GJ (2014) Single-cell genetic analysis reveals the composition of initiating clones and phylogenetic patterns of branching and parallel evolution in myeloma. Leukemia 28:1705–1715

264. Egan JB, Shi CX, Tembe W, Christoforides A, Kurdoglu A, Sinari S, Middha S, Asmann Y, Schmidt J, Braggio E, Keats JJ, Fonseca R, Bergsagel PL, Craig DW, Carpten JD, Stewart AK (2012) Whole-genome sequencing of multiple myeloma from diagnosis to plasma cell leukemia reveals genomic initiating events, evolution, and clonal tides. Blood 120:1060–1066

265. Keats JJ, Chesi M, Egan JB, Garbitt VM, Palmer SE, Braggio E, Van Wier S, Blackburn PR, Baker AS, Dispenzieri A, Kumar S, Rajkumar SV, Carpten JD, Barrett M, Fonseca R, Stewart AK, Bergsagel PL (2012) Clonal competition with alternating dominance in multiple myeloma. Blood 120:1067–1076

266. Schmidt-Hieber M, Gutierrez ML, Perez-Andres M, Paiva B, Rasillo A, Tabernero MD, Sayagues JM, Lopez A, Barcena P, Sanchez ML, Gutierrez NC, San Miguel JF, Orfao A (2013) Cytogenetic profiles in multiple myeloma and monoclonal gammopathy of undetermined significance: a study in highly purified aberrant plasma cells. Haematologica 98:279–287

267. Joshua D, Petersen A, Brown R, Pope B, Snowdon L, Gibson J (1996) The labelling index of primitive plasma cells determines the clinical behaviour of patients with myelomatosis. Br J Haematol 94:76–81

268. Paino T, Paiva B, Sayagues JM, Mota I, Carvalheiro T, Corchete LA, Aires-Mejia I, Perez JJ, Sanchez ML, Barcena P, Ocio EM, San-Segundo L, Sarasquete ME, Garcia-Sanz R, Vidriales MB, Oriol A, Hernandez MT, Echeveste MA, Paiva A, Blade J, Lahuerta JJ, Orfao A, Mateos MV, Gutierrez NC, San-Miguel JF (2014) Phenotypic identification of subclones in multiple myeloma with different chemoresistant, cytogenetic and clonogenic potential. Leukemia

Multiple Myeloma Minimal Residual Disease

Bruno Paiva, Ramón García-Sanz and Jesús F. San Miguel

Abstract

Assessment of minimal residual disease (MRD) is becoming standard diagnostic care for potentially curable neoplasms such as some acute leukemias as well as chronic myeloid and lymphocytic leukemia. Although multiple myeloma (MM) remains as an incurable disease, around half of the patients achieve complete remission (CR), and recent data suggests increasing rates of curability with "total-therapy-like" programs. This landscape is likely to be improved with the advent of new antibodies and small molecules. Therefore, conventional serological and morphological techniques have become suboptimal for sensitive evaluation of highly effective treatment strategies. Although, existing data suggests that MRD could be used as a biomarker to evaluate treatment efficacy, help on therapeutic decisions, and act as surrogate for overall survival, the role of MRD in MM is still a matter of extensive debate. Here, we review the different levels of remission used to define depth of response in MM and their clinical significance, as well as the prognostic value and unique characteristics of MRD detection using immunophenotypic, molecular, and imaging techniques.

B. Paiva · J.F. San Miguel (✉)
Centro de Investigacion Medica Aplicada (CIMA), Clinica
Universidad de Navarra, IDISNA, Pamplona, Spain
e-mail: sanmiguel@unav.es

R. García-Sanz
Hospital Universitario de Salamanca, Centro de Investigación Del Cancer
(IBMCC-USAL, CSIC), Instituto de Investigaion Biomedica de Salamanca (IBSAL),
Salamanca, Spain

© Springer International Publishing Switzerland 2016
A.M. Roccaro and I.M. Ghobrial (eds.), *Plasma Cell Dyscrasias*,
Cancer Treatment and Research 169, DOI 10.1007/978-3-319-40320-5_7

Key facts

The higher efficacy of new treatment strategies for MM demand the incorporation of highly sensitive techniques to monitor treatment efficacy
MRD could be used as a more potent surrogate biomarker for survival than standard CR
We need to understand the pros and cons of the different MRD techniques
The time has come to incorporate highly sensitive, cost-effective, readily available, and standardized MRD techniques into clinical trials to assess its role in therapeutic decisions

Keywords
Myeloma · MRD · Surrogate · Flow · NGS · PET/CT

1 The Definition of Complete Response in MM: An Historical Overview

Changes in the level of the serum paraprotein and/or urinary light-chain excretion form the basis of assessing the response to therapy and monitoring the progress of MM. Response criteria were first developed by the Committee of the Chronic Leukemia and Myeloma Task Force (CLMTF) of the U.S. National Cancer Institute in 1968 and were reviewed by the same group in 1973. The main response parameter was a reduction in the paraprotein of at least 50 %. In 1972 the Southwest Cancer Chemotherapy Study Group, now the Southwest Oncology Group (SWOG), defined 'objective response' as a reduction of at least 75 % in the calculated serum paraprotein synthetic rate (rather than paraprotein concentration) and/or a decrease of at least 90 % in urinary light-chain excretion, sustained for at least 2 months [1].

Neither the CLMTF nor the SWOG response criteria include a definition of complete response (CR) since it was rarely observed with existing treatments. With the introduction of new regimens such as VAD (vincristine, adriamycin, and dexamethasone) and high-dose melphalan (140 mg/m^2) followed by autologous stem cell support (ASCT), measurable paraprotein disappeared in a significant proportion of patients and criteria for complete remission were proposed based on the absence of detectable paraprotein in serum or urine together with a normal number of plasma cells (PCs) in the marrow (i.e., <4–5 %); nevertheless, the initial definition had no consensus on whether the absence of paraprotein should be based on routine electrophoresis alone, or combined with more sensitive methods such as immunofixation [2]. The current definition of CR was introduced by Blade et al. on behalf of the European blood and marrow transplantation (EBMT) more than 15 years ago: negative immunofixation in serum and urine, disappearance of any soft tissue plasmacytomas and <5 % PCs in bone marrow (BM) [2]. The prognostic value of CR has extensively been validated both in transplant-candidate [3–5] and elderly patients [6–8]. A correlation between deeper quality of responses and better outcomes has also been described in the relapse/refractory setting [3]. As expected, different groups have also shown that more important than achieving CR is to maintain it, since those patients that relapse from CR early-on consistently show a dismal outcome [4, 5]. Interestingly, long follow-up observations show that only 1 out of 4 patients in CR remain progression-free at 10 years [6, 7]. All these data together implies that CR is indeed a strong prognostic marker and a clinically relevant end point, but also that similarly to other hematological malignancies, response criteria in MM can be further improved.

Already in 2006, the International Myeloma Working Group (IMWG) highlighted the need for a new definition of CR, and introduced normalization of serum free light-chains (sFLC) and absence of clonal PCs in BM biopsies by immunohistochemistry (IHC) and/or immunofluorescence, as additional requirements to define more stringent CR criteria [8]. Since then, only one large study was able to show the superiority of the stringent over conventional CR criteria to define patients' outcomes [9], while other groups failed to demonstrate the utility of the sFLC assay among immunofixation-negative patients [10–12], maybe because the latter groups did not include simultaneous assessment of PC clonality in BM biopsies. Importantly, the vast majority of CR patients after therapy show recovery of normal PCs that exceeds the percentage of clonal PCs, implying that more sensitive clonality markers are needed such as the clonotypic immunoglobulin (Ig) gene sequences or immunophenoyping. In addition, it has been suggested that the sFLC might be replaced by the heavy-light format [13] and become merely a surrogate for recovery of the immune system rather than an MRD monitoring tool [14]. Overall, it becomes clear that the definition of CR would benefit from an improvement that matches the rapid evolution observed in MM treatment. Such improvement can only be achieved by highly sensitive technologies able to detect MRD at very low levels and accordingly, the notion of immunophenotypic and molecular CR have been slowly integrated into the response criteria in MM [15].

2 The Relationship Between Depth of Response and Survival: Rationale for Implementing MRD Monitoring in MM

At present it is clear that in MM there is a direct correlation between the depth of response, particularly CR, and prolonged progression-free survival (PFS) as well as overall survival (OS). This has been demonstrated in many different individual studies [16–21], and confirmed in meta-analyses among transplant-eligible and non-transplant-eligible patients [22–24]. It has also been demonstrated among newly diagnosed high risk [25, 26] and relapse/refractory MM patients [3, 27]. Albeit the overwhelming amount of data supporting the concept that "the deepest the response, the longer the survival," there is also evidence betraying such correlation: (i) patients in CR with early relapses and dismal survival [4, 5]; (ii) different CR rates that do not translate into different outcomes [28]; (iii) similar CR rates associated with different survival [29]; or (iv) some patients failing to achieve

CR who show excellent outcome (those with an MGUS-like signature at baseline) [30]. Regarding the latter subset, it should be noted that MGUS-like patients in which indeed CR is not a pre-requisite to achieve long-term disease control represent <10 % of the whole MM population [30, 31]; for the vast majority of patients, higher CR rates were indeed needed to prolong survival [7]. Moreover, most of the controversial results described above concerning the value of CR may be (at least partially) related to either (i) heterogeneity in the consolidation or maintenance treatment used in one of the treatment arms but not in the other after response evaluation which may further affect tumor reduction, or (ii) different CR quality reached after different regimens [7], combined with the relatively limited sensitivity of current methods to define CR [15]. Altogether, these observations do not challenge the importance of achieving CR in MM, but unravel the need for further standardization and optimization of MRD detection. Recent data by Rawstron et al. [32] points out that quantitative assessment of tumor load with a cut-off of 10^{-4} (using multiparameter flow cytometry; MFC) would be more informative than a positive versus negative categorization, suggesting that a lower cut-off provided by more sensitive assays (e.g., NGS or high-sensitive MFC) will likely improve outcome prediction further. This has already been confirmed by Martinez-Lopez et al. using NGS [33], who identified three groups of patients with different TTP: patients with high ($<10^{-3}$), intermediate (10^{-3}–10^{-5}), and low ($>10^{-5}$) MRD levels showed significantly different TTP: 27, 48, and 80 months, respectively. Accordingly, these data highlight that beyond CR the deepest the level of MRD eradication the better survival, and that 10^{-5} should be currently considered as the target cut-off level for definition of an improved response category and MRD-negativity. This concept has also been reinforced by data obtained with parallel approaches achieving sensitivity levels beyond 10^{-5} [34].

3 Immunophenotypic CR

Multiparameter flow cytometry (MFC) is particularly well-suited to study biological samples containing PCs, because it allows: (i) simultaneous identification and characterization of normal versus tumors cells at the single-cell-level, (ii) fast evaluation of high-cell numbers (in a few hours), (iii) quantitative assessment of both normal and tumor cells and their corresponding antigen expression levels (e.g., for antibody-based therapy), (iv) combined detection of cell surface and intracellular antigens (e.g., for unequivocal confirmation of clonality within phenotypically aberrant cells), (v) an overview of the whole hematopoiesis through the simultaneous analysis of the different cell lineages [35].

The prognostic value of MFC-based MRD monitoring in MM was introduced in 2002 by the Spanish [36] and British [37] groups; both studies suggesting the utility of monitoring the BM PC compartment among MM patients treated with conventional or high-dose chemotherapy, even if such patients were in CR [37]. This initial positive experience led these groups to implement their corresponding 4- and 6-color flow-MRD methods in large clinical trials. In the PETHEMA/GEM2000 study, flow-MRD was identified as the most relevant prognostic factor in a series of 295 newly diagnosed MM patients receiving HDT/ASCT [38]. MRD-negativity at day 100 after ASCT translated into significantly improved PFS and OS, and the impact of MRD was equally relevant among patients in CR. Similarly, in the intensive-pathway of the MRC Myeloma IX study, MRD-negativity at day 100 after ASCT was predictive of favorable PFS and OS [39]. This outcome advantage was equally demonstrable in patients achieving CR. Furthermore, current data indicate that attaining MRD-negativity is not only relevant for standard but also high-risk patients. In fact, it is important to emphasize that both the PETHEMA/GEM and UK groups have demonstrated that risk assessment by cytogenetics/FISH and flow-MRD monitoring were of independent prognostic value in transplant-eligible patients [38, 39]. Furthermore, it is particularly interesting to observe the benefit of achieving MRD-negativity in high-risk patients, whose outcome becomes similar to that of standard-risk patients [5]. Accordingly, further research on the role of MRD as a surrogate for prolonged OS among high-risk patients is warranted, since it could represent an attractive clinical end point to improve the typical poor prognosis of this patient population. Thus, combined cytogenetic/FISH evaluation at diagnosis plus MRD assessment after HDT/ASCT (day +100), provided powerful risk stratification, which also resulted in a highly effective approach to identify patients with unsustained CR and dismal outcomes [5]. Collectively, these results confirm the superiority of MRD assessment over conventional response criteria to predict outcome in distinct MM genetic subgroups. The effect of maintenance therapy with thalidomide was also assessed in the UK study. Interestingly, MRD-positive patients randomized to the maintenance arm experienced significantly prolonged PFS as compared to the placebo arm; in MRD-negative patients a similar trend was observed [39]. The Spanish myeloma group has also shown that it was possible for elderly patients treated with bortezomib-based induction regimens to achieve MRD-negativity, and that flow-MRD resulted in superior patient prognostication than conventional and stringent CR response criteria [12]. A recent update of this study [40] after a median follow-up >5 years, shows median PFS and OS rates not yet reached for patients in flow-CR after VMP (but not VTP) induction. These results suggest that MRD monitoring is also clinically relevant in elderly patients but MRD-negative cases after two different regimens (VMP and VTP) did not experienced the same outcome. These findings suggest that the level of MRD tumor depletion may have been different between the two regimens, and that the 4-color MFC assay used in this GEM2005 trial was underpowered for ultra-sensitive detection of MRD [40].

The sensitivity of MFC has recently increased due to simultaneous assessment of ≥8 markers and evaluation of greater numbers of cells than what was previously feasible with analogical (4-color) instruments [41]. Thus, the availability of ≥8-color digital flow cytometers coupled to novel sample preparation protocols that allow fast and cost-effective routine evaluation of >5 million nucleated cells, has boosted the sensitivity of modern MFC-based MRD monitoring into that achieved on molecular grounds ($\leq 10^{-5}$) (Table 1). It should be noted that current sensitivity

Table 1 Summary of the most relevant studies based on multiparameter flow cytometry (MFC), allele-specific-oligonucleotide PCR (ASO-PCR), next-generation sequencing (NGS), whole-body magnetic resonance imaging (WB-MRI), and positron emission tomography-computed tomography (PET/CT) detection of minimal residual disease (MRD) in multiple myeloma (MM)

Method	LOD	Setting	Number of patients	Applicability (%)	MRD-negativity (%)	PFS(MRD– vs. MRD+)	P	OS(MRD– vs. MRD+)	P	Reference
4-color MFC	10^{-4}	CT or ASCT	87	NA	26	60 m versus 34 m	0.02	NA	–	San Miguel et al. [36]
3-color MFC	10^{-3}–10^{-4}	ASCT	45	94	56	35 m versus 20 m	0.03	76 % versus 64 % at 5-years	0.28	Rawstron et al. [37]
4-color MFC	10^{-4}	ASCT	295	~95	42	71 m versus 37 m	<0.001	NR versus 89 m	0.002	Paiva et al. [38]
4-color MFC	10^{-4}–10^{-5}	Elderly	102	~95	43	90 % versus 35 % at 3-years	<0.001	94 % versus 70 % at 3-years	0.08	Paiva et al. [12]
4-color MFC	10^{-4}–10^{-5}	ASCT	241 (CR)	~95	74	86 % versus 58 % at 3-years	<0.001	94 % versus 80 % at 3-years	0.001	Paiva et al. [5]
6-color MFC	10^{-4}	ASCT	397	NA	62	29 m versus 16 m	<0.001	81 m versus 59 m	0.02	Rawstron et al. [39]
7-color MFC	10^{-5}	ASCT	31	NA	68	100 % versus 30 % at 3-years	NA	NA	–	Roussel et al. [42]
4-color MFC	10^{-4}	Relapse/refractory	52 (CR)	NA	46	75 m versus 14 m	0.03	NA	–	Paiva [43]
ASO	10^{-5}	ASCT ALLO	50	88	27	110 m versus 35 m	<0.005	NA	–	Martinelli et al. [44]
ASO	10^{-6}	ALLO	70	69	33	100 % versus 0 %[1]	0.001	NA	NS	Bakkus [45]
ASO	10^{-4}	ASCT	87	77	35	64 m versus 16 m	0.001	NA	NA	
fASO	10^{-3}–10^{-5}	ASCT ALLO	20	NA	15 60	NA	–	76 % versus 34 % at 2-years	0.03	Galimberti [46]
ASO	5×10^{-5}	ASCT	24	75	29	34 m versus 15 m	0.042	NA	–	Sarasquete et al. [47]
fASO	10^{-3}–10^{-4}	ASCT	53	91	53	68 % versus 28 %	0.001	86 % versus 68 %	NS	Martinez-Sanchez et al. [48]

(continued)

Table 1 (continued)

Method	LOD	Setting	Number of patients	Applicability (%)	MRD-negativity (%)	PFS(MRD– vs. MRD+)	P	OS(MRD– vs. MRD+)	P	Reference
RQ	$10^{-4}–10^{-5}$	ASCT ALLO	37	86	53 71	70 m versus 19 m	0.003	NR versus NR	0.1	Putkonen et al. [49]
RQ NESTED	10^{-6}	Consolidation	39	51	18	NR versus 38 m	<0.001	72 % versus 48 % at 8-years	0.041	Ladetto et al. [34], Ferrero [50]
RQ-ASO	$10^{-4}–10^{-5}$	ASCT	53	78	48	35 m versus 20 m	0.001	70 m versus 45 m	0.04	Korthals (2012)
RQ-ASO	10^{-5}	ASCT	103	42	46	NR versus 31 m	0.002	NR versus 60 m	0.008	Puig et al. [51]
RQ-ASO	4×10^{-6}	ASCT	22	100	59	48 m versus 13 m	0.004	NA	–	Silvennoinen et al. [52]
NGS	10^{-5}	ASCT Elderly	133	91	27	80 m versus 31 m	<0.001	NR versus 81 m	0.019	Martinez-Lopez et al. [33]
WB-MRI	–	ASCT	100	–	23	–	0.03	100 % (0 focal lesions)	0.001	Hillengass et al. [53]
PET/CT	–	ASCT	192	–	65	47 % versus 32 % at 4-years	0.02	79 % versus 66 % at 4-years	0.02	Zamagni et al. [54]

LOD limit of detection; *NA* not available; *PFS* progression-free survival; *MRD* minimal residual disease; *OS* overall survival; *ASCT* autologous stem cell transplantation; *CR* complete response; *ALLO* allogeneic stem cell transplantation of MFC is at least 1-log superior than that of previous MFC analyses (10^{-4}); therefore, ongoing MFC-based MRD monitoring should result in improved patient' risk stratification versus 4- or 6-color analyses. Accordingly, the Intergroupe Francophone du Myélome has reported on the prognostic value of their 7-color flow-MRD method implemented in a recent phase II study; overall, 68 % of patients achieved MRD-negativity and none of these patients has relapsed so far [42]. Analysis of larger number of cells (i.e., >5 million events) allows visualization of previously undetectable normal PC subsets with more heterogeneous phenotypes, which implies the need for simultaneous evaluation of at least eight parameters and potentially also Kappa and Lambda to improve specificity (and thereby sensitivity). Accordingly, using validated and standardized 8-color panels, clonal PCs are readily and accurately distinguishable from normal PCs according to aberrant phenotypes [35], and their clonality further confirmed by light-chain restriction. Because such analyzes rely on the recognition of aberrant antigenic patterns (i.e., different from normal), flow-MRD is applicable in virtually every MM patient without requiring for patient-specific diagnostic phenotypic profiles (although these are certainly useful). Equally important, the flow-MRD method incorporates a sample quality check of BM cellularity *via* simultaneous detection of B-cell precursors, erythroblasts, myeloid precursors, and/or mast cells. This information is critical to ensure sample quality and to identify hemodiluted BM aspirates that may lead to false-negative results

A potential limitation of MFC is that current strategies could miss hypothetical MM cancer stem cells with more immature phenotypes. However, recent investigations conducted with sensitive ASO-PCR assessment of clonal Ig genes among FACS-sorted peripheral blood B-cell subsets, revealed that such clonotypic cells are either absent, or present below highly sensitive limits of detection [41]. The need for extensive expertise to analyze flow cytometric data, together with the lack of well-standardized flow-MRD methods have been pointed out as additional and perhaps the main limitations of conventional MFC immunophenotyping [55]. However, new software programs have been developed in recent years with improved multidimensional identification and classification of different cell clusters coexisting in a sample (e.g., through principal component analysis and canonical analysis). These tools together with the use of normal and tumor reference databases, would allow for automated detection of normal versus aberrant phenotypic profiles [56]. If such methods become widely adopted, MFC would represent a method of choice for clinically relevant (Table 1), cost-effective yet highly sensitive, standardized MRD monitoring.

4   Molecular CR

Rearrangements of germline V, (D), and J gene segments in the Ig gene complexes (*IGH*, *IGK*, and *IGL*) provide each B-cell with specific V(D)J combinations. The random insertion and deletion of nucleotides at the V(D)J junction sites create highly diverse junctional regions, which represent unique "fingerprint-like" sequences, that are different in each B-cell and thus also in each B-cell malignancy. Since the 90s, these junctional regions (to be identified in each individual patient at diagnosis) have therefore been used as individual tumor-specific targets using Ig allele-specific oligonucleotides (ASO) as primers, initially for nested PCR approaches and later for real-time quantitative PCR-based MRD analysis (ASO-PCR). Such Ig targets can be identified and sequenced with standardized technologies in >95 % of lymphoid malignancies and used for the design of junctional region-specific oligonucleotides, to be applied for sensitive PCR-based detection of low frequencies of malignant cells, down to one malignant cell in 10^4–10^5 normal cells (10^{-4}–10^{-5}) [57]. This time-consuming but sensitive approach has been highly successful for MRD diagnostics in immature B-lineage malignancies, such as acute lymphoblastic leukemia (ALL) and has also been applied in mature B-cell malignancies such as MM, where its clinical relevance has been consistently demonstrated (Table 1).

Initial observations performed in patients undergoing autologous or allogeneic SCT unraveled the prognostic value of reaching molecular remissions [34, 47, 58, 59, 51, 44, 48, 52, 49]. Using nonquantitative approaches, the percentage of molecular remissions observed after allogeneic SCT was significantly higher as compared to patients undergoing autologous SCT, suggesting a role for this technique to evaluate treatment efficacy. Furthermore, Lipinski et al., in a retrospective study performed in 1ññ3 patients undergoing ASCT suggested the potential value of ASO-PCR monitoring to predict progression [60], and this notion of MRD reappearance heralding relapse has been recently confirmed by the GIMEMA group [61].

Semi-quantitative and quantitative approaches have also been used to predict patients' outcome according to MRD levels. Korthals et al. in a cohort of 53 patients undergoing ASCT have shown that different MRD levels by ASO-RQ-PCR before ASCT allowed two discriminate two groups of patients with different PFS and OS (0.2 % 2IgH/βactin) [59]. Putkonen et al. in a series of 37 patients undergoing autologous and allogeneic stem cell transplantation defined 0.01 % as the optimal MRD threshold to distinguish two groups of patients with different PFS and OS [49]. Puig et al., in a recent study that included 103 patients undergoing ASCT also found 10^{-4} as the most significant cut-off level, distinguishing two subgroups with different PFS and, when applied to patients in conventional CR, also different OS [51]. Finally, Ladetto et al. with nested and ASO-RQ-PCR have reported on the significant reduction of residual tumor load after bortezomib, thalidomide and dexamethasone (VTD) consolidation, which translated into prolonged PFS [34]. A recent update of the study showed that MRD monitoring also predicted for different OS: 72 % at 8 years for patients in major MRD response versus 48 % for those with positive MRD [61]. More recent studies have provided similar results [52, 62].

In addition to the well-established clinical value, other advantages of PCR approaches for MRD detection are the bypass for immediate sample processing since it is unaffected by pre-analytical biases such as loss of viable cells over time [47]. This feature makes molecular-based MRD monitoring an attractive approach for studies requiring centralized (or necessarily delayed) analysis. Furthermore, taking advantage of the uniqueness of patient-specific clonal *IGHV* rearrangements,

PCR assays can reach highly sensitive MRD detection levels up to 10^{-6}, although experience from different centers suggests that routine limit of detection stands at 10^{-5} [34, 51]. Importantly, PCR strategies have gone through an extensive validation and standardization process for MRD testing in different hematological neoplasms, such as acute lymphoblastic leukemia, becoming readily standardized and reproducible among different centers [57, 63], although not yet in MM. In contrast to MFC, PCR-based approaches require diagnostic samples to identify patient-specific clonotypic sequences [64]. Furthermore, the high rate of somatic hypermutations both in the heavy- and light-chain immunoglobulins genes [65] prevent the exact annealing of consensus primers, hamper clonal detection, sequencing success rates, and overall ASO performance [51]. To overcome such limitations, additional targets have been tested (e.g.,: *DJH* and *Kde*) [66] and the use of CD138$^+$ positively selected PCs has been shown to significantly increase the applicability of PCR-based MRD monitoring in MM, but still remains in the range of 65–80 % of cases [67]. Accordingly, the technique remains costly, laborious, methodologically complex, and difficult to implement into routine clinical practice.

Sequencing technologies can quickly perform multiple reads of many different DNA fragments and are therefore a natural alternative to overcome some of the limitations of ASO-PCR to monitor MRD in MM. Importantly, this technology allows the detection of previously known tumor-specific sequences within normal DNA fragments (i.e.,: MRD monitoring). Current NGS methods include: (1) pyrosequencing, based on the luminometric detection of the pyrophosphate released when individual nucleotides are added to DNA templates from an emulsion PCR; (2) multiplex sequencing-by-synthesis technology, that rely on light signals emitted during the resynthesis of small DNA fragments previously produced by bridge amplification; and (3) ion semiconductor sequencing, that detects hydrogen ions released during DNA polymerization. Using these techniques, several methods have been developed to sequence rearranged B-cell (BCR) and T-cell receptor (TCR) genes [68–72]. These methods use a consensus PCR to amplify all possible BCR or TCR rearrangements which, at diagnosis, allow to identify clonal rearrangements (arbitrarily defined as those above 5 % among the total sequences identified) [72]. After therapy, clonal Ig rearrangements can be traced among thousands of normal Ig genes through several millions reads, providing high-specificity and sensitivity for MRD detection of BCR and TCR clonal sequences.

One of the greatest advantages of NGS approaches for MRD detection in MM is its sensitivity which, without compromising specificity, is estimated to be in the range of 10^{-5}–10^{-6} [33, 72]. Of note, with NGS it would be possible to detect clonal tiding (i.e., suppression or reemergence of two or more clonal Ig rearrangements following treatment) [73], although subclonality in diagnostic samples is typically below 7 % of all tumor cells patients. Furthermore, in MM the main clonal rearrangement is usually stable from diagnosis to relapse, [74] or if it changes, this problem would not affect a proportion much higher than 5 % of the patients [75]. NGS offers additional advantages, particularly when compared to ASO-PCR, because it is methodologically less complex, and obviates the need to construct dilution standard curves which is the main reason of ASO-PCR failure in MM [51]. Another potential advantage of NGS is the information that it provides about the residual normal B-cell compartment, since it can identify the variability of normal polyclonal B-cells and this information may be of potential prognostic value.

However, there are also some disadvantages. Similarly to ASO-PCR, NGS-based MRD monitoring cannot distinguish hemodiluted from representative BM samples. Albeit the applicability of NGS is superior to that of ASO-PCR, still in around 10 % of patients the clonal rearrangement cannot be identified during the initial PCR step [33, 76]. Similarly to ASO-PCR, the NGS method requires a diagnostic sample to identify the patient-specific clonotypic sequence. In addition, MRD quantitation is only approximate, because the efficacy of amplification is highly variable depending on the specific sequence of the rearrangement [77]. NGS-based MRD monitoring is still centralized on commercial vendors and not yet widely available; if it becomes decentralized, this would require additional validation and standardization within the different centers adopting this technology (similarly to what is being currently done for MFC and ASO-PCR). Finally, NGS is relatively labor-intensive and expensive technology, which are important factors to consider prior to incorporation into routine clinical practice.

Since NGS-based MRD monitoring has only recently been developed, there is yet few clinical data in MM (Table 1). However, the PETHEMA/GEM has already described favorable and promising results in a series of 133 MM patients including both transplant and non-transplant-eligible cases [33]. The applicability of NGS-based MRD monitoring using the LymphoSIGHT® methodology was of 90 %. The median TTP and OS of MRD-negative cases were of 80 months and not reached, respectively [33]. As above mentioned, Martinez-Lopez identified three groups of patients with different TTP: patients with high ($<10^{-3}$), intermediate ($10^{-3}-10^{-5}$), and low ($>10^{-5}$) MRD levels showed significantly different TTP: 27, 48, and 80 months, respectively, which indicates that the deepest the quality of CR, the better the patients outcome [33]. Other studies are providing similar results in MM [78, 79] but these are currently available as abstract, and we should wait for their full publication with all the necessary details.

5 Available Techniques to Monitor Intramedullary and Extramedullary MRD: Towards an Imaging CR in MM?

The possibility of patchy BM infiltration or extramedullary involvement represents a challenge for both immunophenotypic- and molecular-based MRD detection in single BM aspirates. This highlights the potential value of sensitive imaging techniques to redefine CR both at the intramedullary and extra-medullary levels (Table 2).

Table 2 Individual features of currently available techniques to monitor MRD in MM

Technique	Advantages	Disadvantages
MFC (≥8-color)	• Applicable to virtually all patients • Availability in individual laboratories • Reproducibility among centers • Sensitivity (10^{-5}–10^{-6}) • Direct quantitation of MRD levels • Ongoing assessment of sample quality • Diagnostic sample is important but not mandatory • Possibility to standardize (e.g., EuroFlow/IMF) • Turnaround time (2–3 h) • Less expensive technique	• Limited value in patients with patchy BM infiltration and/or extramedullary disease • Requires fresh samples (<36-h) • Requires full implementation of a single, standardized method in multiple individual laboratories for complete standardization • Detection of clonality restricted to the PC compartment
ASO-PCR	• Highly specific detection of clonality • Sensitivity (10^{-5}–10^{-6}) • Detection of all clonal Ig sequences irrespectively of phenotype (i.e., putative CSCs) • Intermediate availability in experienced individual laboratories • Reproducibility among centers • Does not require immediate sample processing • Acquired experienced in standardization (EuroMRD)	• Limited applicability ($\sim$60–70 %) • Limited value in patients with patchy BM infiltration and/or extramedullary disease • Lack of ongoing assessment of sample quality • Requires diagnostic sample • Turnaround time (3–4 weeks for target identification at baseline and ≥5 days during follow-up) • Indirect quantitation of MRD levels • Cost (increased by target identification at baseline)
NGS	• Higher applicability compared to ASO-PCR ($\sim$90 %) • Highly-specific detection of clonality • Sensitivity (10^{-6}) • Detection of all clonal Ig sequences irrespectively of phenotype (i.e.: putative CSCs) • Does not require immediate sample processing • Easy to standardize if confined to commercial services	• Limited availability to commercial services • Limited experience on individual laboratories (with consequent lack of reported reproducibility) • Limited value in patients with patchy BM infiltration and/or extramedullary disease • Lack of ongoing assessment of sample quality • Requires diagnostic sample • Indirect quantitation of MRD levels
PET/CT	• Applicable to virtually all patients • Sensitivity (4 mm) • Detection of extramedullary disease • Not biased by patchy BM infiltration • Diagnostic imaging is important but not mandatory • Turnaround time (2–3 h)	• Intermediate availability Lack of standardization • Moderate reproducibility at MRD assessment • Cost

MFC multiparameter flow cytometry; *ASO-PCR* allele-specific oligonucleotide, polymerase chain reaction; *NGS* next-generation sequencing; *PET/CT* positron emission tomography-computed tomography; *MRD* minimal residual disease; *PC* plasma cell; *CSCs* cancer stem cells; *EuroFlow* see www.EuroFlow.org; *EuroMRD* see www.EuroMRD.org

Magnetic resonance imaging (MRI) is the most sensitive noninvasive imaging technique to detect focal lesions in the spine. However, it should be noted that due to treatment-induced necrosis and inflammation, focal lesions may remain hyperintense for several months after therapy in both responding and non-responding patients. This can explain some inconsistencies found between serological CR and MRI-based CR [53, 80]. Consequently, an interval of at least 3 months has been recommended before MRI monitoring [81]. Although comparative studies are lacking, it can be envisioned that similarly to that found for newly diagnosed patients [82], whole-body MRI (WB-MRI) would be more effective than MRI on the axial skeleton to define full BM imaging response.

In contrast to MRD, positron emission tomography-computed tomography (PET/CT) combines the morphological images provided by CT with the imaging data of a particular metabolic process (e.g., fluorodeoxyglucose–FDG—uptake), and it is probably the technique of choice to detect extramedullary disease. Similarly to MRI, it is important to emphasize that for MRD monitoring (which will pay particular attention to FDG uptake rather than lytic bone lesions), both false positive (e.g., coexisting infectious or inflammatory processes) and false-negative results (e.g., quiescent tumor cells) may occur [83]. A recent comparison between WB-MRI and PET/CT in transplant-eligible patients showed that, against conventional response criteria, PET/CT had the lower sensitivity (50 % vs. 80 %) but higher specificity (85 % vs. 38 %) than WB-MRI. While the utility of other MRI-based techniques is still under investigation (e.g., dynamic contrast-enhanced MRI) [84], the current perception is that PET/CT represents the most promising imaging tool to monitor MRD in MM. That notwithstanding, Zamagni et al. reported that post-ASCT, PET/CT monitoring was also an independent prognostic marker for PFS and OS, even among patients in conventional CR [54]. However, given the sensitivity and specificity observed against traditional response criteria, standardization of PET-CT (including response criteria) and comparison with other sensitive BM-based MRD methods is still needed in order to implement imaging monitoring in the clinical setting [83].

NGS approaches have also been tested in peripheral blood as a promise for MRD detection in MM outside the BM. This approach has provided initial successful results in NHL [85] and it has also been proposed for myeloma [86] but no real correlation has been found in a small study were specific myeloma DNA is lost in most patients after two cycles of therapy despite they conserve the monoclonal protein [87].

6 Conclusions and Future Perspectives: MRD Incorporation into Clinical Trials

So far no clinical trial has randomized MM patients according to their MRD status, in order to investigate the role of MRD to individualize therapy. Overall, the experience of several cooperative groups using different MRD techniques indicates that persistence of MRD is always an adverse prognostic feature (Tables 1 and 2), even among CR patients. Consequently, it would be safer to take clinical decisions based on MRD-positivity rather than on MRD-negativity, since the patchy pattern of BM infiltration typically observed in MM leads to a degree of uncertainty regarding MRD-negative results: does this guarantee absence of tumor cells or is it the result of a nonrepresentative BM sample due to patchy tumor infiltration? Many studies have shown the value of MRD to evaluate the efficacy of specific treatment phases and therefore, to support potential treatment decisions. For example, both the Spanish PETHEMA and the UK MRC study groups have shown that MRD kinetics before and after HDT/ASCT allow identification of chemosensitive versus chemoresistant patients [38, 39]. For the latter, it could be hypothesized that consolidation with alternative therapies would be needed to improve outcomes. Following consolidation physicians face another treatment decision: maintenance versus no maintenance and duration? Ladetto et al. reported PFS rates of 100 % versus 57 % for patients in molecular CR versus MRD-positive cases after consolidation, respectively [34]. Since no maintenance therapy was given in the GIMEMA VEL-03-096 study, one might hypothesize that for those cases failing to reach MRD-negativity despite being in CR/nCR after consolidation, maintenance may represent an effective approach to eradicate MRD levels and improve outcome. Accordingly, Rawstron et al. have shown that one out of four MRD-positive patients randomized to the maintenance arm of the MRC-myeloma IX (intensive) study turned into MRD-negative, and experienced significantly prolonged PFS versus the abstention arm [39]. However, because even MRD-negative patients receiving maintenance continue to show late relapses [39], it may be envisioned that we need to increase the sensitivity of MRD techniques in order to better monitoring "theoretically MRD negative" patients during maintenance therapy; moreover, if treatment decisions are taken according to patients' MRD status, follow-up MRD studies would also become useful to detect MRD reappearance preceding clinical relapse [61]. This approach is likely to imply serial MRD assessment which, at the moment, would require the need of invasive and inconvenient multiple BM aspirates. Most recently, NGS has been evaluated in PB (i.e., plasma) from MM patients after induction and this would represent an attractive minimally invasive approach. However, preliminary data indicates that clonotypic sequences identified at baseline, become undetectable with just a few cycles of chemotherapy, even among electrophoresis positive patients. Thus, further research is warranted to establish the feasibility of PB (e.g., cell- or free DNA-based) MRD monitoring. Furthermore, our knowledge on clonal tiding (i.e., disappearance of pre-existing or occurrence of new clones), during maintenance or progression-free periods without therapy is very limited if exiting at all, and the concept of clonal tiding should also be taken into consideration while designing such treatment strategies.

The choice of MRD technology for monitoring will depend on how individual centers' priorities adjust to the specific advantages that each tool has to offer (Table 2). In turn, extensive research is still warranted to determine how to best integrate medullary and extramedullary MRD monitoring. In other hematological malignancies, baseline risk-factors and MRD monitoring have an established and complementary role to individualize treatment. Over the last two decades, several groups have consistently confirmed the added value of MRD in MM, and the time has come to establish the role of baseline risk-factors plus MRD monitoring for tailored therapy. This requires the introduction of standardized, highly sensitive, cost-effective, and broadly available MRD techniques in clinical trials.

References

1. Alexanian R, Bonnet J, Gehan E, Haut A, Hewlett J, Lane M et al (1972) Combination chemotherapy for multiple myeloma. Cancer 30(2):382–389
2. Blade J, Samson D, Reece D, Apperley J, Bjorkstrand B, Gahrton G et al (1998) Criteria for evaluating disease response and progression in patients with multiple myeloma treated by high-dose therapy and haemopoietic stem cell transplantation. Myeloma Subcommittee of the EBMT. European Group for Blood and Marrow Transplant. Br J Haematol 102(5):1115–1123
3. Harousseau JL, Dimopoulos MA, Wang M, Corso A, Chen C, Attal M et al (2010) Better quality of response to lenalidomide plus dexamethasone is associated with improved clinical outcomes in patients with relapsed or refractory multiple myeloma. Haematologica 95 (10):1738–1744
4. Barlogie B, Anaissie E, Haessler J, van Rhee F, Pineda-Roman M, Hollmig K et al (2008) Complete remission sustained 3 years from treatment initiation is a powerful surrogate for extended survival in multiple myeloma. Cancer 113(2):355–359
5. Paiva B, Gutierrez NC, Rosinol L, Vidriales MB, Montalban MA, Martinez-Lopez J et al (2012) High-risk cytogenetics and persistent minimal residual disease by multiparameter flow cytometry predict unsustained complete response after autologous stem cell transplantation in multiple myeloma. Blood 119(3):687–691
6. Martinez-Lopez J, Blade J, Mateos MV, Grande C, Alegre A, Garcia-Larana J et al (2011) Long-term prognostic significance of response in multiple myeloma after stem cell transplantation. Blood 118(3):529–534
7. Barlogie B, Mitchell A, van Rhee F, Epstein J, Morgan GJ, Crowley J (2014) Curing myeloma at last: defining criteria and providing the evidence. Blood 124(20):3043–3051
8. Durie BG, Harousseau JL, Miguel JS, Blade J, Barlogie B, Anderson K et al (2006) International uniform response criteria for multiple myeloma. Leukemia 20(9):1467–1473
9. Kapoor P, Kumar SK, Dispenzieri A, Lacy MQ, Buadi F, Dingli D et al (2013) Importance of achieving stringent complete response after autologous stem-cell transplantation in multiple myeloma. J Clin Oncol Official J Am Soc Clin Oncol 31(36):4529–4535
10. de Larrea CF, Cibeira MT, Elena M, Arostegui JI, Rosinol L, Rovira M et al (2009) Abnormal serum free light chain ratio in patients with multiple myeloma in complete remission has strong association with the presence of oligoclonal bands: implications for stringent complete remission definition. Blood 114(24):4954–4956
11. Giarin MM, Giaccone L, Sorasio R, Sfiligoi C, Amoroso B, Cavallo F et al (2009) Serum free light chain ratio, total kappa/lambda ratio, and immunofixation results are not prognostic factors after stem cell transplantation for newly diagnosed multiple myeloma. Clin Chem 55 (8):1510–1516
12. Paiva B, Martinez-Lopez J, Vidriales MB, Mateos MV, Montalban MA, Fernandez-Redondo E et al (2011) Comparison of immunofixation, serum free light chain, and immunophenotyping for response evaluation and prognostication in multiple myeloma. J Clin Oncol Official J Am Soc Clin Oncol 29(12):1627–1633
13. Ludwig H, Milosavljevic D, Zojer N, Faint JM, Bradwell AR, Hubl W et al (2013) Immunoglobulin heavy/light chain ratios improve paraprotein detection and monitoring, identify residual disease and correlate with survival in multiple myeloma patients. Leukemia 27(1):213–219

14. Tovar N, Fernandez de Larrea C, Elena M, Cibeira MT, Arostegui JI, Rosinol L et al (2012) Prognostic impact of serum immunoglobulin heavy/light chain ratio in patients with multiple myeloma in complete remission after autologous stem cell transplantation. Biol Blood Marrow Transplant 18(7):1076–1079
15. Rajkumar SV, Harousseau JL, Durie B, Anderson KC, Dimopoulos M, Kyle R et al (2011) Consensus recommendations for the uniform reporting of clinical trials: report of the International Myeloma Workshop Consensus Panel 1. Blood 117(18):4691–4695
16. Cavo M, Tacchetti P, Patriarca F, Petrucci MT, Pantani L, Galli M et al (2010) Bortezomib with thalidomide plus dexamethasone compared with thalidomide plus dexamethasone as induction therapy before, and consolidation therapy after, double autologous stem-cell transplantation in newly diagnosed multiple myeloma: a randomised phase 3 study. Lancet 376(9758):2075–2085
17. Richardson PG, Sonneveld P, Schuster MW, Irwin D, Stadtmauer EA, Facon T et al (2005) Bortezomib or high-dose dexamethasone for relapsed multiple myeloma. N Engl J Med 352 (24):2487–2498
18. Dimopoulos M, Spencer A, Attal M, Prince HM, Harousseau JL, Dmoszynska A et al (2007) Lenalidomide plus dexamethasone for relapsed or refractory multiple myeloma. N Engl J Med 357(21):2123–2132
19. Facon T, Mary JY, Hulin C, Benboubker L, Attal M, Pegourie B et al (2007) Melphalan and prednisone plus thalidomide versus melphalan and prednisone alone or reduced-intensity autologous stem cell transplantation in elderly patients with multiple myeloma (IFM 99-06): a randomised trial. Lancet 370(9594):1209–1218
20. San Miguel JF, Schlag R, Khuageva NK, Dimopoulos MA, Shpilberg O, Kropff M et al (2008) Bortezomib plus melphalan and prednisone for initial treatment of multiple myeloma. N Engl J Med 359(9):906–917
21. Rosinol L, Oriol A, Teruel AI, Hernandez D, Lopez-Jimenez J, de la Rubia J et al (2012) Superiority of bortezomib, thalidomide, and dexamethasone (VTD) as induction pretransplantation therapy in multiple myeloma: a randomized phase 3 PETHEMA/GEM study. Blood 120(8):1589–1596
22. Sonneveld P, Goldschmidt H, Rosinol L, Blade J, Lahuerta JJ, Cavo M et al (2013) Bortezomib-based versus nonbortezomib-based induction treatment before autologous stem-cell transplantation in patients with previously untreated multiple myeloma: a meta-analysis of phase III randomized, controlled trials. J Clin Oncol Official J Am Soc Clin Oncol 31(26):3279–3287
23. Gay F, Larocca A, Wijermans P, Cavallo F, Rossi D, Schaafsma R et al (2011) Complete response correlates with long-term progression-free and overall survival in elderly myeloma treated with novel agents: analysis of 1175 patients. Blood 117(11):3025–3031
24. van de Velde HJ, Liu X, Chen G, Cakana A, Deraedt W, Bayssas M (2007) Complete response correlates with long-term survival and progression-free survival in high-dose therapy in multiple myeloma. Haematologica 92(10):1399–1406
25. Usmani SZ, Crowley J, Hoering A, Mitchell A, Waheed S, Nair B et al (2013) Improvement in long-term outcomes with successive Total Therapy trials for multiple myeloma: are patients now being cured? Leukemia 27(1):226–232
26. Nooka AK, Kaufman JL, Muppidi S, Langston A, Heffner LT, Gleason C et al (2014) Consolidation and maintenance therapy with lenalidomide, bortezomib and dexamethasone (RVD) in high-risk myeloma patients. Leukemia 28(3):690–693
27. Stewart AK, Rajkumar SV, Dimopoulos MA, Masszi T, Spicka I, Oriol A et al (2015) Carfilzomib, lenalidomide, and dexamethasone for relapsed multiple myeloma. N Engl J Med 372(2):142–152
28. Morgan GJ, Davies FE, Gregory WM, Russell NH, Bell SE, Szubert AJ et al (2011) Cyclophosphamide, thalidomide, and dexamethasone (CTD) as initial therapy for patients with multiple myeloma unsuitable for autologous transplantation. Blood 118(5):1231–1238

29. Palumbo A, Cavallo F, Gay F, Di Raimondo F, Ben Yehuda D, Petrucci MT et al (2014) Autologous transplantation and maintenance therapy in multiple myeloma. N Engl J Med 371 (10):895–905

30. Paiva B, Vidriales MB, Rosinol L, Martinez-Lopez J, Mateos MV, Ocio EM et al (2013) A multiparameter flow cytometry immunophenotypic algorithm for the identification of newly diagnosed symptomatic myeloma with an MGUS-like signature and long-term disease control. Leukemia 27(10):2056–2061

31. Zhan F, Barlogie B, Arzoumanian V, Huang Y, Williams DR, Hollmig K et al (2007) Gene-expression signature of benign monoclonal gammopathy evident in multiple myeloma is linked to good prognosis. Blood 109(4):1692–1700

32. Rawstron AC, Gregory WM, de Tute RM, Davies FE, Bell SE, Drayson MT et al (2015) Minimal residual disease in myeloma by flow cytometry: independent prediction of survival benefit per log reduction. Blood 125(12):1932–1935

33. Martinez-Lopez J, Lahuerta JJ, Pepin F, Gonzalez M, Barrio S, Ayala R et al (2014) Prognostic value of deep sequencing method for minimal residual disease detection in multiple myeloma. Blood 123(20):3073–3079

34. Ladetto M, Pagliano G, Ferrero S, Cavallo F, Drandi D, Santo L et al (2010) Major tumor shrinking and persistent molecular remissions after consolidation with bortezomib, thalidomide, and dexamethasone in patients with autografted myeloma. J Clin Oncol 28 (12):2077–2084

35. Paiva B, Puig N, Garcia-Sanz R, San Miguel JF (2015) Is this the time to introduce minimal residual disease in multiple myeloma clinical practice? Clin Cancer Res

36. San Miguel JF, Almeida J, Mateo G, Blade J, Lopez-Berges C, Caballero D et al (2002) Immunophenotypic evaluation of the plasma cell compartment in multiple myeloma: a tool for comparing the efficacy of different treatment strategies and predicting outcome. Blood 99 (5):1853–1856

37. Rawstron AC, Davies FE, DasGupta R, Ashcroft AJ, Patmore R, Drayson MT et al (2002) Flow cytometric disease monitoring in multiple myeloma: the relationship between normal and neoplastic plasma cells predicts outcome after transplantation. Blood 100(9):3095–3100

38. Paiva B, Vidriales MB, Cervero J, Mateo G, Perez JJ, Montalban MA et al (2008) Multiparameter flow cytometric remission is the most relevant prognostic factor for multiple myeloma patients who undergo autologous stem cell transplantation. Blood 112(10): 4017–4023

39. Rawstron AC, Child JA, de Tute RM, Davies FE, Gregory WM, Bell SE et al (2013) Minimal residual disease assessed by multiparameter flow cytometry in multiple myeloma: impact on outcome in the Medical Research Council Myeloma IX Study. J Clin Oncol Official J Am Soc Clin Oncol 31(20):2540–2547

40. Mateos MV, Oriol A, Martinez-Lopez J, Teruel AI, Lopez de la Guia A, Lopez J et al (2014) Update of the GEM2005 trial comparing VMP/VTP as induction in elderly multiple myeloma patients: do we still need alkylators? Blood

41. Thiago LS, Perez-Andres M, Balanzategui A, Sarasquete ME, Paiva B, Jara-Acevedo M et al (2014) Circulating clonotypic B cells in multiple myeloma and monoclonal gammopathy of undetermined significance. Haematologica 99(1):155–162

42. Roussel M, Lauwers-Cances V, Robillard N, Hulin C, Leleu X, Benboubker L et al (2014) Front-line transplantation program with lenalidomide, bortezomib, and dexamethasone combination as induction and consolidation followed by lenalidomide maintenance in patients with multiple myeloma: a phase II study by the Intergroupe Francophone du Myelome. J Clin Oncol 32(25):2712–2717

43. Paiva (2014) Haematologica. 2015 Feb 100(2):e53–5. Epub 2014 Nov 7. No abstract available. PMID: 25381128 . doi: 10.3324/haematol.2014.115162

44. Martinelli G, Terragna C, Zamagni E, Ronconi S, Tosi P, Lemoli RM et al (2000) Molecular remission after allogeneic or autologous transplantation of hematopoietic stem cells for multiple myeloma. J Clin Oncol 18(11):2273–2281

45. Bakkus (2004) Br J Haematol. 2004 Sept 126(5):665–74. PMID: 15327517
46. Galimberti (2005) Leuk Res. 2005 Aug 29(8):961–6. PMID: 15978948
47. Sarasquete ME, Garcia-Sanz R, Gonzalez D, Martinez J, Mateo G, Martinez P et al (2005) Minimal residual disease monitoring in multiple myeloma: a comparison between allelic-specific oligonucleotide real-time quantitative polymerase chain reaction and flow cytometry. Haematologica 90(10):1365–1372
48. Martinez-Sanchez P, Montejano L, Sarasquete ME, Garcia-Sanz R, Fernandez-Redondo E, Ayala R et al (2008) Evaluation of minimal residual disease in multiple myeloma patients by fluorescent-polymerase chain reaction: the prognostic impact of achieving molecular response. Br J Haematol 142(5):766–774
49. Putkonen M, Kairisto V, Juvonen V, Pelliniemi TT, Rauhala A, Itala-Remes M et al (2010) Depth of response assessed by quantitative ASO-PCR predicts the outcome after stem cell transplantation in multiple myeloma. Eur J Haematol 85(5):416–423
50. Ferrero (2014) Leukemia. 2015 Mar 29(3):689–95. Epub 2014 Jul 16. PMID: 25027515. doi: 10.1038/leu.2014.219
51. Puig N, Sarasquete ME, Balanzategui A, Martinez J, Paiva B, Garcia H et al (2014) Critical evaluation of ASO RQ-PCR for minimal residual disease evaluation in multiple myeloma. A comparative analysis with flow cytometry. Leukemia 28(2):391–397
52. Silvennoinen R, Lundan T, Kairisto V, Pelliniemi TT, Putkonen M, Anttila P et al (2014) Comparative analysis of minimal residual disease detection by multiparameter flow cytometry and enhanced ASO RQ-PCR in multiple myeloma. Blood Cancer J 10(4):e250
53. Hillengass J, Ayyaz S, Kilk K, Weber MA, Hielscher T, Shah R et al (2012) Changes in magnetic resonance imaging before and after autologous stem cell transplantation correlate with response and survival in multiple myeloma. Haematologica 97(11):1757–1760
54. Zamagni E, Patriarca F, Nanni C, Zannetti B, Englaro E, Pezzi A et al (2011) Prognostic relevance of 18-F FDG PET/CT in newly diagnosed multiple myeloma patients treated with up-front autologous transplantation. Blood 118(23):5989–5995
55. Flanders A, Stetler-Stevenson M, Landgren O (2013) Minimal residual disease testing in multiple myeloma by flow cytometry: major heterogeneity. Blood 122(6):1088–1089
56. Pedreira CE, Costa ES, Lecrevisse Q, van Dongen JJ, Orfao A (2013) EuroFlow consortium. Overview of clinical flow cytometry data analysis: recent advances and future challenges. Trends Biotechnol 31(7):415–425
57. van der Velden VH, Hochhaus A, Cazzaniga G, Szczepanski T, Gabert J, van Dongen JJ (2003) Detection of minimal residual disease in hematologic malignancies by real-time quantitative PCR: principles, approaches, and laboratory aspects. Leukemia 17(6):1013–1034
58. Corradini P, Carniti C (2014) Molecular methods for detection of minimal residual disease following transplantation in lymphoid and plasma cell disorders. Methods Mol Biol 1109:209–237
59. Korthals M, Sehnke N, Kronenwett R, Schroeder T, Strapatsas T, Kobbe G et al (2013) Molecular monitoring of minimal residual disease in the peripheral blood of patients with multiple myeloma. Biol Blood Marrow Transplant 19(7):1109–1115
60. Lipinski E, Cremer FW, Ho AD, Goldschmidt H, Moos M (2001) Molecular monitoring of the tumor load predicts progressive disease in patients with multiple myeloma after high-dose therapy with autologous peripheral blood stem cell transplantation. Bone Marrow Transplant 28(10):957–962
61. Ferrero S, Ladetto M, Drandi D, Cavallo F, Genuardi E, Urbano M et al (2015) Long-term results of the GIMEMA VEL-03-096 trial in MM patients receiving VTD consolidation after ASCT: MRD kinetics' impact on survival. Leukemia 29(3):689–695
62. Gambella M, Omedè P, Oliva S, Gilestro M, Muccio VE, Drandi D et al (2014) In Multiple Myeloma, Minimal Residual Disease (MRD) Is an Early Predictor of Progression and Is Modulated By Maintenance Therapy with Lenalidomide. Blood Am Soc Hematol 124 (21):3394–3394

63. Langerak AW, Groenen PJ, Bruggemann M, Beldjord K, Bellan C, Bonello L et al (2012) EuroClonality/BIOMED-2 guidelines for interpretation and reporting of Ig/TCR clonality testing in suspected lymphoproliferations. Leukemia 26(10):2159–2171

64. Biran N, Ely S, Chari A (2014) Controversies in the assessment of minimal residual disease in multiple myeloma: clinical significance of minimal residual disease negativity using highly sensitive techniques. Curr Hematol Malign Rep 9(4):368–378

65. Garcia-Sanz R, Lopez-Perez R, Langerak AW, Gonzalez D, Chillon MC, Balanzategui A et al (1999) Heteroduplex PCR analysis of rearranged immunoglobulin genes for clonality assessment in multiple myeloma. Haematologica 84(4):328–335

66. Gonzalez D, Garcia-Sanz R (2005) Incomplete DJH rearrangements. Methods Mol Med 113:165–173

67. Puig N, Sarasquete ME, Alcoceba M, Balanzategui A, Chillon MC, Sebastian E et al (2013) The use of CD138 positively selected marrow samples increases the applicability of minimal residual disease assessment by PCR in patients with multiple myeloma. Ann Hematol 92 (1):97–100

68. Boyd SD, Gaeta BA, Jackson KJ, Fire AZ, Marshall EL, Merker JD et al (2010) Individual variation in the germline Ig gene repertoire inferred from variable region gene rearrangements. J Immunol 184(12):6986–6992

69. Freeman JD, Warren RL, Webb JR, Nelson BH, Holt RA (2009) Profiling the T-cell receptor beta-chain repertoire by massively parallel sequencing. Genome Res 19(10):1817–1824

70. Robins H, Desmarais C, Matthis J, Livingston R, Andriesen J, Reijonen H et al (2012) Ultra-sensitive detection of rare T cell clones. J Immunol Methods 375(1–2):14–19

71. Logan AC, Zhang B, Narasimhan B, Carlton V, Zheng J, Moorhead M et al (2013) Minimal residual disease quantification using consensus primers and high-throughput IGH sequencing predicts post-transplant relapse in chronic lymphocytic leukemia. Leukemia 27(8):1659–1665

72. Faham M, Zheng J, Moorhead M, Carlton VE, Stow P, Coustan-Smith E et al (2012) Deep-sequencing approach for minimal residual disease detection in acute lymphoblastic leukemia. Blood 120(26):5173–5180

73. Boyd SD, Marshall EL, Merker JD, Maniar JM, Zhang LN, Sahaf B et al (2009) Measurement and clinical monitoring of human lymphocyte clonality by massively parallel VDJ pyrosequencing. Sci Transl Med 1(12):12ra23

74. Puig N, Conde I, Jimenez C, Sarasquete ME, Balanzategui A, Alcoceba M et al (2015) The predominant myeloma clone at diagnosis, CDR3 defined, is constantly detectable across all stages of disease evolution. Leukemia

75. Munshi NC, Minvielle S, Tai Y, Fulciniti M, Richardson PG, Attal M et al (2014) Deep sequencing of immunoglobulin loci reveals evolution of IgH clone in multiple myeloma patients over the course of treatment. Blood Am Soc Hematol 124(21):2005–2005

76. Avet-Loiseau H, Corre J, Maheo S, Zheng J, Faham M, Richardson PG et al (2014) Identification rate of myeloma-specific clonotypes in multiple diagnostic sample types from patients with multiple myeloma using next-generation sequencing method. Blood Am Soc Hematol 124(21):2036–2036

77. van Dongen JJ, Langerak AW, Bruggemann M, Evans PA, Hummel M, Lavender FL et al (2003) Design and standardization of PCR primers and protocols for detection of clonal immunoglobulin and T-cell receptor gene recombinations in suspect lymphoproliferations: report of the BIOMED-2 Concerted Action BMH4-CT98-3936. Leukemia 17(12):2257–2317

78. Takamatsu H, Murata R, Zheng J, Moorhead M, Takezako N, Ito S et al (2014) Prognostic value of sequencing-based minimal residual disease detection in multiple myeloma. Blood Am Soc Hematol 124(21):2003–2003

79. Jasielec J, Dytfeld D, Griffith KA, McDonnell K, Lebovic D, Kandarpa M et al (2014) Minimal residual disease status predicts progression-free survival in Newly Diagnosed Multiple Myeloma (NDMM) patients treated with carfilzomib, lenalidomide, and low-dose dexamethasone (KRd). Blood Am Soc Hematol 124(21):2127–2127

80. Bartel TB, Haessler J, Brown TL, Shaughnessy JD Jr, van Rhee F, Anaissie E et al (2009) F18-fluorodeoxyglucose positron emission tomography in the context of other imaging techniques and prognostic factors in multiple myeloma. Blood 114(10):2068–2076

81. Zamagni E, Cavo M (2012) The role of imaging techniques in the management of multiple myeloma. Br J Haematol 159(5):499–513

82. Bauerle T, Hillengass J, Fechtner K, Zechmann CM, Grenacher L, Moehler TM et al (2009) Multiple myeloma and monoclonal gammopathy of undetermined significance: importance of whole-body versus spinal MR imaging. Radiology 252(2):477–485

83. Caers J, Withofs N, Hillengass J, Simoni P, Zamagni E, Hustinx R et al (2014) The role of positron emission tomography-computed tomography and magnetic resonance imaging in diagnosis and follow up of multiple myeloma. Haematologica 99(4):629–637

84. Hillengass J, Bauerle T, Bartl R, Andrulis M, McClanahan F, Laun FB et al (2011) Diffusion-weighted imaging for non-invasive and quantitative monitoring of bone marrow infiltration in patients with monoclonal plasma cell disease: a comparative study with histology. Br J Haematol 153(6):721–728

85. Roschewski M, Dunleavy K, Pittaluga S, Moorhead M, Pepin F, Kong K et al (2015) Circulating tumour DNA and CT monitoring in patients with untreated diffuse large B-cell lymphoma: a correlative biomarker study. Lancet Oncol

86. Kubiczkova-Besse L, Drandi D, Sedlarikova L, Oliva S, Gambella M, Omedè P et al (2014) Cell-free DNA for minimal residual disease monitoring in multiple myeloma patients. Blood Am Soc Hematol 124(21):3423–3423

87. Korde N, Mailankody S, Roschewski M, Faham M, Kotwaliwale C, Moorhead M et al (2014) Minimal Residual Disease (MRD) Testing in newly diagnosed multiple myeloma (MM) patients: a prospective head-to-head assessment of cell-based, molecular, and molecular-imaging modalities

Treatment of Newly Diagnosed Elderly Multiple Myeloma

Guillemette Fouquet, Francesca Gay, Eileen Boyle,
Sara Bringhen, Alessandra Larocca, Thierry Facon,
Xavier Leleu and Antonio Palumbo

Abstract

Multiple myeloma (MM) is a disease of the elderly, with a median age at diagnosis of approximately 70 years old, and more than 30 % of patients aged >75 years. This latter and very elderly population is going to significantly rise in the near future given the increase in life expectancy in Western countries, and, most importantly, global health status of elderly patients is improving, justifying appropriate treatments. Changes in treatment paradigm from the old melphalan-prednisone regimen used since the 1970s to its use as a backbone in a nontransplant setting since the late 1990s have highlighted different subgroups in elderly MM. Some "elderly" patients could be treated like transplant eligible patients, more likely those aged between 65 and the early 70; while a second group would rather be referred to current approved treatment regimens for the non-transplant setting. A dose-intensity approach seems reasonable for this group, aiming for the best response, eventually the complete response (CR) or even minimal residual disease (MRD). The advent of novel agents such as thalidomide, bortezomib, and most recently lenalidomide have allowed a major improvement in outcome as compared to historical combinations, and soon the novel class of monoclonal antibodies should help to further improve these patients' survival. Nonetheless, elderly patients are more

G. Fouquet · E. Boyle · T. Facon
Service des maladies du sang, Hôpital Huriez, CHRU, Lille, France

X. Leleu (✉)
Service d'Hématologie et Thérapie Cellulaire, CHU, La Milétrie, Poitiers, France
e-mail: xavier.leleu@chu-poitiers.fr

F. Gay · S. Bringhen · A. Larocca · A. Palumbo
Myeloma Unit, Division of Hematology, University of Torino, Turin, Italy

© Springer International Publishing Switzerland 2016
A.M. Roccaro and I.M. Ghobrial (eds.), *Plasma Cell Dyscrasias*,
Cancer Treatment and Research 169, DOI 10.1007/978-3-319-40320-5_8

123

susceptible to side effects and are often unable to tolerate full drug doses, and thus require lower dose intensity regimens, or novel drugs or combinations with more favourable safety profile. Recent developments in MM have focused on identifying these vulnerable patients through geriatric assessment and novel myeloma scoring system, including the notions of frailty, disability and comorbidities. Eventually, we have reached an era in which we should be able to provide individualized treatment strategies and drug doses—"tailored therapy"—to improve tolerability and optimize efficacy and ultimately survival for most elderly MM patients.

Keyword

Newly diagnosed · Elderly · Multiple myeloma

1 Introduction

Multiple myeloma (MM) is a malignant neoplasia characterized by clonal plasma cell proliferation, driven by intrinsic genomic abnormalities and extrinsic bone marrow stromal cell support, associated with a monoclonal protein present in the blood and/or urine [1]. In Western countries, MM represents 1.5 % of all malignant diseases, with an annual age-adjusted incidence of 5.6 cases per 100,000 people [2].

MM is a disease of the elderly: median age at diagnosis is close to 70 years, with about two-third aged ≥ 65 years—including 34.8 % of patients diagnosed after 75 years, and 9.6 % after 85 years [2]. The number of elderly MM patients is expected to increase over time, thanks to the increased life expectancy of the general population, but also to the improved survival enabled by the increase use of potent novel agents.

However, MM remains a fatal disease and its prognosis remains poor in elderly patients, with a median overall survival of 24 months in patients aged over 75 years at diagnosis in the US [2], and a 5-year overall survival of 26 % for the 70–79 years old, and 14 % for the 80–99 year old in the UK [3]. There still is an unmet medical need in this population, as early as the first relapse setting for most of them, and even at diagnosis for the very elderly and frail; progress is therefore needed for these patients. Still, despite the efforts in drug development and progress in understanding the physiopathology of MM, management of elderly patients with MM will remain challenging, because of specific clinical and biological features but essentially because of frailty, comorbidities, financial, and psychosocial factors.

We will review current treatments, discuss various improvements in global appreciation of the health status, and display future perspectives.

2 Geriatric Assessment

Frailty. A precise clinical assessment is essential when treating elderly patients, as age alone is obviously very insufficient, knowing this population is characterized by an important heterogeneity. Several studies have showed that the "in the ballpark" geriatric assessment drove to a certain failure in many elderly patients. The notion of frailty has therefore been introduced to help qualify these patients characterized by a certain risk of significant side effects during treatment—and shorter survival due to these safety issues. It is now a consensual term, but no single sign of symptom is sufficient to define it [4]. Indexes of frailty have been developed according to several factors such as weakness, poor endurance, weight loss, low physical activity, and slow gait speed. At least three factors should be present in order to define a "clinically frail elderly patient", and the presence of this "frailty" has been identified as an independent pejorative factor in elderly adults [5]. The different degrees of frailty are summarized in Table 1.

Comorbidities also have to be taken into account, formally defined as the concurrent presence of at least two diseases diagnosed in the same person [4]. The frequency of individual chronic conditions, along with the incidence of comorbid conditions, rises with age. Comorbidity is associated with polymedication and increased risk of drug interactions. Many prognostic indices for the elderly incorporating comorbidity are available [6–8], but these scores are often complicated.

Disability. Disability is an important notion in geriatric assessment, and can include both physical and mental impairments. It is defined as the difficulty or dependency in carrying out activities essential to independent living, including both essential personal care and household tasks, and activities that are important to maintain a person's quality of life [9]. Disability, independent of its causes, is associated with a higher risk of mortality; disabled adults are more likely to become hospitalized [10]. In patients with MM, disability can be caused by orthopaedic problems and pain; otherwise, the main causes of physical disability in the elderly are chronic diseases such as cardiovascular disease, stroke or arthritis [10].

Table 1 Levels of frailty and disability in elderly patients [9]

Frailty grade	Description
Very fit	Active, energetic patients, who exercise regularly or occasionally
Moderately fit	Patients not regularly active beyond routinely walking
Vulnerable	Patients who can perform limited activities but yet do not need help from other people
Mildly frail	Patients who need help for household tasks (shopping, walking several blocks, managing their finances, and medications)
Moderately frail	Patients who need partial help for their personal care (dressing, bathing, toileting, eating)
Severely frail	Patients completely dependent on other people for their personal care

Scoring system. It should therefore be mandatory to perform a geriatric assessment to all elderly patients with MM, at least over the age of 70, and/or suffering from any kind of frailty, comorbidities or disability. One might consider that these patients should be seen and assessed by geriatricians which expertise is indisputable, but unfortunately this ideal assessment is rarely feasible due to the lack of geriatricians and the increased number of elderly MM patients.

Very recently, **a frailty score** that combines age, comorbidities and functional status (disability) has been proposed for elderly patients with MM [11]. In addition to age, three tools were used: the Katz Activity of Daily Living (ADL), the Lawton Instrumental Activity of Daily Living (IADL), and the Charlson Comorbidity Index (CCI). In a multivariate analysis, adjusted for ISS, chromosome abnormalities and type of therapy, a higher risk of death was observed for patients aged 75–80 years (score -1), and over 80 years (score $= 2$), and for those with an ADL score ≤ 4 (score $= 1$), an IADL ≤ 5 (score $= 1$) or a CCI ≥ 2 (score $= 1$). By combining the risk scores (range, 0–5) for these variables, patients were stratified into three distinctive risk groups for overall survival: fit (score $= 0$), intermediate fitness (score $= 1$) and frail (score ≥ 2). This frailty score could predict survival and toxicity, as the "frail" group displayed an increased risk of death, progression, non-hematologic adverse events and treatment discontinuation, regardless of ISS stage, chromosome abnormalities and type of treatment [11]. The authors even proposed an association of this frailty score with the ISS score.

Several questions remain unanswered; for instance, whether all patients should benefit from this evaluation or only patients selected according to their age and comorbidities. In routine practice, geriatric assessment is performed especially for patients aged over 70–75 years and identified with comorbidities. However, if geriatric assessment can help to better understand the precise geriatric risk that fits each elderly patient, it could thus also be useful to identify elderly patients (65–70 years, or even over 70) that could benefit from a "young" patient-based therapy, if they are deemed fit enough.

3 Biologic and Cytogenetic Features

Biologic and cytogenetic features in MM are quite similar amongst the young and the elderly. Most of the cytogenetic data collected in the past few years came from younger, transplant-eligible newly diagnosed patients. Recently, the Intergroupe Francophone du Myélome (IFM) group reported on a series of 1890 elderly patients (>65 years) [12]. Patients were classified in two groups: 66–75 years ($n = 1{,}239$), and >75 years ($n = 651$), and incidence and clinical impact of three chromosomal aberrations [del(13), $t(4;14)$, or del(17p)] were analyzed. Interestingly, they found a lower incidence of $t(4; 14)$ and del(13) in the oldest patients, whereas incidence of del(17p) was remarkably stable. Regardless of treatment, both $t(4; 14)$ and del(17p) were associated with a worse clinical outcome in this cohort of elderly patients with MM, highlighting the importance of cytogenetic analysis at diagnosis in all MM patients.

However, even if some data seem to suggest that VMP (melphalan-prednisone-bortezomib) may overcome the adverse prognosis associated with certain high-risk cytogenetic abnormalities [13], there is no certainty yet about the optimal management of these patients.

4   Response to Therapy as Primary Goal in Elderly Patients

The primary goal in MM has always been to improve survival across all age categories, as MM remains lethal for the vast majority of patients in a median of 5–7 years. In elderly patients, things are not always as simple: even if prolongation of disease-free survival and overall survival remains the ultimate goal, achieving prolonged treatment-free intervals and good quality of life have indeed also become important aims, along with avoiding complications—especially bone disease and thromboembolic events.

A surrogate marker to survival has long been to obtain at least VGPR (very good partial response). More recently, deeper responses such as CR (complete response) or even MRD (minimal residual disease) have become the optimal short-term endpoint, highly correlated to prolonged survival, including in elderly patients. The role of CR has indeed been evaluated in a retrospective analysis of 1175 elderly patients with newly diagnosed MM treated with novel agents and MP [14]. In this study, achieving CR was associated with improved progression-free survival (PFS) and overall survival (OS). Moreover, upon using more sensitive parameters such as serum free light-chain and multiparameter flow cytometry to define the depth of response, the Spanish group's prospective analysis of elderly patients receiving novel agents showed that achieving an immunophenotypic response translated into better PFS compared with conventional CR or stringent CR [15].

However, in older patients, settling for a lower degree of response may be reasonable from case to case as treatment-related toxicities could outshine any benefit derived from the achievement of a CR. Despite improvement in overall survival, novel agents are indeed associated with adverse events that may impair quality of life (QOL) [16], which tempers down the benefit in improvement of MM-related symptoms such as skeletal-related events. This impairment in QOL can, however, be transient—as seen in the VISTA trial where Bortezomib was associated with a deterioration of the QOL indices for the first four cycles only [17]. In the absence of difference in treatment efficacy, the choice of initial treatment should thus be based on QOL indicators in elderly patients.

5   Supportive Care

Besides specific therapies, supportive care is essential in MM and especially in elderly patients. These patients need special attention in terms of management of anemia, pain (with a special focus on painkillers' adverse effects), hypercalcemia, bone disease (especially use of intravenous bisphosphonates), infections prophylaxis (crucial in elderly patients) and nutrition.

Occurrence of adverse events during treatment should also be carefully taken into account to adjust doses and schedule.

6 Review of Current Approved First-Line Therapy

Melphalan-prednisone (MP) remained the gold standard for many years since its first description by Alexanian in [18]. Combining MP with conventional agents such as anthracyclines and vincristine did not improve outcome [19]; but combinations to novel agents such as Thalidomide and Bortezomib finally led to an improvement in overall survival. The current standards of care upfront in elderly MM patients ineligible for autologous stem cells transplantation are thus MPT (melphalan-prednisone-thalidomide) and VMP (bortezomib-melphalan-prednisone), with derivatives in the alkylating agent-based backbone, with either cyclophosphamide (CTD: cyclophosphamide-thalidomide-dexamethasone) [20], and bendamustine.

6.1 Thalidomide-Based Therapy

Thalidomide is particularly appealing in the elderly because of its lack of myelosuppression and its simple use in case of renal insufficiency, but will probably become more and more outshined by the advent of novel generation drugs. Ludwig et al. first showed the superiority of thalidomide-dexamethasone compared with MP in elderly patients, and especially in the over 75 subgroup [21]. Hulin et al. in the IFM 01/01 then reported the superiority of MPT (melphalan-prednisone-thalidomide) over MP-placebo in patients older than 75 years with newly diagnosed MM [22]. A significant benefit in progression-free survival and overall survival was indeed observed, and toxicity was acceptable with however more grade 2–4 neuropathy and grade 3–4 neutropenia in the MPT arm. A meta-analysis of published data from six randomized trials confirmed the improvement in progression-free survival (PFS) and overall survival (OS) with MPT (melphalan-prednisone-thalidomide) compared with MP [23]. The longer the treatment was continued, the better the outcome was. The reported median PFS and OS with MPT were 20.3 and 39.3 months, respectively. Toxicity, nevertheless, was always higher in the MPT arm [22, 24, 25], and this regimen is likely to be dethroned by less-toxic associations.

The combination of cyclophosphamide, thalidomide and dexamethasone (CTD) also improved response rates compared with MP. Evidence from the Myeloma IX trial suggested a survival benefit in CTD-treated patients with favourable cytogenetics, although early deaths from infections related to high-dose dexamethasone were significant [26, 27].

6.2 Bortezomib-Based Therapy

Bortezomib has excellent activity in MM at any stage of the disease and is synergistic with other agents, which led to several combination strategies.

First developed in the VISTA trial [17, 28], the addition of twice-weekly intravenous bortezomib to MP (VMP) is now a well-established regimen. VMP was proven superior to MP in response rate, CR rate, median TTP (time to progression) and OS, even over all cytogenetic and renal failure subgroups [29]. This superiority was sustained after a median follow-up of 60 months, in terms of median time to second-line antimyeloma therapy (31 months with VMP versus 20.5 months with MP) and median OS (56 months versus 43 months, respectively).

Neuropathy was the major side effect of this regimen. Changes in schedule and administration have then been made in order to reduce toxicity: the twice-weekly schedule was replaced by a weekly schedule in 2010 based on new clinical evidence [30–33] and from intravenous to subcutaneous administration in 2012 [28, 34]. Once weekly regimens are better tolerated especially in the elderly, and are associated with reduced toxicity such as neuropathy, diarrhea, constipation and thrombocytopenia [35]. Two schedules can however be discussed: a once weekly regimen from the start [31], or a twice weekly regimen for the first cycle ("VISTA" regimen) followed by a once weekly regimen for the remaining cycles [33]. It has been shown that a higher cumulative bortezomib dose, resulting from an increased dose/intensity or a prolonged treatment duration, is associated with improved OS [36]. The authors propose that dose/schedule modifications—and for instance beginning with a twice-weekly schedule, continuing therapy in responding patients, proactive management of adverse events, and subcutaneous administration of bortezomib, could help to achieve higher cumulative doses and maximize treatment duration and outcomes. The subcutaneous administration of bortezomib is indeed associated with a reduced toxicity (especially neuropathy) and similar activity [34].

Given its known efficacy and its improved safety profile, plus its easiness and in dose adaptation, VMP has now become the most prescribed regimen worldwide upfront for elderly MM.

6.3 Bendamustine Upfront in Elderly MM

The data on bendamustine are scarcer, but this drug is approved upfront with prednisone in elderly patients that could not benefit from MPT or MPV because of peripheral neuropathy. The rationale for this approval was based on a randomized trial in which bendamustine-prednisone has been proven superior to MP [37], with respect to CR rate (32 % vs. 13 %, $p = 0.007$), and with a benefit in terms of time-to-treatment failure (14 months vs. 10 months; $p = 0.020$), but without any benefit on overall survival. Bendamustine-prednisone is now an interesting option for patients ineligibile for autologous stem cell transplantation, and ineligible for VMP or MPT regimens.

Bendamustine plus prednisone in combination with bortezomib is currently being evaluated in several pilot clinical trials.

6.4 Autologous Stem Cell Transplantation (ASCT)

Although age does not affect the outcome of ASCT [38], the 65-year-old cut-off was commonly used to determine ASCT eligibility in patients with MM for safety reasons. However, the feasibility of ASCT is now well-established in fit patients up to the age of 70, although it should remain a "case-per-case" decision [39]. Even if evidence from the IFM 99-06 trial did not suggest any benefit of ASCT in this population [24], early ASCT may nevertheless be appropriate in selected fit patients between 65 and 70 years of age. Intermediate-dose melphalan (140 mg/m^2) should be preferred to high-dose melphalan (200 mg/m^2) in this population, as retrospective data suggests a better safety profile and a similar efficacy [40]. Lower doses (100–140 mg/m^2) can be used for older patients.

Tandem ASCT with melphalan 100 mg/m^2 (MEL100) is another option: Palumbo et al. indeed showed that tandem MEL100 ASCT was superior to conventional MP therapy, especially in patients aged 65–70 [41]. They then reported another valuable option including tandem MEL100 ASCT for elderly patients with MM, especially for those aged <70: 4 cycles of bortezomib-pegylated liposomal doxorubicin-dexamethasone, tandem MEL100 ASCT, 4 cycles of lenalidomide-prednisone consolidation, and lenalidomide maintenance until disease progression. After a median follow-up of 66 months, this sequential approach resulted in a median time-to-progression of 55 months, a median PFS of 48 months, a median OS not reached and 5-year OS of 63 % [42].

ASCT in elderly patients with significantly compromised renal function should however be avoided.

6.5 A New Standard of Care, Lenalidomide-Based

Recently, lenalidomide plus low-dose dexamethasone (Rd) has emerged as a promising new option especially in relapsed MM, or upfront in elderly patients. It is an attractive option for elderly patients because of its excellent tolerability, convenience and efficacy: amongst the patients 70 and older from the ECOG study, the 3-year OS rate was indeed 70 % [43].

The IFM2007-01/MM020/FIRST study [44] compared lenalidomide-low dose dexamethasone upfront in elderly MM patients, to the standard of care MPT. This phase 3 multicenter trial randomized 1623 newly diagnosed elderly MM patients aged 65 years or older and ineligible for ASCT, between three treatment arms: melphalan-prednisone-thalidomide (MPT) administered for 12 cycles so 18 months, versus lenalidomide-dexamethasone given either for 18 cycles so 18 months (Rd18) or until progression or intolerance (continuous Rd). Lenalidomide was given at 25 mg/day for 21 days out of 28, and dexamethasone at 20 or 40 mg per week.

Approximately, 35 % of patients included were aged over 75 years, 47–50 % had a creatinine clearance <60 mL/min and 8–10 % <30 mL/min.

Compared with MPT, continuous Rd significantly improved PFS, and even showed an OS benefit at the interim analysis. With a median follow-up of 37 months, median PFS was 25.5 months for Rd, compared with 20.7 months for Rd 18 and 21.2 months for MPT. Improvement in OS was significant when comparing continuous Rd with MPT (estimated 4-year OS, 59.4 % vs. 51.4 %, $p = 0.0168$), but not when comparing continuous Rd with Rd18 (4-year OS, 59.4 % vs. 55.7 %, $p = 0.307$). In addition, Rd was superior to MPT across all other efficacy endpoints, including response rate, TTP, time to treatment failure, time to second-line antimyeloma therapy and duration of response.

Moreover, median PFS and OS achieved with MPT in the FIRST study compare favourably with those reported in published data: median PFS of 21.2 months versus 20.3 months in the meta-analysis, and median OS of about 46 months versus 39.3 months, respectively [23]. Rd was thus superior to MPT intrinsically, and not because MPT was less efficient than expected in this study.

It is worth noting that evaluation of PFS2 (PFS on second-line therapy), which is now adopted as a surrogate marker for OS and was a secondary endpoint in the FIRST study, also showed improvement in favour of continuous Rd as compared with MPT (HR = 0.78, $p = 0.0051$).

Bahlis et al. recently reported that duration of response was remarkably longer in patients treated with continuous Rd (35 months) versus Rd18 (22.18 months, $p < 0.01$) or MPT (22.3 months, $p < 0.01$) regardless of the depth of response, but the benefits of continuous Rd were even more pronounced in patients who achieved a greater depth of response. When comparing continuous Rd versus Rd18 and MPT, median PFS was indeed not reached versus 31 and 34.7 months, respectively, for patients in VGPR, and median PFS not reached versus 45.2 and 44.6 months, respectively, for patients in CR [45].

Concerning the safety profile, Rd was also generally better tolerated than MPT [44]. Interestingly, most of the adverse events—and especially infections—were mainly imputable to dexamethasone, more than to lenalidomide itself. The incidence of thromboembolic events was slightly higher in the continuous Rd arm: 8 %, versus 6 % in Rd18, and 5 % in the MPT arm. Second primary malignancies were higher with MPT (5 %) than with continuous Rd (3 %), which is consistent with reports suggesting that the increased risk of a second primary cancer among patients treated with lenalidomide may be related to prior or concurrent melphalan use. Quality of life was also assessed, and was improved in all three arms of treatment.

Lenalidomide plus low-dose dexamethasone is thus becoming a new standard of care upfront for MM patients ineligible for ASCT, and has been recently approved by the EMA in this indication.

This FIRST study has pushed the boundaries of MM treatment at least twice, defining not one but 2 new changes in treatment paradigm in elderly MM patients upfront: for the first time an alkylator-free option is suitable for first-line therapy, and a doublet-based regimen, supposedly safer, could prove more effective than a triplet-based regimen. One could foresee that some patients might never be exposed to alkylators throughout their MM disease history in the near future. On the other hand, one would also find of interest to compare Rd to VMP to validate the superiority of Rd not only over MPT but over all MP-triplet-based regimens. Indeed, the FIRST results should be interpreted with caution, as the benefit was mainly observed in the continuous Rd arm once the continuous phase started (while no treatment was then proposed to the other arms), and especially for responding patients. Available data are insufficient for now to firmly recommend continuous Rd over Rd18.

7   Continuous Treatment or Maintenance Therapy

Several studies have recently evaluated the role of continuous therapy in the form of maintenance or continuous treatment for elderly MM patients upfront. These approaches included:

7.1   Bortezomib-Based Treatments

- Bortezomib-thalidomide (VT) maintenance, following VMPT induction [32, 33],
- VT or VP (bortezomib-prednisone) maintenance, following VMP or VTP (bortezomib-thalidomide-prednisone) induction [30].

7.2   Lenalidomide-Based Treatments

- Lenalidomide maintenance after MPR (melphalan-prednisone-lenalidomide) in MM015 study [46, 47],
- Continuous Rd in the FIRST study [44].

   Taken together, these studies support the role of continuous/maintenance therapy in elderly MM patients, at least in terms of PFS and time to second-line anti-myeloma therapy. These survival end points indeed are almost systematically prolonged by more than one year for patients exposed to maintenance versus no treatment.

- With a bortezomib-based maintenance, median PFS varies from 31 to 39 months, versus 27 months without maintenance. No significant OS benefit has been proven for now. Amongst patients achieving CR (38–42 % of patients), results are impressive, with a median PFS of 54 months and a 5-years OS of 78 % [30].
- With a lenalidomide-based maintenance, median PFS varies from 25.5 to 31 months, versus 13–21.2 months without maintenance, and 3-years OS is estimated to be 70 % versus 62–66 % without maintenance.

Maintenance therapy did not manage to overcome the adverse prognosis of cytogenetic abnormalities in these studies, but no increased toxicity was seen as compared to standard therapy.

For now, lenalidomide maintenance is the only regimen that has proven safe enough for long-term use, bortezomib having been studied only intravenously for now. The role of subcutaneous bortezomib, novel generation proteasome inhibitors particularly of oral form, or monoclonal antibodies in this setting is currently under study and should pave the way for novel strategies.

Whether all elderly patients should receive a maintenance therapy, what type (for instance monotherapy or combination), and for how long, remains an important question that future studies should address.

7.3 Sequential Versus Alternating Therapy, Two Keywords in One Trial: Continuous and Switch

- If VMP and Rd are now considered the two most effective regimens in the first-line treatment of elderly MM patients, one way to further improve outcome might be to find a way to combine all these drugs. However, this would probably result toxic if used simultaneously. Mateos et al. recently reported preliminary results for the GEM2010MAS65 trial, which compared a sequential arm consisting of 9 cycles of VMP followed by 9 cycles of Rd, to an alternating arm consisting on one cycle of VMP alternating with one Rd, up to 18 cycles, in elderly MM patients with newly diagnosed MM [48]. These two approaches were both very effective, and no difference was seen between the two arms: median PFS 30 months, median OS not reached, and 3-years OS was 67 and 68 %. The safety profile was acceptable, although in a much lesser extent above 75 years old.

This study provided the best results ever reported in elderly patients upfront compared to any other treatment approach in elderly MM; and depict what may very much look like the introduction of continuous treatment in elderly MM upfront. One may foresee either VMP followed by R(d) or Rd ±X followed by R(X)(d) or R(X) or X as the very likely next most used regimens for countries with access to all drugs and able to prescribe continuous treatment. Nonetheless, so many questions lay upon us, still.

8 Future Perspectives

Future perspectives in the treatment of elderly patients with MM include improvement in treatment decision with geriatric assessment and optimization of tailored therapy, favouring all-oral regimens with progress in safety profile, and new families of drugs such as monoclonal antibodies.

8.1 Tailored Therapy

Tailored therapy in elderly patients should begin by a geriatric assessment; for instance using the new frailty score recently published which includes evaluation of age, disability and comorbidities [11]. The therapy decision based on frailty should help us propose the optimal therapy—the safer and most efficient regimen—for each category of patients with the help of specific end-points, dose adjustments and toxicity management recommendations.

Consensual options for first-line therapy now include VMP and the newcomer Rd, whereas the use of MPT should decline in the near future. It is not yet possible to officially recommend one regimen over another, although several patient- and disease-related characteristics may suggest one approach over the other. For instance, VMP does not lead to a risk of thrombosis but instead favours neuropathy. Rd is an all-oral regimen, compared to VMP that needs an hospital stay for the subcutaneous administration of bortezomib.

An important concern is also to try and improve the survival of the poor risk elderly MM patients who currently have a very short survival, and ideally overcome their adverse risk profile. Indeed, while we have a clear understanding of the adverse events of each therapy and thus know which patients we should avoid exposure to a particular treatment, little is known about efficient tailored therapy based on the risk profile, either good or poor. In the same vein, we also need to propose appropriate treatments options to patients with a very good risk MM, who could benefit from an intensive treatment and tend to a prolonged survival similar to that of matched age-related normal individuals.

8.2 Lenalidomide, a New Platform onto Which New Regimens Are Developed, Especially in the Elderly MM

Since the FIRST study reported the impressive results obtained with lenalidomide-low dose dexamethasone, a two-drug based regimen, one wondered about the efficacy of a three-drug regimen using Rd as a platform. This aspect has actually already been anticipated, and we should soon start to contemplate the results of the first phase 3 trials with Rd used as a platform for the studied arm, mostly in the context of triplet-based regimens, in the upfront setting.

Ongoing studies developed in this setting include:

- Rd + proteasome inhibitor bortezomib: SWOG-SO777, versus Rd
- Rd + proteasome inhibitor carfilzomib: ECOG E1A11, versus Bortezomib +Rd
- Rd + novel generation proteasome inhibitor: Tourmaline MM2: Ixazomib, versus Rd
- Rd + novel class of monoclonal antibodies, elotuzumab: Eloquent 1, versus Rd
- Rd + novel class of monoclonal antibodies, daratumumab: MAIA, versus Rd.

Other lenalidomide-based combinations have already been studied, such as lenalidomide-melphalan-prednisone (MPR), which despite a clear efficacy was proven too toxic in elderly patients [46]. Dose-adjusted cyclophosphamide-lenalidomide-dexamethasone (CRDa) is also under investigation by the UK group (MRC-XI), with promising results in terms of early response and toxicity [49].

If one of these Rd-based regimens is proven effective and is approved in first-line therapy for elderly MM patients, the choice of upfront therapy between Rd + X compared to VMP will still have to be clarified.

8.3   Monoclonal Antibodies

Monoclonal antibodies finally arrived in the therapeutic arsenal of MM, even if none was approved in MM so far. The recent very positive results with at least two of them represent a major step forward in the management of MM. Two targets are particularly promising: anti-CD38 (daratumumab and more recently SAR650984) and anti-CS1/SLAMF7 (elotuzumab).

Great hopes are based on these antibodies, in terms of their expected ability to strengthen the efficacy of current regimens and combinations, and also because they are known for their very good safety profiles in the short and long term. Interestingly, it is not expected for tumour cells to develop mechanisms of resistance to these agents, which makes them even more attractive. Finally, monoclonal antibodies will almost naturally combine to IMiDs (including thalidomide, lenalidomide and the last in line pomalidomide), the second most effective class of agents in MM, whom immunomodulatory effect should reinforce significantly the action of monoclonal antibodies towards tumour cells.

- CD38 is a transmembrane glycoprotein which plays a role in adhesion, signalling and intracellular calcium mobilization via enzymatic activity. It is overexpressed on the surface of malignant plasma cells in MM, making it an ideal therapeutic target. Daratumumab is a promising anti-CD38 monoclonal antibody which effectively mediates destruction of CD38-expressing malignant plasma cells. It was first tested as single agent in the GEN501 trial with remarkable tolerance but rather modest efficacy, with an overall response rate of 35 % a median PFS of 23 weeks [50]. In the GEN503 trial, daratumumab was tested in combination with lenalidomide and dexamethasone in relapsed or refractory MM (RRMM). Tolerance was excellent and efficacy was outstanding, as 75 % of patients obtained at least a very good partial response [51]. Daratumumab was also tested in combination with various platforms (VD, VMP, VTP, POM-D), which led to an overall response rate of 100 % for newly diagnosed MM patients, and 50 % in relapsed MM [52]. Moreover, the addition of Daratumumab was well tolerated in all evaluable patients and did not result in significant additional toxicity.

- SAR650984 is another anti-CD38 antibody whose association with lenalidomide and dexamethasone allowed an overall response rate of 64.5 % in heavily treated patients with RRMM, and a median PFS of 6.2 months [53]. This combination was well tolerated with impressive durable responses and warrants further evaluation.
- Elotuzumab is an anti-CS1/SLAMF7 antibody. The exact function of CS1 (also called SLAMF7) in MM cells is not completely understood; however, previous reports suggest that CS1 may be involved in cell adhesion (MM cells and bone marrow stromal cells), cell cycle regulation and other growth and survival pathways [54]. Targeting of SLAMF7 by elotuzumab on NK cells activate NK cells. As a single agent, Elotuzumab did not show any activity in MM despite plasma cell target saturation at the higher elotuzumab doses studied [55]. Encouraging response rates have been observed in combination with lenalidomide [56] in phase 1/2 trials, and in a much lesser extent with bortezomib [57]. Impressive response rate (92 %) and median PFS (not reached at a median follow-up of 20.8 months) have been described with elotuzumab at 10 mg/kg in combination with lenalidomide and low-dose dexamethasone in RRMM patients in a phase II trial [58]. Ongoing phase 3 trials are testing elotuzumab in combination with lenalidomide and low-dose dexamethasone both in the relapse (Eloquent 2) and the frontline setting (Eloquent 1 and 2).

Monoclonal antibodies thus seem very promising agents in MM therapy, and their very favourable safety profile makes them ideal candidates for elderly patients. Their exact place however remains to be determined, whether they should be used in addition to known regimens, and/or in consolidation or maintenance setting, as an add-on or even a backbone onto which to build upon.

8.4   Other Drugs

Other proteasome inhibitors (such as carfilzomib or ixazomib), IMIDs (pomalidomide), and novel families of drugs like HDAC inhibitors (panobinostat, vorinostat) or kinesin spindle inhibitors (Filanesib) are currently under investigation in the relapse setting, and for some of them in the upfront setting as well already, and could become valuable options in MM management in the future.

9   Conclusion

Management of elderly patients with MM remains challenging. The availability of novel agents such as thalidomide, lenalidomide and bortezomib has improved the treatment options and outcome of these patients, but has also taught us about the frailty of some of these elderly patients. For the first time achievement of CR was not necessarily followed by a prolonged survival, if the treatment was stopped in relation to drug toxicity profile. Out of the "battlefield" that drug development looks like in MM, the standards of care in first-line therapy of elderly MM patients are VMP, and Rd for the very near future.

Other combinations, including the second and third generation of novel classes and monoclonal antibodies, are under clinical development. Maintenance treatment with novel agents is emerging as a new strategy to sustain disease control and delay disease progression; however, the optimal maintenance regimen or molecule has yet to be determined, and longer follow-up is needed to assess the optimal duration and the OS benefit.

The optimal treatment strategy should allow a good efficacy but also a favourable safety profile, and quality of life needs to be taken into account especially in elderly patients. No data are available that assess screening for vulnerability before choosing and starting therapy for MM, but geriatric assessment should help to develop tailored therapies for these patients in the future.

10   Disclosures of Potential Conflicts of Interest

XL and TF have received honorarium from Janssen, Celgene, Takeda, Amgen, LeoPharma, Novartis, BMS, TEVA, Pierre Fabre

AP has received honorarium from Janssen, Celgene, Takeda, Amgen, Novartis, BMS,

SB has received honorarium from Janssen, Celgene, Mundifarma; AL has received honorarium from Janssen, Celgene, FG has received honorarium from Janssen, Celgene, Sanofi, Mundifarma

References

1. Fonseca R, Bergsagel PL, Drach J, Shaughnessy J, Gutierrez N, Stewart AK, Morgan G, Van Ness B, Chesi M, Minvielle S, Neri A, Barlogie B, Kuehl WM, Liebisch P, Davies F, Chen-Kiang S, Durie BG, Carrasco R, Sezer O, Reiman T, Pilarski L, Avet-Loiseau H, International Myeloma Working G (2009) International myeloma working group molecular classification of multiple myeloma: spotlight review. Leukemia: official journal of the Leukemia Society of America. Leuk Res Fund 23(12):2210–2221. doi:10.1038/leu.2009.174
2. SEER data,. US Population data (1969–2012) SEER Datasets [Internet]. [cited 2015 Jan 4]. http://seer.cancer.gov/data/citation.html
3. ONS. Office for National Statistics (ONS) [Internet]. Office for National Statistics (2010) [cited 2015 Jan 4]. http://www.ons.gov.uk/ons/index.html
4. Fried LP, Ferrucci L, Darer J, Williamson JD, Anderson G (2004) Untangling the concepts of disability, frailty, and comorbidity: implications for improved targeting and care. J Gerontol A Biol Sci Med Sci 59(3):255–263
5. Fried LP, Tangen CM, Walston J, Newman AB, Hirsch C, Gottdiener J, Seeman T, Tracy R, Kop WJ, Burke G, McBurnie MA, Cardiovascular Health Study Collaborative Research G (2001) Frailty in older adults: evidence for a phenotype. J Gerontol A Biol Sci Med Sci 56(3): M146–156
6. Charlson M, Szatrowski TP, Peterson J, Gold J (1994) Validation of a combined comorbidity index. J Clin Epidemiol 47(11):1245–1251

7. Walter LC, Brand RJ, Counsell SR, Palmer RM, Landefeld CS, Fortinsky RH, Covinsky KE (2001) Development and validation of a prognostic index for 1-year mortality in older adults after hospitalization. JAMA 285(23):2987–2994

8. Lee SJ, Lindquist K, Segal MR, Covinsky KE (2006) Development and validation of a prognostic index for 4-year mortality in older adults. JAMA 295(7):801–808. doi:10.1001/jama.295.7.801

9. Palumbo A, Bringhen S, Ludwig H, Dimopoulos MA, Blade J, Mateos MV, Rosinol L, Boccadoro M, Cavo M, Lokhorst H, Zweegman S, Terpos E, Davies F, Driessen C, Gimsing P, Gramatzki M, Hajek R, Johnsen HE, Leal Da Costa F, Sezer O, Spencer A, Beksac M, Morgan G, Einsele H, San Miguel JF, Sonneveld P (2011) Personalized therapy in multiple myeloma according to patient age and vulnerability: a report of the European Myeloma Network (EMN). Blood 118(17):4519–4529. doi:10.1182/blood-2011-06-358812

10. Fried LP, Guralnik JM (1997) Disability in older adults: evidence regarding significance, etiology, and risk. J Am Geriatr Soc 45(1):92–100

11. Palumbo A, Bringhen S, Mateos MV, Larocca A, Facon T, Kumar SK, Offidani M, McCarthy P, Evangelista A, Lonial S, Zweegman S, Musto P, Terpos E, Belch A, Hajek R, Ludwig H, Stewart AK, Moreau P, Anderson K, Einsele H, Durie BG, Dimopoulos MA, Landgren O, San Miguel JF, Richardson P, Sonneveld P, Rajkumar SV (2015) Geriatric assessment predicts survival and toxicities in elderly myeloma patients: an International Myeloma Working Group report. Blood 125(13):2068–2074. doi:10.1182/blood-2014-12-615187

12. Avet-Loiseau H, Hulin C, Campion L, Rodon P, Marit G, Attal M, Royer B, Dib M, Voillat L, Bouscary D, Caillot D, Wetterwald M, Pegourie B, Lepeu G, Corront B, Karlin L, Stoppa AM, Fuzibet JG, Delbrel X, Guilhot F, Kolb B, Decaux O, Lamy T, Garderet L, Allangba O, Lifermann F, Anglaret B, Moreau P, Harousseau JL, Facon T (2013) Chromosomal abnormalities are major prognostic factors in elderly patients with multiple myeloma: the intergroupe francophone du myelome experience. J Clin Oncol Official J Am Soc Clin Oncol 31(22):2806–2809. doi:10.1200/jco.2012.46.2598

13. Hideshima T, Richardson PG, Anderson KC (2011) Mechanism of action of proteasome inhibitors and deacetylase inhibitors and the biological basis of synergy in multiple myeloma. Mol Cancer Ther 10(11):2034–2042. doi:10.1158/1535-7163.mct-11-0433

14. Gay F, Larocca A, Wijermans P, Cavallo F, Rossi D, Schaafsma R, Genuardi M, Romano A, Liberati AM, Siniscalchi A, Petrucci MT, Nozzoli C, Patriarca F, Offidani M, Ria R, Omede P, Bruno B, Passera R, Musto P, Boccadoro M, Sonneveld P, Palumbo A (2011) Complete response correlates with long-term progression-free and overall survival in elderly myeloma treated with novel agents: analysis of 1175 patients. Blood 117(11):3025–3031. doi:10.1182/blood-2010-09-307645

15. Paiva B, Martinez-Lopez J, Vidriales MB, Mateos MV, Montalban MA, Fernandez-Redondo E, Alonso L, Oriol A, Teruel AI, de Paz R, Larana JG, Bengoechea E, Martin A, Mediavilla JD, Palomera L, de Arriba F, Blade J, Orfao A, Lahuerta JJ, San Miguel JF (2011) Comparison of immunofixation, serum free light chain, and immunophenotyping for response evaluation and prognostication in multiple myeloma. J Clin Oncol Official J Am Soc Clin Oncol 29(12):1627–1633. doi:10.1200/jco.2010.33.1967

16. Sonneveld P, Verelst SG, Lewis P, Gray-Schopfer V, Hutchings A, Nixon A, Petrucci MT (2013) Review of health-related quality of life data in multiple myeloma patients treated with novel agents. Leukemia: official journal of the Leukemia Society of America. Leuk Res Fund 27(10):1959–1969. doi:10.1038/leu.2013.185

17. San Miguel JF, Schlag R, Khuageva NK, Dimopoulos MA, Shpilberg O, Kropff M, Spicka I, Petrucci MT, Palumbo A, Samoilova OS, Dmoszynska A, Abdulkadyrov KM, Schots R, Jiang B, Mateos MV, Anderson KC, Esseltine DL, Liu K, Cakana A, van de Velde H, Richardson PG, Investigators VT (2008) Bortezomib plus melphalan and prednisone for initial treatment of multiple myeloma. New Engl J Med 359(9):906–917. doi:10.1056/NEJMoa0801479

18. Alexanian R, Bergsagel DE, Migliore PJ, Vaughn WK, Howe CD (1968) Melphalan therapy for plasma cell myeloma. Blood 31(1):1–10

19. Cavo M, Benni M, Ronconi S, Fiacchini M, Gozzetti A, Zamagni E, Cellini C, Tosi P, Baccarani M, Tura S, Writing Committee of the "Bologna 90" Clinical T (2002) Melphalan-prednisone versus alternating combination VAD/MP or VND/MP as primary therapy for multiple myeloma: final analysis of a randomized clinical study. Haematologica 87 (9):934–942

20. Ludwig H, Miguel JS, Dimopoulos MA, Palumbo A, Garcia Sanz R, Powles R, Lentzsch S, Ming Chen W, Hou J, Jurczyszyn A, Romeril K, Hajek R, Terpos E, Shimizu K, Joshua D, Hungria V, Rodriguez Morales A, Ben-Yehuda D, Sondergeld P, Zamagni E, Durie B (2014) International Myeloma Working Group recommendations for global myeloma care. Leukemia: official journal of the Leukemia Society of America. Leuk Res Fund 28(5):981–992. doi:10. 1038/leu.2013.293

21. Ludwig H, Hajek R, Tothova E, Drach J, Adam Z, Labar B, Egyed M, Spicka I, Gisslinger H, Greil R, Kuhn I, Zojer N, Hinke A (2009) Thalidomide-dexamethasone compared with melphalan-prednisolone in elderly patients with multiple myeloma. Blood 113(15):3435–3442. doi:10.1182/blood-2008-07-169565

22. Hulin C, Facon T, Rodon P, Pegourie B, Benboubker L, Doyen C, Dib M, Guillerm G, Salles B, Eschard JP, Lenain P, Casassus P, Azais I, Decaux O, Garderet L, Mathiot C, Fontan J, Lafon I, Virion JM, Moreau P (2009) Efficacy of melphalan and prednisone plus thalidomide in patients older than 75 years with newly diagnosed multiple myeloma: IFM 01/01 trial. J Clin Oncol Official J Am Soc Clin Oncol 27(22):3664–3670. doi:10.1200/jco. 2008.21.0948

23. Fayers PM, Palumbo A, Hulin C, Waage A, Wijermans P, Beksac M, Bringhen S, Mary JY, Gimsing P, Termorshuizen F, Haznedar R, Caravita T, Moreau P, Turesson I, Musto P, Benboubker L, Schaafsma M, Sonneveld P, Facon T, Nordic Myeloma Study G, Italian Multiple Myeloma N, Turkish Myeloma Study G, Hemato-Oncologie voor Volwassenen N, Intergroupe Francophone du M, European Myeloma N (2011) Thalidomide for previously untreated elderly patients with multiple myeloma: meta-analysis of 1685 individual patient data from 6 randomized clinical trials. Blood 118(5):1239–1247. doi:10.1182/blood-2011-03-341669

24. Facon T, Mary JY, Hulin C, Benboubker L, Attal M, Pegourie B, Renaud M, Harousseau JL, Guillerm G, Chaleteix C, Dib M, Voillat L, Maisonneuve H, Troncy J, Dorvaux V, Monconduit M, Martin C, Casassus P, Jaubert J, Jardel H, Doyen C, Kolb B, Anglaret B, Grosbois B, Yakoub-Agha I, Mathiot C, Avet-Loiseau H (2007) Melphalan and prednisone plus thalidomide versus melphalan and prednisone alone or reduced-intensity autologous stem cell transplantation in elderly patients with multiple myeloma (IFM 99-06): a randomised trial. Lancet 370(9594):1209–1218. doi:S0140-6736(07)61537-2 [pii] 10.1016/S0140-6736(07) 61537-2

25. Palumbo A, Bringhen S, Liberati AM, Caravita T, Falcone A, Callea V, Montanaro M, Ria R, Capaldi A, Zambello R, Benevolo G, Derudas D, Dore F, Cavallo F, Gay F, Falco P, Ciccone G, Musto P, Cavo M, Boccadoro M (2008) Oral melphalan, prednisone, and thalidomide in elderly patients with multiple myeloma: updated results of a randomized controlled trial. Blood 112(8):3107–3114. doi:10.1182/blood-2008-04-149427

26. Morgan GJ, Davies FE, Gregory WM, Russell NH, Bell SE, Szubert AJ, Navarro Coy N, Cook G, Feyler S, Byrne JL, Roddie H, Rudin C, Drayson MT, Owen RG, Ross FM, Jackson GH, Child JA, Group NHOS (2011) Cyclophosphamide, thalidomide, and dexamethasone (CTD) as initial therapy for patients with multiple myeloma unsuitable for autologous transplantation. Blood 118(5):1231–1238. doi:10.1182/blood-2011-02-338665

27. Morgan GJ, Davies FE, Gregory WM, Bell SE, Szubert AJ, Cook G, Drayson MT, Owen RG, Ross FM, Jackson GH, Child JA (2013) Long-term follow-up of MRC Myeloma IX trial: Survival outcomes with bisphosphonate and thalidomide treatment. Clin Cancer Res Official J Am Associa Cancer Res 19(21):6030–6038. doi:10.1158/1078-0432.ccr-12-3211

28. San Miguel JF, Schlag R, Khuageva NK, Dimopoulos MA, Shpilberg O, Kropff M, Spicka I, Petrucci MT, Palumbo A, Samoilova OS, Dmoszynska A, Abdulkadyrov KM, Delforge M, Jiang B, Mateos MV, Anderson KC, Esseltine DL, Liu K, Deraedt W, Cakana A, van de Velde H, Richardson PG (2013) Persistent overall survival benefit and no increased risk of second malignancies with bortezomib-melphalan-prednisone versus melphalan-prednisone in patients with previously untreated multiple myeloma. J Clin Oncol Official J Am Soc Clin Oncol 31(4):448–455. doi:10.1200/jco.2012.41.6180
29. San-Miguel JF, Richardson PG, Sonneveld P, Schuster MW, Irwin D, Stadtmauer EA, Facon T, Harousseau JL, Ben-Yehuda D, Lonial S, Goldschmidt H, Reece D, Blade J, Boccadoro M, Cavenagh JD, Neuwirth R, Boral AL, Esseltine DL, Anderson KC (2008) Efficacy and safety of bortezomib in patients with renal impairment: results from the APEX phase 3 study. Leukemia: official journal of the Leukemia Society of America. Leuk Res Fund 22(4):842–849. doi:10.1038/sj.leu.2405087
30. Mateos MV, Oriol A, Martinez-Lopez J, Gutierrez N, Teruel AI, Lopez de la Guia A, Lopez J, Bengoechea E, Perez M, Polo M, Palomera L, de Arriba F, Gonzalez Y, Hernandez JM, Granell M, Bello JL, Bargay J, Penalver FJ, Ribera JM, Martin-Mateos ML, Garcia-Sanz R, Lahuerta JJ, Blade J, San-Miguel JF (2012) Maintenance therapy with bortezomib plus thalidomide or bortezomib plus prednisone in elderly multiple myeloma patients included in the GEM2005MAS65 trial. Blood 120(13):2581–2588. doi:10.1182/blood-2012-05-427815
31. Palumbo A, Bringhen S, Larocca A, Rossi D, Di Raimondo F, Magarotto V, Patriarca F, Levi A, Benevolo G, Vincelli ID, Grasso M, Franceschini L, Gottardi D, Zambello R, Montefusco V, Falcone AP, Omede P, Marasca R, Morabito F, Mina R, Guglielmelli T, Nozzoli C, Passera R, Gaidano G, Offidani M, Ria R, Petrucci MT, Musto P, Boccadoro M, Cavo M (2014) Bortezomib-melphalan-prednisone-thalidomide followed by maintenance with bortezomib-thalidomide compared with bortezomib-melphalan-prednisone for initial treatment of multiple myeloma: updated follow-up and improved survival. J Clin Oncol Official J Am Soc Clin Oncol 32(7):634–640. doi:10.1200/jco.2013.52.0023
32. Palumbo A, Bringhen S, Rossi D, Cavalli M, Larocca A, Ria R, Offidani M, Patriarca F, Nozzoli C, Guglielmelli T, Benevolo G, Callea V, Baldini L, Morabito F, Grasso M, Leonardi G, Rizzo M, Falcone AP, Gottardi D, Montefusco V, Musto P, Petrucci MT, Ciccone G, Boccadoro M (2010) Bortezomib-melphalan-prednisone-thalidomide followed by maintenance with bortezomib-thalidomide compared with bortezomib-melphalan-prednisone for initial treatment of multiple myeloma: a randomized controlled trial. J Clin Oncol Official J Am Soc Clin Oncol 28(34):5101–5109. doi:10.1200/jco.2010.29.8216
33. Mateos MV, Oriol A, Martinez-Lopez J, Gutierrez N, Teruel AI, de Paz R, Garcia-Larana J, Bengoechea E, Martin A, Mediavilla JD, Palomera L, de Arriba F, Gonzalez Y, Hernandez JM, Sureda A, Bello JL, Bargay J, Penalver FJ, Ribera JM, Martin-Mateos ML, Garcia-Sanz R, Cibeira MT, Ramos ML, Vidriales MB, Paiva B, Montalban MA, Lahuerta JJ, Blade J, Miguel JF (2010) Bortezomib, melphalan, and prednisone versus bortezomib, thalidomide, and prednisone as induction therapy followed by maintenance treatment with bortezomib and thalidomide versus bortezomib and prednisone in elderly patients with untreated multiple myeloma: a randomised trial. Lancet Oncol 11(10):934–941. doi:10.1016/s1470-2045(10)70187-x
34. Moreau P, Pylypenko H, Grosicki S, Karamanesht I, Leleu X, Grishunina M, Rekhtman G, Masliak Z, Robak T, Shubina A, Arnulf B, Kropff M, Cavet J, Esseltine DL, Feng H, Girgis S, van de Velde H, Deraedt W, Harousseau JL (2011) Subcutaneous versus intravenous administration of bortezomib in patients with relapsed multiple myeloma: a randomised, phase 3, non-inferiority study. Lancet Oncol 12(5):431–440. doi:10.1016/s1470-2045(11)70081-x
35. Richardson PG, Sonneveld P, Schuster M, Irwin D, Stadtmauer E, Facon T, Harousseau JL, Ben-Yehuda D, Lonial S, Goldschmidt H, Reece D, Miguel JS, Blade J, Boccadoro M, Cavenagh J, Alsina M, Rajkumar SV, Lacy M, Jakubowiak A, Dalton W, Boral A, Esseltine DL, Schenkein D, Anderson KC (2007) Extended follow-up of a phase 3 trial in

relapsed multiple myeloma: final time-to-event results of the APEX trial. Blood 110 (10):3557–3560. doi:10.1182/blood-2006-08-036947

36. Mateos MV, Richardson PG, Dimopoulos MA, Palumbo A, Anderson KC, Shi H, Elliott J, Dow E, van de Velde H, Niculescu L, San Miguel JF (2015) Effect of cumulative bortezomib dose on survival in multiple myeloma patients receiving bortezomib-melphalan-prednisone in the phase III VISTA study. Am J Hematol 90(4):314–319. doi:10.1002/ajh.23933

37. Ponisch W, Mitrou PS, Merkle K, Herold M, Assmann M, Wilhelm G, Dachselt K, Richter P, Schirmer V, Schulze A, Subert R, Harksel B, Grobe N, Stelzer E, Schulze M, Bittrich A, Freund M, Pasold R, Friedrich T, Helbig W, Niederwieser D, East German Study Group of H, Oncology (2006) Treatment of bendamustine and prednisone in patients with newly diagnosed multiple myeloma results in superior complete response rate, prolonged time to treatment failure and improved quality of life compared to treatment with melphalan and prednisone–a randomized phase III study of the East German Study Group of Hematology and Oncology (OSHO). J Cancer Res Clin Oncol 132(4):205–212. doi:10.1007/s00432-005-0074-4

38. Siegel DS, Desikan KR, Mehta J, Singhal S, Fassas A, Munshi N, Anaissie E, Naucke S, Ayers D, Spoon D, Vesole D, Tricot G, Barlogie B (1999) Age is not a prognostic variable with autotransplants for multiple myeloma. Blood 93(1):51–54

39. Gertz MA, Dingli D (2014) How we manage autologous stem cell transplantation for patients with multiple myeloma. Blood 124(6):882–890. doi:10.1182/blood-2014-03-544759

40. Badros A, Barlogie B, Siegel E, Morris C, Desikan R, Zangari M, Fassas A, Anaissie E, Munshi N, Tricot G (2001) Autologous stem cell transplantation in elderly multiple myeloma patients over the age of 70 years. Br J Haematol 114(3):600–607

41. Palumbo A, Bringhen S, Petrucci MT, Musto P, Rossini F, Nunzi M, Lauta VM, Bergonzi C, Barbui A, Caravita T, Capaldi A, Pregno P, Guglielmelli T, Grasso M, Callea V, Bertola A, Cavallo F, Falco P, Rus C, Massaia M, Mandelli F, Carella AM, Pogliani E, Liberati AM, Dammacco F, Ciccone G, Boccadoro M (2004) Intermediate-dose melphalan improves survival of myeloma patients aged 50 to 70: results of a randomized controlled trial. Blood 104 (10):3052–3057. doi:10.1182/blood-2004-02-0408

42. Gay F, Magarotto V, Crippa C, Pescosta N, Guglielmelli T, Cavallo F, Pezzatti S, Ferrari S, Liberati AM, Oliva S, Patriarca F, Offidani M, Omede P, Montefusco V, Petrucci MT, Giuliani N, Passera R, Pietrantuono G, Boccadoro M, Corradini P, Palumbo A (2013) Bortezomib induction, reduced-intensity transplantation, and lenalidomide consolidation-maintenance for myeloma: updated results. Blood 122(8):1376–1383. doi:10.1182/blood-2013-02-483073

43. Jacobus S, Callander NS, Siegel D, Abonour R, David P, Fonseca R et al (2010) Outcome of elderly patients 70 years and older with newly diagnosed myeloma in the ECOG randomized trial of lenalidomide/high-dose dexamethasone (RD versus lenalidomide/low-dose dexamethasone (RD). (abs.0370). Haematologica 95(s2):149

44. Benboubker L, Dimopoulos MA, Dispenzieri A, Catalano J, Belch AR, Cavo M, Pinto A, Weisel K, Ludwig H, Bahlis N, Banos A, Tiab M, Delforge M, Cavenagh J, Geraldes C, Lee JJ, Chen C, Oriol A, de la Rubia J, Qiu L, White DJ, Binder D, Anderson K, Fermand JP, Moreau P, Attal M, Knight R, Chen G, Van Oostendorp J, Jacques C, Ervin-Haynes A, Avet-Loiseau H, Hulin C, Facon T, Team FT (2014) Lenalidomide and dexamethasone in transplant-ineligible patients with myeloma. New Engl J Med 371(10):906–917. doi:10.1056/NEJMoa1402551

45. Bahlis NJ, Corso A, Mugge L, Shen Z, Desjardins P, Stoppa A, Decaux O, De Revel T, Granell M, Marit G, Nahi H, Demuynck H, Huang S, Basu S, Guthrie TH, Ervin-Haynes A, Leupin N, Marek J, Chen G, Facon T (2014) Impact of response quality on survival outcomes in transplant-ineligible newly diagnosed multiple myeloma (NDMM) patients (Pts): results from the first trial. Blood (ASH Annual Meeting Abstract) Abstract 3458

46. Falco P, Cavallo F, Larocca A, Rossi D, Guglielmelli T, Rocci A, Grasso M, Siez ML, De Paoli L, Oliva S, Molica S, Mina R, Gay F, Benevolo G, Musto P, Omede P, Freilone R, Bringhen S, Carella AM, Gaidano G, Boccadoro M, Palumbo A (2013) Lenalidomide-prednisone induction followed by lenalidomide-melphalan-prednisone consolidation and lenalidomide-prednisone maintenance in newly diagnosed elderly unfit myeloma patients. Leukemia: official journal of the Leukemia Society of America. Leuk Res Fund 27(3):695–701. doi:10.1038/leu.2012.271

47. Palumbo A, Hajek R, Delforge M, Kropff M, Petrucci MT, Catalano J, Gisslinger H, Wiktor-Jedrzejczak W, Zodelava M, Weisel K, Cascavilla N, Iosava G, Cavo M, Kloczko J, Blade J, Beksac M, Spicka I, Plesner T, Radke J, Langer C, Ben Yehuda D, Corso A, Herbein L, Yu Z, Mei J, Jacques C, Dimopoulos MA, Investigators MM (2012) Continuous lenalidomide treatment for newly diagnosed multiple myeloma. New Engl J Med 366 (19):1759–1769. doi:10.1056/NEJMoa1112704

48. Mateos M, Martinez-Lopez J, Hernandez M, Martinez R, Rosiñol L, Ocio EM, Echeveste MA, Pérez de Oteyza J, Oriol A, Bargay J, Gironella M, Martín J, Cabrera C, De La Rubia J, Gutiérrez NC, Martin M, Paiva B, Montalbán MA, Bladé J, Lahuerta JJ, San Miguel JF (2014) Comparison of sequential vs alternating administration of bortezomib, melphalan, prednisone (VMP) and lenalidomide plus dexamethasone (Rd) in elderly pts with newly diagnosed multiple myeloma (MM) patients: GEM2010MAS65 trial. Blood (ASH Annual Meeting Abstract) Abstract 178

49. Pawlyn C, Brioli A, Gregory W, Hinsley S, Lindsay J, Cook G, Milligan D, Chapman C, Owen RG, Drayson MT, Russell N, Jackson GH, Davies FE, Morgan GJ (2014) Lenalidomide combined with cyclophosphamide and dexamethasone is effective and well tolerated induction treatment for newly diagnosed myeloma patients of all ages. Blood (ASH Annual Meeting Abstracts) Abstract 540

50. Lokhorst HM, Plesner T, Gimsing P, Nahi H, Lisby S, Richardson P (2013) Daratumumab, a CD38 monoclonal antibody study in advanced multiple myeloma—An open-label, dose escalation followed by open-label extension in a single-arm Phase I/II study. Proc EHA 2013 Abstract S576

51. Plesner T, Arkenau H, Lokhorst HM, Gimsing P, Krejcik J, Lemech C, Minnema MC, Lassen U, Laubach JP, Ahmadi T, Yeh H, Guckert ME, Feng H, Brun NC, Lisby S, Basse L, Palumbo A, Richardson PG (2014) Safety and Efficacy of Daratumumab with Lenalidomide and Dexamethasone in relapsed or relapsed, refractory multiple myeloma. Blood (ASH Annual Meeting Abstract) Abstract 84

52. Moreau P, Mateos M, Bladé J, Benboubker L, de la Rubia J, Facon T, Comenzo RL, Fay JW, Qin X, Masterson T, Schecter J, Ahmadi T, San Miguel J (2014) An open-label, multicenter, phase 1b study of daratumumab in combination with backbone regimens in patients with multiple myeloma. Blood (ASH Annual Meeting Abstract) Abstract 176

53. Martin TG, Baz R, Benson Jr. DM, Lendvai N, Campana F, Charpentier E, Vij R (2014) A phase Ib dose escalation trial of SAR650984 (Anti-CD-38 mAb) in combination with lenalidomide and dexamethasone in relapsed/refractory multiple myeloma. Blood (ASH Annual Meeting Abstracts) Abstract 83

54. Moreau P, Touzeau C (2014) Elotuzumab for the treatment of multiple myeloma. Future Oncol (London, England) 10(6):949–956. doi:10.2217/fon.14.56

55. Zonder JA, Mohrbacher AF, Singhal S, van Rhee F, Bensinger WI, Ding H, Fry J, Afar DE, Singhal AK (2012) A phase 1, multicenter, open-label, dose escalation study of elotuzumab in patients with advanced multiple myeloma. Blood 120(3):552–559. doi:10.1182/blood-2011-06-360552

56. Lonial S, Vij R, Harousseau JL, Facon T, Moreau P, Mazumder A, Kaufman JL, Leleu X, Tsao LC, Westland C, Singhal AK, Jagannath S (2012) Elotuzumab in combination with lenalidomide and low-dose dexamethasone in relapsed or refractory multiple myeloma. J Clin Oncol Official J Am Soc Clin Oncol 30(16):1953–1959. doi:10.1200/jco.2011.37.2649

57. Jakubowiak AJ, Benson DM, Bensinger W, Siegel DS, Zimmerman TM, Mohrbacher A, Richardson PG, Afar DE, Singhal AK, Anderson KC (2012) Phase I trial of anti-CS1 monoclonal antibody elotuzumab in combination with bortezomib in the treatment of relapsed/refractory multiple myeloma. J Clin Oncol Official J Am Soc Clin Oncol 30 (16):1960–1965. doi:10.1200/jco.2011.37.7069
58. Lonial S, Jagannath S, Moreau P, Jakubowiak AJ, Raab MS, Facon T, Vij R, Bleickardt E, Reece DE, Benboubker L, Zonder JA, Deng W, Singhal AK, Richardson PG (2013) Phase (Ph) I/II study of elotuzumab (Elo) plus lenalidomide/dexamethasone (Len/dex) in relapsed/refractory multiple myeloma (RRMM), updated Ph II results and Ph I/II long-term safety. J Clin Oncol 31(Suppl.), Abstract 8542 (2013)

Management of Transplant-Eligible Patients with Newly Diagnosed Multiple Myeloma

Jacob Laubach and Shaji Kumar

Abstract

Treatment approaches for newly diagnosed myeloma have changed considerably during the past decade, along with a better understanding of the disease heterogeneity. Availability of new drug classes such as proteasome inhibitors and immunomodulatory drugs, and use of these drugs in combinations have led to higher response rates and deeper responses in the vast majority of patients with newly diagnosed myeloma. In addition to improved efficacy, these regimens are tolerated better than those with conventional chemotherapy drugs, which have reduced the early mortality seen in MM, while allowing for successful stem cell collection in patients undergoing stem cell transplant consolidation. Ongoing clinical trials with newer drugs such as monoclonal antibodies are being explored as options for newly diagnosed MM. The optimal regimen continues to evolve and is often dictated by the intent to transplant, age and comorbidities. Despite the increasing response rates seen with the new regimens, autologous stem cell transplantation remains an effective modality for consolidation, further deepening the responses seen with the initial therapy. Post-transplant approaches have further added to the efficacy of this platform with both post-transplant consolidation and maintenance demonstrating value in clinical trials. Currently, the combination of an effective initial therapy followed by one or two autologous stem cell transplants, with or without consolidation followed by maintenance appear to provide the maximum benefit in terms of duration of disease control for patients with newly diagnosed MM.

J. Laubach (✉)
Dana-Farber Cancer Institute, Boston, MA, USA
e-mail: jacobp_laubach@dfci.harvard.edu

S. Kumar (✉)
Mayo Clinic, Rochester, MN, USA
e-mail: Kumar.Shaji@mayo.edu

© Springer International Publishing Switzerland 2016
A.M. Roccaro and I.M. Ghobrial (eds.), *Plasma Cell Dyscrasias*,
Cancer Treatment and Research 169, DOI 10.1007/978-3-319-40320-5_9

145

Keywords
Multiple myeloma · Risk stratification · Immunomodulatory drugs · Proteasome
inhibitors · Stem cell transplantation

1 Introduction

Multiple myeloma (MM) management has evolved rapidly in recent years due to
the availability of new, more effective, chemotherapeutic agents and drug combinations for this disease, and as a result of these developments patient outcomes have
improved considerably. In spite of significant progress in the field, however, MM
remains incurable and most patients ultimately succumb to the disease. This
highlights the need for ongoing efforts in drug development and optimization of
clinical management at each phase of the disease, from the time of diagnosis to first
and subsequent relapses. The management of newly diagnosed disease is particularly important in this respect, as this phase in the disease typically represents the
point in which the deepest and most durable response to therapy can be achieved.

2 Diagnosis and Risk Assessment

The diagnosis of multiple myeloma is based on clinical, laboratory, bone marrow,
and radiographic findings that establish the presence of a clonal population of
plasma cells in the bone marrow and/or extramedullary sites and characterize the
burden of disease. Decisions regarding therapy are predicated on the presence of
symptoms and/or organ dysfunction (hypercalcemia, renal impairment, anemia, and
bone lesions). Patients with monoclonal gammopathy of undetermined significance
(MGUS) or smoldering multiple myeloma (SMM) have traditionally been observed
without systemic chemotherapy.

Risk assessment is a critical aspect of the diagnostic evaluation as it informs
prognostication and influences treatment decisions. Chromosomal analysis using
metaphase cytogenetics and fluorescence in situ hybridization (FISH) [1] and the
International staging system stage [2] are at present the most important determinants of prognosis. Chromosomal abnormalities t(4;14), t(14;16), t(14;20), del17p,
gain (1q), and del(1p) have been associated with high-risk disease, as has ISS stages
II and III [3, 4]. Other factors associated with high risk include plasma cell leukemia, plasmablastic myeloma, renal failure, and extramedullary disease. Gene
expression profiling (GEP), where available, is useful in risk assessment as well [5,
6].

3 General Approach to Newly Diagnosed MM in Transplant-Eligible Patients

Systemic therapy is initiated with the intent of reducing tumor burden to a minimal state and preserving organ function while minimizing toxicities associated with chemotherapy. Induction regimens typically incorporate two to four agents with distinct and synergistic mechanisms of anti-myeloma activity. Chemotherapy is preceded in certain situations such as pathologic fracture of a long bone or spinal plasmacytoma by surgical intervention or radiation therapy.

Induction therapy is typically administered over a 3–5 month period prior to stem cell mobilization and harvest. Following stem cell collection, the patient can proceed with consolidation with high-dose therapy and autologous stem cell transplantation (ASCT) or, alternatively, store stem cells, and defer transplant until a later point. Patients who opt against immediate ASCT typically resume induction therapy to complete 6–8 months of induction therapy in total, at which point the patient can proceed with maintenance therapy until disease progression or be observed without systemic therapy until time of disease progression.

4 Treatment Options for NDMM in Transplant-Eligible Patients

4.1 Two-Drug Regimens

4.1.1 Thalidomide-Dexamethasone

Thalidomide (thal) has been largely supplanted in the United States by the second generation Immunomodulatory Drug (IMiD) lenalidomide (len) in newly diagnosed MM due to lenalidomide's greater potency and more favorable side effect profile. However, thalidomide remains an important option for management of newly diagnosed patients in regions of the world where lenalidomide is not available for frontline therapy.

Thalidomide-dexamethasone (thal-dex) was evaluated in a randomized, phase III trial comparing this combination to dexamethasone alone [7]. Thal was given continuously and dose escalated from 50 to 100 mg in cycle 1 and to 200 mg at cycle 2 and beyond, while dex was given in both arms at 40 mg in 4-day pulses days 1–4, 9–12, and 17–20 of each 28 day cycle. Thal-dex was associated with superior overall response rate (ORR = partial response or better) (63 vs. 46 %) and time to progression (TTP) (22.6 vs. 6.5 months). Grade 3/4 toxicities were more common with the combination, and included deep venous vein thrombosis (DVT) (11.5 vs. 1.7 %), pulmonary embolism (6.8 vs. 1.7 %), and peripheral neuropathy (3.4 vs. 0 %). With appropriate supportive care, including anticoagulation and dose reduction for neuropathy, the thalidomide-dexamethasone regimen can, as noted previously, be considered a suitable regimen for upfront therapy in regions where lenalidomide is not available.

4.1.2 Lenalidomide-Dexamethasone

Lenalidomide-dexamethasone (len-dex) is an effective and well-tolerated regimen for newly diagnosed MM. In a phase II trial involving 34 patients who received len 25 mg daily on days 1–21 of a 28 day cycle plus dex 40 mg on days 1–4, 9–12, and 17–20, the ORR among evaluable patients was 91 %, the 2-year time to progression (TTP) 71 %, and 2-year TTP among patients who proceeded to transplant following len-dex induction was 83 %. Stem cell collection was adequate in all patients who underwent stem cell harvest, with a median CD34 cell count of 7.9×10^6. Grade 3/4 toxicities included fatigue, neutropenia, and pneumonitis.

A subsequent, randomized phase III trial compared len plus high-dose dex (len-Dex) (40 mg given in 4 day pulses over 28 day cycle) to len-low-dose dex (len-dex) (40 mg once weekly). The primary endpoint was response rate after four cycles. Although the ORR was superior in the high-dose dexamethasone group (81 vs. 70 %), overall survival (OS) was superior in the low-dose dex arm (96 vs. 87 %) owing to a lower incidence of high-grade toxicities as well as deaths on therapy in the group who received low-dose dex.

The rate of peripheral neuropathy associated with len is low, making the agent an attractive option for patients with significant preexisting neuropathy. Aspirin is administered in conjunction with len to decrease the incidence of therapy-associated venous thromboembolic events (VTE), while anticoagulation is recommended for individuals who are at high risk for or have a prior history of DVT/VTE. Prolonged exposure to len prior to stem cell mobilization is not advised, as this can impair stem cell collection [8, 9]. Rash related to len is relatively common but typically is mild and responds to brief interruption of therapy and use of supportive measures such as topical corticosteroid and antihistamine [10].

4.1.3 Bortezomib-Dexamethasone

The efficacy of bortezomib (bortez) plus dex was demonstrated in a randomized phase III study comparing it to what had previously been a standard of care for induction therapy in transplant-eligible patients with newly diagnosed MM, vincristine plus doxorubicin and dexamethasone (VAD) [11]. Bortez-dex was superior to VAD with respect to post-induction ORR (78.5 vs. 62.8 %), very good partial response (VGPR) or better (37.7 vs. 15.1 %), and complete response (CR) plus near CR (nCR) (14.8 vs. 6.4 %). Of note, a higher rate and depth of response was observed with bortez-dex in high-risk subgroups, including patients with ISS 2 or 3 disease, where there was a higher rate of VGPR or better as well as CR/nCR, and patients with high-risk cytogenetics (either t(4;14) or del17p), where there was a higher rate of VGPR or better.

The well-known neurotoxicity of bortez is dose dependent and typically affects long, thinly myelinated sensory nerves, although motor and autonomic neuropathy can occur as well. Herpes zoster reactivation is also a known complication of bortez, and antiviral prophylaxis is strongly recommended for patients receiving the agent. Thrombocytopenia occurs frequently in association with bortez, is cyclical and thus predictable, and typically resolves prior to a subsequent cycle of therapy.

It is feasible to administer subcutaneous (SC) rather than intravenous (IV) bortez in combination with dex as induction therapy based on data from a phase III clinical trial comparing the two formulations in the setting of relapsed MM that showed non-inferior efficacy and a more favorable toxicity profile associated with SC bortez [12].

4.2 Three- and Four-Drug Regimens

The rationale for regimens that incorporate three or more agents derives from preclinical studies demonstrating synergy between the various drug classes employed in the treatment of MM, namely the IMiDs, proteasome inhibitors, alkylating agents, and anthracylines [13]. Clinical trial experience suggests such regimens improve the overall rate of response as well as depth of response to therapy. However, the improvement in response associated with these regimens may come with the cost of greater toxicity, a factor that likewise influences decisions regarding therapy for NDMM.

4.2.1 Cyclophosphamide-Bortezomib-Dexamethasone

Cyclophosphamide-bortezomib-dexamethasone (cy-bortez-dex) is an active, well tolerated, and widely used regimen for induction therapy for patients with newly diagnosed MM. In a phase II study, 33 patients with NDMM received oral cy 300 mg/m^2 days 1, 8, and 15; IV bortez 1.3 mg/m^2 days 1, 4, 8, and 11; and dex 40 mg days 1–4, 9–12, and 17–20 in a 28 day cycle [14]. The rate of PR or better was 88 %, VGPR or better 61 %, and CR/nCR 39 %. Responses were rapid, evidenced by a mean 80 % decline in M-protein concentration after two cycles of therapy. Stem cell collection was successful in all patients who proceeded with stem cell harvest following induction. Grade 3/4 toxicies included thrombocytopenia (25 %), neutropenia (13 %), anemia (12 %), thrombosis (7 %), and neuropathy (7 %).

The randomized, phase II EVOLUTION trial compared cy-bortez-dex to len-bortez-dex and cy-len-bortez-dex. Patients in the cy-bortez-dex arm received cy 500 mg/m^2 days 1 and 8; IV bortez 1.3 mg/m^2 days 1, 4, 8, and 11; and dex 40 mg days 1, 8, and 15 in a 21 day cycle during induction. The schedule was modified during the study to add an additional dose of cy on day 15. In the original cohort of 33 patients, the ORR of PR or better across all cycles was 75 %, rate of VGPR or better 41 %, and CR rate 22 %. Among the 17 patients who received cy-bortez-dex on modified schedule, the ORR across all cycles was 100 %, rate of VGPR or better 53 %, and CR rate 47 %. The rate of grade 3/4 neutropenia was 24–30 %, thrombocytopenia 12 %, and neuropathy 9–18 %.

4.2.2 Bortezomib-Thalidomide-Dexamethasone

The bortezomib-thalidomide-dexamethasone (bortez-thal-dex) regimen has been evaluated in two phase III trials. In one study, patients with newly diagnosed disease were randomized to thal 100/200 mg daily and dex 40 mg days 1, 2, 4, 5, 8, 9, 11, and 12 of a 28 day cycle with or without IV bortez 1.3 mg/m^2 days 1, 4, 8, and 11 followed by tandem autologous transplantation, two cycles of consolidation with the same regimen received during the induction phase, and long-term term dex maintenance therapy [15]. The three-drug regimen was associated with superior rates of overall response, VGPR, nCR/CR, and CR at all phases of treatment. PFS at 3 years was 68 % with bortez-thal-dex and 56 % in the arm that received thal-dex. The 3-year overall survival rate was 86 % with bortez-thal-dez and 84 % with thal-dex. Grade 3/4 adverse events occurred in 56 % of patients receiving 3-drug therapy versus 33 % among patients receiving thalidomide-dexamethasone. The rate of grade 3/4 neuropathy with the bortez-thal-dex combination was 10 %.

In another phase III trial, bortez-thal-dex was compared to thal-dex and vincristine, BCNU, melphalan, cy, prednisone/vincristine, BCNU, doxorubicin, dex/bortezomib (VBMCP/VBAD/B) in patients with NDMM who received induction therapy followed by autologous transplantation and maintenance therapy [16]. Bortez-thal-dex produced the highest ORR (85 %) and CR rate (35 %), as well as the longest median PFS (56.2 months).

4.2.3 Lenalidomide-Bortezomib-Dexamethasone

Lenalidomide-bortezomib-dexamethasone (len-bortez-dex) is also highly active and widely utilized in newly diagnosed patients. In a phase I/II study, the maximum tolerated dose (MTD) was established at len 25 mg days 1–14; IV bortez 1.3 mg/m^2 days 1, 4, 8, and 11; and dex 20 mg on the day of and day following bortez in a 21 day cycle [17]. In the phase II portion of the study, the rates of PR, VGPR, and nCR/CR were 100, 74, and 52 %, respectively. Important adverse events included neuropathy, rash, neutropenia, and thrombocytopenia. The rate of thrombotic events was 11 %.

In a subsequent phase II study, 31 patients with newly diagnosed MM received three cycles of len-bortez-dex induction with len 25 mg days 1–14; IV bortez 1.3 mg/m^2 day 1, 4, 8, and 11; and dex 40 mg days 1, 8, and 15 of a 21 day cycle, followed by autologous transplantation, two cycles of len-bortez-dex consolidation, and thereafter lenalidomide maintenance. The ORR after induction was 93 %, including a nCR/CR rate of 23 %. Rates of nCR/CR after autologous transplantation and consolidation were 47 and 50 %, respectively. The estimated 3-year rates of PFS and OS were 77 and 100 %. None of the 21 patients who received MRD negativity progressed during the 3-year follow-up period. The rate of treatment-related neuropathy was 55 %, although there were no instances of grade 3 or 4 neuropathy. Stem cell collection was successful in all but one patient. Five patients in the study required a second collection with plerixafor and G-CSF to achieve the 2×10^6 CD34 cells/kg required for transplantation.

4.2.4 Carfilzomib-Lenalidomide-Dexamethasone

Carfilzomib-lenalidomide-dexamethasone (Carfilz-len-dex) is a potent combination for which there is expanding experience in the management of newly diagnosed MM. In a phase I/II trial, patients received four cycles of induction with carfilz 20/27/36 mg/m^2 days 1, 2, 8, 9, 15, and 16; len 25 mg days 1–21; and dex 40/20 mg weekly in a 28 day cycle, followed by stem cell mobilization and harvest.

Patients then continued with induction therapy to complete 8 cycles of therapy followed by maintenance, noting that patients had the option to proceed with transplant after four cycles [18]. Carfilzomib 36 mg/m^2 was utilized in the phase II portion of the study. The rates of overall response and nCR or better after four cycles were 100 and 67 %, and the rate of nCR or better improved to 78 % after eight cycles. The quality and depth of response appeared similar in patients with standard and high-risk disease. Grade 3/4 adverse events included thrombocytopenia, anemia, neutropenia, hypophosphatemia, elevated liver function tests, and dyspnea. While peripheral neuropathy occurred in 23 % of patients, there were no instances of grade 3/4 neuropathy.

In a subsequent phase II study, patients with previously untreated smoldering or overt MM received eight cycles of induction therapy with carfilz 20/36 mg/m^2; len 25 mg days 1–21; and dex 20/10 mg days 1, 2, 8, 9, 15, 16, 22, and 23 of 28 day treatment cycles, followed by maintenance with lenalidomide for 2 years [19]. Transplant-eligibile patients underwent stem cell collection after four cycles of therapy. Among patients with overt MM, the ORR was 98 % after eight cycles, with a rate of CR or sCR of 43 %. Among 30 patients who achieved CR and underwent minimal residual disease (MRD) assessment, the rate of MRD negativity was 97 %. In addition to expected hematologic toxicities, there was a significant degree of pulmonary, cardiac, and vascular toxicity, as 58 % of patients experienced pulmonary toxicity (including 16 % grade 3/4), 38 % experienced cardiac toxicity (including 11 % grade 3), and 56 % experienced vascular toxicity (including 13 % grade 3/4).

4.2.5 Bortezomib-Doxorubicin-Dexamethasone

The efficacy of this regimen was established in a phase III study in which 827 patients were randomized to either bortez-doxorubicin-dex or vincristine-doxorubicin-dex induction followed by autologous transplant with high-dose melphalan conditioning [20]. Patients randomized to bortez-doxorubicin-dex received post-transplant maintenance with bortezomib every other week for 2 years, while patients randomized to vincristine-doxorubicin-dex received maintenance with thalidomide 50 mg daily for 2 years. The bortezomib-containing treatment arm was associated with a higher rate of CR plus nCR after induction (31 vs. 15 %) and following bortezomib maintenance (49 vs. 34 %); superior PFS (35 vs. 28 months); and improved OS. Notably, significant benefit with bortezomib-containing therapy was observed in high-risk patients, including those with renal impairment defined as serum creatinine greater than 2 mg/dl and those harboring deltion 17p13. High-grade peripheral neuropathy occurred more frequently in patients who received bortezomib.

4.2.6 Cyclophosphamide-Bortezomib-Lenalidomide-Dexamethasone

The four-drug cy-len-bortez-dex regimen is typically reserved for patients with high-risk MM. Doses and schedule of the agents included can be based on the aforementioned EVOLUTION trial, in which treatment was given in 21 day cycles with cy 500 mg/m^2 on days 1 and 8; len 25 mg days 1–14; bortez 1.3 mg/m^2 days 1, 4, 8, and 11; and dex 40 mg days 1, 8, and 15 [21]. Reduction in the frequency of bortez to weekly on days 1, 8, and 15 as well as subcutaneous administration enhance tolerability of the regimen.

It is noted that although the EVOLUTION trial was not powered to formally compare response rates between the regimens evaluated, response rates appeared similar among patients who received cy-len-bortez-dex versus those who received the three drug regimens of either len-bortez-dex or cy-bortez-dex. Moreover, hematologic toxicities—particularly neutropenia and febrile neutropenia—were more frequent with cy-len-bortez-dex. In addition, two patients died during the course of the study, both were in the four-drug cy-len-bortez-dex group and resulted from renal failure.

5 Choice of Initial Therapy

Given the increasingly broad range of options for induction therapy in patients with newly diagnosed disease, the choice of initial treatment has become more complex. Choice of therapy must take into account various factors, including prognostic factors, such as ISS stage, cytogenetics, and, if available, genomic findings; the nature and extent of MM-associated organ impairment; the presence of extensive extramedullary disease; the presence of comorbid conditions such as peripheral neuropathy, diabetes, or heart failure; as well as patient preferences regarding the mode of treatment administration.

Patients with high-risk disease based on ISS stage or genetic analysis are best treated with a three-drug regimen such as cy-bortez-dex, len-bortez-dex, or carfilz-len-dex. Highest risk patients such as those with 17p deletion are ideally treated with a regimen that incorporates agents with the highest degree of anti-myeloma activity, namely a proteasome inhibitor and IMiD. Currently available data indicate carfilz-len-dex may be an ideal choice for the patient with ultra-high-risk disease-based depth of response to therapy, although prospective data from randomized trials evaluating this regimen in the upfront setting are not yet available. Other three-drug regimens incorporating proteasome inhibitor and IMiD such as len-bortez-dex or bortezomib-thal-dex are also very appropriate choices in this context.

Bortezomib-containing regimens such as bortez-dex and cy-bortez-dex are appropriate for patients with significant renal dysfunction at the time of diagnosis, including those who have documented AL amyloidosis occurring in association with MM, as bortezomib is generally well tolerated and effective in terms of reversing renal impairment [22]. Len can be employed in patients with renal impairment as well but requires dose modification in this context. Carfilzomib can likewise be administered to individuals with renal impairment, including those receiving dialysis, with dose reduction to 15 mg/m^2 in cycle 1 and increase in dose to 20 and 27 mg/m^2 in subsequent cycles of the agent is tolerated [23].

Patients with significant preexisting peripheral neuropathy benefit from regimens that are minimally neurotoxic. Ideal options in this respect include len-dex and carfilz-len-dex, as both len and carfilz are associated with a relatively modest degree of neurotoxicity in comparison to agents such as bortezomib and thalidomide.

The presence of extensive extramedullary involvement poses a significant clinical challenge, and warrants use of a three-or four-drug regimen. Several reports have suggested that bortezomib is effective in this context [24, 25], though other reports have described instances of bortezomib resistance [26] highlighting the rationale for multi-drug combination regimens in this context.

Individuals with primary plasma cell leukemia (PCL) are treated with three-or four-drug regimens that incorporate bortezomib, a practice based on several studies demonstrating benefit with this approach [27–29]. Options in this regard include bortez-thal-dex, len-bortez-dex, and bortez-doxorubicin-dex. Regimens incorporating carfilzomib such as carfilz-len-dex are likely to be effective as induction therapy in cases of primary PCL. Such patients should proceed rapidly from induction therapy to intensification with high-dose therapy and autologous transplant followed by consolidation and maintenance.

6 Stem Cell Transplantation in MM

High-dose therapy and autologous stem cell transplantation (ASCT), is a widely accepted consolidation approach in myeloma following initial therapy of newly diagnosed disease in patients eligible to undergo the procedure. Several randomized trials have demonstrated an advantage for SCT compared to conventional therapy alone and formed the basis for this approach [30, 31]. As has been described in the earlier sections, use of these new drugs in combinations has led to response depth that rivals those seen with ASCT [32–34]. These results have led to an intense debate regarding the current role of SCT [35].

High-dose therapy for management of MM was introduced over two decades ago based on the ability of high doses of chemotherapy to overcome innate and acquired drug resistance, albeit primarily alkylator resistance. Based on the favorable results from several randomized trials, this modality was rapidly incorporated into the treatment algorithm of the younger patients [30, 31, 36]. While the initial trials laid the foundation for ASCT approaches for myeloma, subsequent trials and large single arm studies have systematically refined the role of this approach. The initial French trials and the MRC VII trial demonstrated an increased response depth and duration and overall survival for ASCT compared to conventional therapies used at that time, mostly alkylator and steroid-based combination regimens. The details of the trials comparing SCT to conventional therapy are detailed in Table 1. However, the randomized trials that allowed for delayed use of ASCT following failure of conventional therapies and those limited to chemo sensitive patient populations failed to demonstrate a benefit for ASCT. Furthermore, a randomized trial specifically asking the question of timing of ASCT suggested

Table 1 Clinical trials comparing ASCT to conventional therapies

Study	Randomization	Patients (N)	ORR (%)	CR (%)	PFS	OS
Attal et al. (IFM 90) [30]	ASCT: (4–6 alternating cycles of VMCP and BVAP followed by Mel (140 mg/m^2) and TBI (8 Gy)	100	81	22	28 month	57 month
	CCT (alternating cycles VMCP and BVAP for 12 months)	100	57	5	18 month	44 month
Child et al. (MRC VII) [31]	ASCT: melphalan (200 mg/m^2) or melphalan (140 mg/m^2) + TBI; IFN maintenance	200	86	44	31.6 month	54.1 month
	CCT (4–12 cycles): ACMC; IFN maintenance	201	48	8	19.6 month	42.3 month
Fermand et al. (MAG90) [40]	ASCT: lomustine, VP16, cyclophosphamide, melphalan + TBI	91	78	57	39 month	65 month
	CCT: VMCP to plateau	94	58	20	13 month	64 month
Fermand et al. (MAG91) [37]	ASCT: melphalan (200 mg/m^2) or melphalan + busulfan	94	59	6	25.3 month	47.8 month
	CCT: VMCP	96	56	4	18.7 month	47.6 month
Barlogie et al. (S9321) [38]	ASCT: melphalan (140 mg/m^2) + TBI, followed by randomization to IFN maintenance	261	93	17	17 % (7 year)	38 % (7 year)
	CCT: VMCP followed by randomization to IFN maintenance	255	90	15	14 % (7 year)	38 % (7 year)
Blade et al. (PETHEMA) [39]	ASCT: melphalan (200 mg/m^2) or melphalan (140 mg/m^2) + TBI; IFN maintenance	81	82	30	42 month	66 month
	CCT: VBMCP alternating with VBAD; IFN maintenance	83	83	11	33 month	61 month
Palumbo et al. (MMSG) [36]	ASCT: melphalan (100 mg/m^2) × 2	95	72	25	28	58
	CCT: melphalan + prednisone	99	66	6	16	42

ASCT autologous stem cell transplantation; *CCT* conventional chemotherapy; *CR* complete remission; *ORR* overall response rate; *OS* overall survival; *PFS* progression-free survival; *TBI* total body irradiation
VMCP vincristine, melphalan, cyclophosphamide, prednisone; *BVAP* vincristine, carmustine, doxorubicin, prednisone; *ACMC* Adriamycin, cyclophosphamide, melphalan, carmustine
VBMCP-BCNU, vincristine, melphalan, prednisone; *VBAD* vincristine, *BCNU* doxorubicin, dexamethasone

that frontline ASCT and ASCT used at the time of first relapse were associated with similar overall survival [37–40]. However, use of early ASCT was associated with a longer time without therapy and symptoms, a good surrogate for improved quality of life. This paradigm appears to hold true today as was shown in a single institution study comparing outcomes of patients getting novel agent-based induction followed by early or delayed stem cell transplant. This question is being prospectively addressed in a large phase 3 trial. While the overall utility of ASCT continue to be debated in the current era, a recent Italian trial showed better outcome with transplant-based approach compared with non-transplant consolidation, both in the setting of IMiD-based induction therapy [41]. Palumbo et al. randomly assigned 273 patients 65 years of age or younger to high-dose melphalan plus stem cell transplantation or MPR consolidation therapy after induction, and 251 of the patients to lenalidomide maintenance therapy or no maintenance therapy after ASCT. Both progression-free and overall survivals were significantly longer with high-dose melphalan plus stem cell transplantation than with MPR.

Subsequent clinical trials and retrospective studies further allowed us to define the selection of patients, conditioning therapy and post-transplant consolidation, and maintenance strategies. The question of the ideal conditioning therapy was specifically addressed in an IFM trial, which showed better outcome when high-dose melphalan was used alone (without TBI) and has led to this being the current standard [42]. Other smaller trials have explored alternate approaches to conditioning such as BuCy, but concerns regarding toxicity remain. Recent studies are exploring the potential benefit of integrating novel agents into the conditioning regimens pre-ASCT. In a phase 2 trial the French added four doses of bortezomib to standard high-dose melphalan, which was well tolerated, and when compared with historical controls had deeper responses. Another phase 2 trial also explored the same approach, though with a slightly different bortezomib schedule and demonstrated excellent efficacy. Carfilzomib also has been integrated into the conditioning regimen with no safety issues. While the randomized trials included patients younger than 65, studies suggest similar benefits for older patients who are considered eligible to undergo the procedure [43, 44]. Renal insufficiency is common at diagnosis and patients with compromised renal function also can benefit from ASCT, if they are otherwise considered eligible [45]. Unlike other malignancies, response to preceding chemotherapy is not a prerequisite for consideration of ASCT in myeloma. In fact patients, refractory to initial therapy of their disease can derive comparable benefits from ASCT as those responding to the pre-ASCT regimen [46]. Given this scenario, ASCT has been considered the standard of care for patients with myeloma who are eligible. Single institution studies as well as population-based studies suggest that ASCT played a significant role in the improved survival seen among patients with myeloma in the recent two decades.

7 Role of Second ASCT

A second ASCT can be considered for management of MM either as consolidation therapy soon after the first ASCT (Tandem ASCT) or as salvage therapy in patients relapsing after previous ASCT. Investigators at the University of Arkansas initially reported on the use of sequential ASCT in their Total Therapy I protocol, which consisted of a series of induction regimens and two cycles of high-dose therapy.

Table 2 Clinical trials comparing double ASCT to single ASCT

Study	Randomization	Patients (N)	ORR (%)	CR (%)	EFS	OS
Barlogie et al. [83]	Total therapy	123	86	40	49 months	62 months
	Single ASCT (Historical controls)	116	52	NA	22 months	48 months
Attal et al. [47]	Double (VAD followed by ASCT1 with Mel 140 mg/m^2, ASCT2 with Mel 140 mg/m^2 and TBI)	200	88	50 (CR + VGPR)	30 months	58 months
	Single (VAD followed by ASCT with Mel 140 mg/m^2)	199	84	42 (CR + VGPR)	25 months	48 months
Cavo et al. [48]	Double (VAD followed by ASCT1 with Mel 200 mg/m^2, ASCT2 with Mel 120 mg/m^2 with busulfan (12 mg/kg))	158	NA	47 (CR + nCR)	35 months	71 months
	Single (VAD followed by ASCT with Mel 140 mg/m^2)	163	NA	33 (CR + nCR)	23 months	65 months
Sonneveld et al. [49]	Double: VAD followed by IDM (Mel 70 mg/m^2 × 2) followed by CT × 120 mg/Kg +TBI	155	90	13	22 months	55 months
	Single: VAD followed by IDM (Mel 70 mg/m^2 × 2)	148	86	28	20 months	50 months
Fermand et al. [50]	Double: VAD followed by ASCT1 with Mel 140 mg/m^2, followed by ASCT2 with Mel 140 mg/m^2, Etoposide 30 mg/kg, TBI (12 Gy)	99	NA	39 (CR + VGPR)	ND	ND
	Single: VAD followed by ASCT 1 carmustine, etoposide, Mel 140 mg/m^2, CT × 60 mg/kg, TBI (12 Gy)	94	NA	37 (CR + VGPR)	ND	ND

ASCT autologous stem cell transplantation; *CR* complete remission; *ORR* overall response rate; *OS* overall survival; *EFS* event-free survival; *TBI* total body irradiation

Total Therapy VAD followed by HDCTX (high-dose cyclophosphamide) and GM-CSF for PBSC collection, EDAP (etoposide, dexamethasone, cytarabine, cisplatin) followed by first ASCT with MEL 200. If sustained partial remission (PR) or CR, a second ASCT with MEL 200 was performed followed by Interferon (IFN) maintenance

Several randomized trials have since directly addressed the question of single versus double upfront transplants (Table 2). In the IFM-94 trial the event-free survival (20 vs. 10 %) and the overall survival (42 vs. 21 %) at 7 years post-transplant doubled with addition of the second ASCT, despite no major improvement in the combined CR and VGPR rate with double transplant (50 vs. 42 %) [47]. The benefit was mostly restricted to those not achieving a VGPR with the first ASCT. In the Bologna, 96 trial addition of a second HDT prolonged time to progression by 17 months with no clear OS improvement [48]. As with IFM94, patients failing to achieve a CR or nCR after the first HDT obtained the maximum benefit. Similarly, the HOVON24 trial also showed prolonged EFS for double ASCT without any improvement in the OS, while the MAG95 trial did not have improvement in either EFS or OS with the double ASCT [49, 50]. A meta-analysis of the tandem trials, tandem AHCT did not improve OS or event-free survival despite a significant increase in response rate and was associated with a statistically significant increase in TRM [51].

The role of a second transplant as salvage therapy after previous transplants has been reported in single institution studies and in a small prospective trial from UK [52, 53]. In a report of 172 patients relapsing after one ASCT, 54 patients received a second ASCT and the rest received salvage chemotherapy. While there was a trend toward improved OS with repeat ASCT, there was no benefit for those relapsing <18 months from the initial ASCT with median survival <6 months compared to 3 years for those with a longer response from first ASCT. An EBMTR analysis of "planned" sequential transplants (presumed tandem) or "unplanned" (presumed salvage) showed a median survival from ASCT of 60 months for the planned group versus 51 months for the rest ($P = 0.05$) [54]. We recently examined the outcomes in 98 patients undergoing salvage auto-SCT (auto-SCT2) for relapsed MM after receiving an initial transplant (auto-SCT1) between 1994 and 2009. The median PFS from auto-SCT2 was 10.3 months and the median OS from auto-SCT2 was 33 months. Only a shorter TTP after auto-SCT1 predicted for a shorter OS post auto-SCT2. It is clearly a reasonable approach for patients with relapsed disease, especially those who had an excellent response and disease stabilization with their initial ASCT.

8 Post-Transplant Maintenance Approaches in MM

The majority of patients undergoing ASCT will eventually have disease progression and in particular patients with high-risk genetic abnormalities are likely to relapse even faster. Multiple approaches have been explored for improving the risk of relapse post-ASCT and have been termed as either consolidation or maintenance, with the distinction between the two approaches remaining unclear.

Initial attempts in the 1960s to early 1980s with single agent corticosteroids, continuous conventional chemotherapy or interferon often improved progression-free survival but with inconsistent impact on overall survival [55–62]. The Myeloma Trialists' Collaborative Group subsequently performed a meta-analysis which evaluated the benefits of interferon as an induction and maintenance therapy; including 24 trials and 4012 patients [63]. During induction, response rates were slightly better with interferon (57.5 vs. 53.1 %). PFS was better with interferon (33 vs. 24 % at 3 years), an effect seen in both induction and maintenance portions. Median time to progression was increased by about 6 months in both settings. OS was also better with interferon (53 vs. 49 % at 3 years) with median survival improvement of 4 months. This benefit was however restricted to the smaller trials and was associated with considerable toxicity. With the introduction of new drugs such as IMiDs and proteasome inhibitors, attention was turned towards exploring the potential of these drugs for maintenance therapy.

8.1 Thalidomide

Thalidomide was the first immunomodulatory agent that showed efficacy in the treatment of MM [32, 64]. It has been studied as a maintenance therapy in clinical trials, either as a single agent or combined with corticosteroids or other agents with varying efficacy. Attal et al. conducted a randomized trial of maintenance treatment with thalidomide and pamidronate. In the IFM trial (IFM 99-02), 2 months after high-dose therapy, 597 patients younger than age 65 years were randomly assigned to receive no maintenance (arm A), pamidronate (arm B), or pamidronate plus thalidomide (arm C). Overall, 55 % of patients in arm A, 57 % in arm B, and 67 % in arm C achieved a complete or very good partial response. Both 3-year event free survival and 4-year overall survival rates were significantly better in thalidomide maintenance group compared to other two groups [65]. Barlogie et al. randomized 668 patients to receive thalidomide until disease progression or unacceptable side effects. After a median follow-up of 42 months the thalidomide and control groups had 5-year event-free survival rates of 56 and 44 %. The 5-year rate of overall survival was approximately similar in both groups. Severe peripheral neuropathy and deep-vein thrombosis was seen more often in thalidomide group [66]. In MRC IX trial, 820 newly diagnosed MM patients were randomized to open-label thalidomide maintenance until progression, or no maintenance. Median PFS was significantly longer with thalidomide maintenance, but median OS was similar between regimens. Patients with favorable FISH showed improved PFS and a trend toward a late survival benefit. In contrast, those with adverse FISH abnormalities receiving thalidomide showed no significant PFS benefit and "worse" OS [67, 68]. In the HOVON-50 trial, 556 patients was randomly assigned to three cycles of vincristine, Adriamycin, and dexamethasone (VAD), or arm thalidomide 200 mg orally, continuously, plus Adriamycin and dexamethasone (TAD). After induction therapy and stem cell mobilization, patients received high-dose melphalan, 200 mg/m^2, followed by maintenance with alpha-interferon or thalidomide 50 mg daily. Thalidomide significantly improved overall response rate and significantly prolonged progression-free survival from median 25 to 34 months. Median overall survival was longer in the thalidomide arm, although not statistically significant (73 vs. 60 months) [69]. Stewart et al. reported a randomized, controlled trial comparing thalidomide-prednisone as maintenance therapy with observation in 332 patients who had undergone autologous stem cell transplantation with melphalan 200 mg/m^2 (MY 10 trial). With a median follow-up of 4.1 years, no differences in

OS between thalidomide-prednisone and observation were detected; thalidomide-prednisone was associated with superior myeloma-specific progression-free survival and progression-free survival (4-year estimates were 32 vs. 14 %) and more frequent venous thromboembolism (7.3 % vs. none). Those allocated to thalidomide-prednisone reported worse HRQoL with respect to cognitive function, dyspnea, constipation, thirst, leg swelling, numbness, dry mouth, and balance problems [70]. Spencer et al. examined if the addition of 12 months thalidomide consolidation following AHSCT would improve the durability of responses achieved and overall survival. Post-ASCT, 129 patients were randomly assigned to receive indefinite prednisolone maintenance therapy (control group) and 114 to receive the same in addition to 12 months of thalidomide consolidation (thalidomide group). After a median follow-up of 3 years, 3-year PFS rates were 42 and 23 %and the OS rates were 86 and 75 % in the thalidomide and control groups, respectively. There was no difference in survival between groups 12 months after disease progression (79 vs. 77 %) [71]. Krishnan A et al. integrated thalidomide maintenance to their randomized trial comparing the effectiveness of allogeneic HSCT with non-myeloablative conditioning after autologous HSCT with tandem autologous HSCT. In the auto-auto group 217 patients received maintenance treatment, 77 % of who completed planned maintenance. Use of maintenance had no effect on PFS or OS [72]. Maiolino et al. examined the efficacy of thalidomide plus dexamethasone as a maintenance therapy after autologous hematopoietic stem cell transplantation. 108 patients were randomized to receive maintenance with dexamethasone or dexamethasone with thalidomide (200 mg daily) for 12 months or until disease progression. After a median follow-up of 27 months, 2-year progression-free survival was 30 % in dexamethasone arm and 64 % in thalidomide and dexamethasone arm. Overall survival at 2 years was not significantly improved with the addition of thalidomide (70 vs. 85 % in respectively) [73]. Kagoya et al. performed another meta-analysis, which included 6 trials and 2786 patients to assess the efficacy of thalidomide maintenance. While thalidomide improved progression-free survival no significant benefit was seen for overall survival and had more frequent venous thrombosis and peripheral neuropathy. The improvement was especially prominent in a subgroup of studies using corticosteroids with thalidomide [74].

8.1.1 Bortezomib

Bortezomib is a proteasome inhibitor, which has efficacy in treatment of both newly diagnosed and relapsed MM [33, 75]. It has been studied as a maintenance therapy in clinical trials, either as a single agent or combined with corticosteroids or other agents with varying efficacy. It was evaluated as a maintenance therapy after autologous HSCT in the HOVON-65/GMMG-HD4 trial, where 827 eligible patients with newly diagnosed symptomatic MM were randomly assigned to receive induction therapy with vincristine, doxorubicin, and dexamethasone (VAD) or bortezomib, doxorubicin, and dexamethasone (PAD) followed by high-dose melphalan and autologous stem cell transplantation. Maintenance consisted of thalidomide 50 mg after VAD induction once per day or bortezomib

1.3 mg/m^2 after PAD induction once every 2 weeks for 2 years. Complete response rate (CR) was superior after PAD induction (15 vs. 31 %) and bortezomib maintenance (34 vs. 49 %). After a median follow-up of 41 months, PFS was superior in the PAD arm (median of 28 vs. 35 months). In multivariate analysis, overall survival was better in the PAD arm. In high-risk patients presenting with increased creatinine more than 2 mg/dL, bortezomib significantly improved PFS from a median of 13 to 30 months and OS from a median of 21 to 54 months. A benefit was also observed in patients with deletion 17p13 (median PFS, 12 vs. 22 months; median OS, 24 months vs. not reached at 54 months). In the thalidomide arm, 64 % of the patients discontinued maintenance therapy because of progressive disease (PD), toxicity, and other reasons (31, 31, and 2 %, respectively). In the bortezomib arm, 47 % discontinued maintenance therapy because of PD, toxicity, and other reasons (29, 9, and 9 %, respectively). Grade 3–4 PNP rate was significantly greater in the PAD group (16 vs. 7 %) [20]. However given the study design, it is hard to differentiate if the benefit came from the introduction of bortezomib as part of induction or maintenance or both. Rosinol et al. reported a PETHEMA group phase III randomized trial where after induction, patients underwent a melphalan-based single ASCT with a randomization to maintenance therapy for 3 years with bortezomib plus thalidomide (VT), T alone or IFN-α alone. At a median follow-up of 24 months from the initiation of maintenance, the VT arm had a significantly longer PFS than T or IFN-a (78 vs. 63 vs. 49 %). There was no OS benefit seen across the three maintenance arms [16].

8.1.2 Lenalidomide

Given the significantly better toxicity profile lenalidomide has been evaluated as a maintenance treatment in several clinical trials. In the IFM 05-02 study, patients having received previous induction therapy with either vincristine-doxorubicin-dexamethasone or bortezomib-dexamethasone (VD) followed by one or two ASCT were treated with 2 cycles of lenalidomide consolidation therapy and were thereafter randomized to lenalidomide maintenance (10–15 mg daily) or placebo until disease progression. After a median follow-up of 45 months from randomization, the 4-year estimates of PFS were 43 % for the lenalidomide group and 22 % for the placebo group, while no difference in OS was seen between the two groups (73 vs. 75 %). The lenalidomide group had an increased incidence of hematological toxicities (primarily neutropenia) and an increase in SPMs (Hematologic malignancies 13 vs. 5 patients and solid organ malignancies 10 vs. 4 patients consecutively for lenalidomide and no maintenance groups. The median EFS were 40 months for the lenalidomide group and 23 months for the placebo group. With a longer follow-up of 60 months, lenalidomide maintenance improved PFS (42 %) compared with placebo (18 %). OS was similar in both groups (68 % at 5 years for the lenalidomide group vs. 67 % for the placebo group) [76, 77]. The CALGB 100104 study randomly assigned 614 patients younger than 65 years of age who had no progressive disease after first-line transplantation to maintenance treatment with either lenalidomide (10 mg per day for the first 3 months, increased to 15 mg if tolerated) or placebo until relapse. With a median follow-up of 48 months, and the OS was

80 % for the lenalidomide group and 70 % for the placebo group. The lenalidomide group had an increased incidence of hematological toxicities (primarily neutropenia) and an increase in second primary malignancies (SPMs). The cumulative incidence risk for the development of SPM was greater for the lenalidomide group compared with the placebo group [78, 79].

In another phase 3 study, Palumbo et al. randomized 273 newly diagnosed transplant-eligible patients to high-dose melphalan plus stem cell transplantation or MPR after initial induction therapy with lenalidomide-dexamethasone. After stem cell transplantation or MPR consolidation, 251 of 273 patients were re-randomized to either maintenance or no maintenance. Maintenance therapy with lenalidomide (10 mg on days 1–21 of each 28-day cycle) was administered until disease progression or development of unacceptable adverse effects. Among these 251 patients, median progression free survival was significantly longer with lenalidomide maintenance therapy than with no maintenance therapy (41.9 vs. 21.6 months). Lenalidomide maintenance therapy, as compared with no maintenance therapy, had no significant effect on the 3-year overall survival rate (88 vs. 79.2 %). Beneficial effect of maintenance therapy on progression free survival was similar in both stem cell transplantation and MPR consolidation arms. 11 patients (2.8 %) had a second primary cancer in various phases of study. 3 out of these 11 patients developed second primary cancer during the lenalidomide maintenance therapy [41].

Given the contradictory data, definitive conclusions remain difficult to make. However, given the benefit in the CALGB phase 3 trial among those not achieving a CR/VGPR, it is reasonable to consider offering maintenance to those individuals. However, in the high-risk patients prolonged treatment with bortezomib-based regimens appear to be justified based on the data from the HOVON trial. For the remaining patients, once could consider a short consolidation as shown in the French trial; namely two cycles of lenalidomide-Dex, given that this trial failed to show any difference in OS.

9 Allogeneic Stem Cell Transplant for MM

There has been limited success with allogeneic stem cell transplant (Allo-SCT) for treatment of myeloma, largely a result of high treatment-related mortality in this patient population. There is little doubt that a graft versus myeloma effect exists and is obvious from the higher rate of molecular responses following allo-SCT compared to ASCT which in turn translates into longer remissions [80]. Several trials have compared the allogeneic approach with ASCT, with enrichment for patients with high-risk disease.

The IFM 99-03/99-04 clinical trials studied patients with high-risk myeloma (beta2-microglobulin >3 mg/L and chromosome 13 deletion) [81]. Sixty-five patients with an HLA-identical sibling donor were assigned to receive RIC allogeneic stem cell transplantation (IFM99-03 trial), and 219 patients without an

HLA-identical sibling donor were assigned to undergo second ASCT (IFM99-04 protocol). The incidence of acute GVHD was 32 %, chronic GVHD was 43 % and TRM was 10 %. On an intent-to-treat basis, the median OS and EFS did not differ significantly between the groups (35 and 25 months in the IFM99-03 trial vs. 41 and 30 months in the IFM99-04 trial, respectively). When the 166 patients randomly assigned in the tandem ASCT protocol was compared to those undergoing allogeneic transplant the EFS was similar (35 vs. 31.7 months), with a trend for better OS with tandem ASCT (median, 47.2 vs. 35 months; $P = 0.07$). In the Italian trial, 108 patients <65 years, with newly diagnosed MM received standard ASCT followed by low-dose TBI conditioning and HLA-matched sibling PBSCT (median of 2–4 months from ASCT) or went on to receive a second ASCT [82]. At a median follow-up of 3 years, TRM was 11 % with allo-SCT vs. 4 % with double ASCT; CR rate was 46 versus 16 %; OS was 84 versus 62 % and PFS was 75 versus 41 %, all significant differences. More recently, the BMT CTN performed a randomized trial, where patients were assigned to receive an ASCT followed by an allo-SCT (auto-allo group) or tandem ASCTs (auto-auto group) on the basis of the availability of an HLA-matched sibling donor. Patients in the auto-auto group subsequently underwent a random allocation (1:1) to maintenance therapy (thalidomide plus dexamethasone) or observation. There was no difference in the PFS or OS between the auto-auto and the auto-allo approaches. At this time, the role of allo-SCT in myeloma remain undefined, while the majority believe that a small group of high-risk patients may benefit from this procedure, they should preferably be done in the context of clinical trials.

References

1. Avet-Loiseau H (2007) Role of genetics in prognostication in myeloma. Best Pract Res Clin Haematol 20(4):625–635
2. Greipp PR, San Miguel J, Durie BG et al (2005) International staging system for multiple myeloma. J Clin Oncol 23(15):3412–3420
3. Munshi NC, Anderson KC, Bergsagel PL et al (2011) Consensus recommendations for risk stratification in multiple myeloma: report of the International Myeloma Workshop Consensus Panel 2. Blood 117(18):4696–4700
4. Boyd KD, Ross FM, Chiecchio L et al (2012) A novel prognostic model in myeloma based on co-segregating adverse FISH lesions and the ISS: analysis of patients treated in the MRC Myeloma IX trial. Leukemia 26(2):349–355
5. Zhan F, Hardin J, Kordsmeier B et al (2002) Global gene expression profiling of multiple myeloma, monoclonal gammopathy of undetermined significance, and normal bone marrow plasma cells. Blood 99(5):1745–1757
6. Decaux O, Lode L, Magrangeas F et al (2008) Prediction of survival in multiple myeloma based on gene expression profiles reveals cell cycle and chromosomal instability signatures in high-risk patients and hyperdiploid signatures in low-risk patients: a study of the Intergroupe Francophone du Myelome. J Clin Oncol 26(29):4798–4805
7. Rajkumar SV, Rosinol L, Hussein M et al (2008) Multicenter, randomized, double-blind, placebo-controlled study of thalidomide plus dexamethasone compared with dexamethasone as initial therapy for newly diagnosed multiple myeloma. J Clin Oncol 26(13):2171–2177

8. Kumar S, Dispenzieri A, Lacy MQ et al (2007) Impact of lenalidomide therapy on stem cell mobilization and engraftment post-peripheral blood stem cell transplantation in patients with newly diagnosed myeloma. Leukemia 21(9):2035–2042

9. Paripati H, Stewart AK, Cabou S et al (2008) Compromised stem cell mobilization following induction therapy with lenalidomide in myeloma. Leukemia 22(6):1282–1284

10. Sviggum HP, Davis MD, Rajkumar SV, Dispenzieri A (2006) Dermatologic adverse effects of lenalidomide therapy for amyloidosis and multiple myeloma. Arch Dermatol 142(10):1298–1302

11. Harousseau JL, Attal M, Avet-Loiseau H et al (2010) Bortezomib plus dexamethasone is superior to vincristine plus doxorubicin plus dexamethasone as induction treatment prior to autologous stem-cell transplantation in newly diagnosed multiple myeloma: results of the IFM 2005-01 phase III trial. J Clin Oncol 28(30):4621–4629

12. Moreau P, Pylypenko H, Grosicki S et al (2011) Subcutaneous versus intravenous administration of bortezomib in patients with relapsed multiple myeloma: a randomised, phase 3, non-inferiority study. Lancet Oncol 12(5):431–440

13. Mitsiades N, Mitsiades CS, Richardson PG et al (2003) The proteasome inhibitor PS-341 potentiates sensitivity of multiple myeloma cells to conventional chemotherapeutic agents: therapeutic applications. Blood 101(6):2377–2380

14. Reeder CB, Reece DE, Kukreti V et al (2009) Cyclophosphamide, bortezomib and dexamethasone induction for newly diagnosed multiple myeloma: high response rates in a phase II clinical trial. Leukemia 23(7):1337–1341

15. Cavo M, Tacchetti P, Patriarca F et al (2010) Bortezomib with thalidomide plus dexamethasone compared with thalidomide plus dexamethasone as induction therapy before, and consolidation therapy after, double autologous stem-cell transplantation in newly diagnosed multiple myeloma: a randomised phase 3 study. Lancet 376(9758):2075–2085

16. Rosinol L, Oriol A, Teruel AI et al (2012) Superiority of bortezomib, thalidomide, and dexamethasone (VTD) as induction pretransplantation therapy in multiple myeloma: a randomized phase 3 PETHEMA/GEM study. Blood 120(8):1589–1596

17. Richardson PG, Weller E, Lonial S et al (2010) Lenalidomide, bortezomib, and dexamethasone combination therapy in patients with newly diagnosed multiple myeloma. Blood 116(5):679–686

18. Jakubowiak AJ, Dytfeld D, Griffith KA et al (2012) A phase 1/2 study of carfilzomib in combination with lenalidomide and low-dose dexamethasone as a frontline treatment for multiple myeloma. Blood 120(9):1801–1809

19. Korde N, Roschewski M, Zingone A et al (2015) Treatment with carfilzomib-lenalidomide-dexamethasone with lenalidomide extension in patients with smoldering or newly diagnosed multiple myeloma. JAMA Oncol 1(6):746–754

20. Sonneveld P, Schmidt-Wolf IG, van der Holt B et al (2012) Bortezomib induction and maintenance treatment in patients with newly diagnosed multiple myeloma: results of the randomized phase III HOVON-65/ GMMG-HD4 trial. J Clin Oncol 30(24):2946–2955

21. Kumar S, Flinn I, Richardson PG et al (2012) Randomized, multicenter, phase 2 study (EVOLUTION) of combinations of bortezomib, dexamethasone, cyclophosphamide, and lenalidomide in previously untreated multiple myeloma. Blood 119(19):4375–4382

22. Chanan-Khan AA, Kaufman JL, Mehta J et al (2007) Activity and safety of bortezomib in multiple myeloma patients with advanced renal failure: a multicenter retrospective study. Blood 109(6):2604–2606

23. Badros AZ, Vij R, Martin T et al (2013) Carfilzomib in multiple myeloma patients with renal impairment: pharmacokinetics and safety. Leukemia 27(8):1707–1714

24. Laura R, Cibeira MT, Uriburu C et al (2006) Bortezomib: an effective agent in extramedullary disease in multiple myeloma. Eur J Haematol 76(5):405–408

25. Hughes M, Micallef-Eynaud P (2006) Bortezomib in relapsed multiple myeloma complicated by extramedullary plasmacytomas. Clin Lab Haematol 28(4):267–269

26. Ali R, Ozkalemkas F, Ozkan A et al (2007) Bortezomib and extramedullary disease in multiple myeloma: the shine and dark side of the moon. Leuk Res 31(8):1153–1155
27. D'Arena G, Valentini CG, Pietrantuono G et al (2012) Frontline chemotherapy with bortezomib-containing combinations improves response rate and survival in primary plasma cell leukemia: a retrospective study from GIMEMA Multiple Myeloma Working Party. Ann Oncol 23(6):1499–1502
28. Libby E, Candelaria-Quintana D, Moualla H, Abdul-Jaleel M, Rabinowitz I (2010) Durable complete remission of primary plasma cell leukemia with the bortezomib plus melphalan and prednisone (VMP) regimen. Am J Hematol 85(9):733–734
29. Al-Nawakil C, Tamburini J, Bardet V et al (2008) Bortezomib, doxorubicin and dexamethasone association is an effective option for plasma cell leukemia induction therapy. Leuk Lymphoma 49(10):2012–2014
30. Attal M, Harousseau JL, Stoppa AM et al (1996) A prospective, randomized trial of autologous bone marrow transplantation and chemotherapy in multiple myeloma. Intergroupe Francais du Myelome. N Engl J Med 335(2):91–97
31. Child JA, Morgan GJ, Davies FE et al (2003) High-dose chemotherapy with hematopoietic stem-cell rescue for multiple myeloma. N Engl J Med 348(19):1875–1883
32. Rajkumar SV, Blood E, Vesole D, Fonseca R, Greipp PR (2006) Phase III clinical trial of thalidomide plus dexamethasone compared with dexamethasone alone in newly diagnosed multiple myeloma: a clinical trial coordinated by the Eastern Cooperative Oncology Group. J Clin Oncol 24(3):431–436
33. Richardson PG, Sonneveld P, Schuster MW et al (2005) Bortezomib or high-dose dexamethasone for relapsed multiple myeloma. N Engl J Med 352(24):2487–2498
34. Rajkumar SV, Jacobus S, Callander N et al (2007) A randomized trial of lenalidomide plus high-dose dexamethasone (RD) versus lenalidomide plus low-dose dexamethasone (Rd) in newly diagnosed multiple myeloma (E4A03): a trial coordinated by the Eastern Cooperative Oncology Group. Blood 110(11):74
35. Kumar SK, Rajkumar SV, Dispenzieri A et al (2008) Improved survival in multiple myeloma and the impact of novel therapies. Blood 111(5):2516–2520
36. Palumbo A, Bringhen S, Petrucci MT et al (2004) Intermediate-dose melphalan improves survival of myeloma patients aged 50 to 70: results of a randomized controlled trial. Blood 104 (10):3052–3057
37. Fermand JP, Katsahian S, Divine M et al (2005) High-dose therapy and autologous blood stem-cell transplantation compared with conventional treatment in myeloma patients aged 55 to 65 years: long-term results of a randomized control trial from the Group Myelome-Autogreffe. J Clin Oncol 23(36):9227–9233
38. Barlogie B, Kyle RA, Anderson KC et al (2006) Standard chemotherapy compared with high-dose chemoradiotherapy for multiple myeloma: final results of phase III US Intergroup Trial S9321. J Clin Oncol 24(6):929–936
39. Blade J, Rosinol L, Sureda A et al (2005) High-dose therapy intensification compared with continued standard chemotherapy in multiple myeloma patients responding to the initial chemotherapy: long-term results from a prospective randomized trial from the Spanish cooperative group PETHEMA. Blood 106(12):3755–3759
40. Fermand JP, Ravaud P, Chevret S et al (1998) High-dose therapy and autologous peripheral blood stem cell transplantation in multiple myeloma: up-front or rescue treatment? Results of a multicenter sequential randomized clinical trial. Blood 92(9):3131–3136
41. Palumbo A, Cavallo F, Gay F et al (2014) Autologous transplantation and maintenance therapy in multiple myeloma. N Engl J Med 371(10):895–905
42. Moreau P, Facon T, Attal M et al (2002) Comparison of 200 mg/m(2) melphalan and 8 Gy total body irradiation plus 140 mg/m(2) melphalan as conditioning regimens for peripheral blood stem cell transplantation in patients with newly diagnosed multiple myeloma: final analysis of the Intergroupe Francophone du Myelome 9502 randomized trial. Blood 99 (3):731–735

43. Siegel DS, Desikan KR, Mehta J et al (1999) Age is not a prognostic variable with autotransplants for multiple myeloma. Blood 93(1):51–54

44. Kumar SK, Dingli D, Lacy MQ et al (2008) Autologous stem cell transplantation in patients of 70 years and older with multiple myeloma: Results from a matched pair analysis. Am J Hematol 83(8):614–617

45. Gertz MA, Lacy MQ, Dispenzieri A et al (2007) Impact of age and serum creatinine value on outcome after autologous blood stem cell transplantation for patients with multiple myeloma. Bone Marrow Transplant 39(10):605–611

46. Kumar S, Lacy MQ, Dispenzieri A et al (2004) High-dose therapy and autologous stem cell transplantation for multiple myeloma poorly responsive to initial therapy. Bone Marrow Transplant 34(2):161–167

47. Attal M, Harousseau JL, Facon T et al (2003) Single versus double autologous stem-cell transplantation for multiple myeloma. N Engl J Med 349(26):2495–2502

48. Cavo M, Tosi P, Zamagni E et al (2007) Prospective, randomized study of single compared with double autologous stem-cell transplantation for multiple myeloma: Bologna 96 clinical study. J Clin Oncol 25(17):2434–2441

49. Sonneveld P, van der Holt B, Vellenga E et al (2005) Intensive Versus Double Intensive Therapy in Untreated Multiple Myeloma: Final Analysis of the HOVON 24 Trial. Blood 106 (11):2545

50. JP F, C A, JP M. Single versus tandem high dose therapy (HDT) supported with autologous blood stem cell (ABSC) transplantation using unselected or CD34-enriched ABSC: results of a two by two designed randomized trial in 230 young patients with multiple myeloma (MM). Hematol J. 2003;4(Suupl 1):S59

51. Kumar A, Kharfan-Dabaja MA, Glasmacher A, Djulbegovic B (2009) Tandem versus single autologous hematopoietic cell transplantation for the treatment of multiple myeloma: a systematic review and meta-analysis. J Natl Cancer Inst 101(2):100–106

52. Tricot G, Jagannath S, Vesole DH, Crowley J, Barlogie B (1995) Relapse of multiple myeloma after autologous transplantation: survival after salvage therapy. Bone Marrow Transplant 16(1):7–11

53. Elice F, Raimondi R, Tosetto A et al (2006) Prolonged overall survival with second on-demand autologous transplant in multiple myeloma. Am J Hematol 81(6):426–431

54. Morris C, Iacobelli S, Brand R et al (2004) Benefit and timing of second transplantations in multiple myeloma: clinical findings and methodological limitations in a European Group for Blood and Marrow Transplantation registry study. J Clin Oncol 22(9):1674–1681

55. Alexanian R, Balcerzak S, Bonnet JD et al (1975) Prognostic factors in multiple myeloma. Cancer 36(4):1192–1201

56. Treatment comparisons in the third MRC myelomatosis trial (1980) Medical research council's working party on leukaemia in adults. Br J Cancer 42(6):823–830

57. Cohen HJ, Bartolucci AA, Forman WB, Silberman IIR (1986) Consolidation and maintenance therapy in multiple myeloma: randomized comparison of a new approach to therapy after initial response to treatment. J Clin Oncol 4(6):888–899

58. Belch A, Shelley W, Bergsagel D et al (1988) A randomized trial of maintenance versus no maintenance melphalan and prednisone in responding multiple myeloma patients. Br J Cancer 57(1):94–99

59. Berenson JR, Crowley JJ, Grogan TM et al (2002) Maintenance therapy with alternate-day prednisone improves survival in multiple myeloma patients. Blood 99(9):3163–3168

60. Shustik C, Belch A, Robinson S et al (2007) A randomised comparison of melphalan with prednisone or dexamethasone as induction therapy and dexamethasone or observation as maintenance therapy in multiple myeloma: NCIC CTG MY.7. Br J Haematol 136(2):203–211

61. Mellstedt H, Aahre A, Bjorkholm M et al (1979) Interferon therapy in myelomatosis. Lancet 2 (8144):697

62. Fritz E, Ludwig H (2000) Interferon-alpha treatment in multiple myeloma: meta-analysis of 30 randomised trials among 3948 patients. Ann Oncol 11(11):1427–1436

63. Interferon as therapy for multiple myeloma (2001) an individual patient data overview of 24 randomized trials and 4012 patients. Br J Haematol 113(4):1020–1034
64. Singhal S, Mehta J, Desikan R et al (1999) Antitumor activity of thalidomide in refractory multiple myeloma. N Engl J Med 341(21):1565–1571
65. Attal M, Harousseau JL, Leyvraz S et al (2006) Maintenance therapy with thalidomide improves survival in patients with multiple myeloma. Blood 108(10):3289–3294
66. Barlogie B, Tricot G, Anaissie E et al (2006) Thalidomide and hematopoietic-cell transplantation for multiple myeloma. N Engl J Med 354(10):1021–1030
67. Morgan GJ, Davies FE, Gregory WM et al (2013) Long-term follow-up of MRC Myeloma IX trial: survival outcomes with bisphosphonate and thalidomide treatment. Clin Cancer Res 19 (21):6030–6038
68. Morgan GJ, Gregory WM, Davies FE et al (2012) The role of maintenance thalidomide therapy in multiple myeloma: MRC Myeloma IX results and meta-analysis. Blood 119 (1):7–15
69. Lokhorst HM, van der Holt B, Zweegman S et al (2010) A randomized phase 3 study on the effect of thalidomide combined with adriamycin, dexamethasone, and high-dose melphalan, followed by thalidomide maintenance in patients with multiple myeloma. Blood 115(6):1113–1120
70. Stewart AK, Trudel S, Bahlis NJ et al (2013) A randomized phase 3 trial of thalidomide and prednisone as maintenance therapy after ASCT in patients with MM with a quality-of-life assessment: the National Cancer Institute of Canada Clinicals Trials Group Myeloma 10 Trial. Blood 121(9):1517–1523
71. Spencer A, Prince HM, Roberts AW et al (2009) Consolidation therapy with low-dose thalidomide and prednisolone prolongs the survival of multiple myeloma patients undergoing a single autologous stem-cell transplantation procedure. J Clin Oncol 27(11):1788–1793
72. Krishnan A, Pasquini MC, Logan B et al (2011) Autologous haemopoietic stem-cell transplantation followed by allogeneic or autologous haemopoietic stem-cell transplantation in patients with multiple myeloma (BMT CTN 0102): a phase 3 biological assignment trial. Lancet Oncol. 12(13):1195–1203
73. Maiolino A, Hungria VT, Garnica M et al (2012) Thalidomide plus dexamethasone as a maintenance therapy after autologous hematopoietic stem cell transplantation improves progression-free survival in multiple myeloma. Am J Hematol 87(10):948–952
74. Kagoya Y, Nannya Y, Kurokawa M (2012) Thalidomide maintenance therapy for patients with multiple myeloma: meta-analysis. Leuk Res 36(8):1016–1021
75. Richardson PG, Barlogie B, Berenson J et al (2003) A phase 2 study of bortezomib in relapsed, refractory myeloma. N Engl J Med 348(26):2609–2617
76. Attal M, Lauwers-Cances V, Marit G et al (2012) Lenalidomide maintenance after stem-cell transplantation for multiple myeloma. N Engl J Med 366(19):1782–1791
77. Attal M, Lauwers-Cances V, Marit G et al (2013) Lenalidomide maintenance after stem-cell transplantation for multiple myeloma: follow-up analysis of the IFM 2005-02 trial. Blood 122 (21):406
78. McCarthy PL, Owzar K, Hofmeister CC et al (2012) Lenalidomide after stem-cell transplantation for multiple myeloma. N Engl J Med 366(19):1770–1781
79. McCarthy P, Owzar K, Hofmeister CC et al (2013) Analysis of overall survival (OS) in the context of cross-over from placebo to lenalidomide and the incidence of second primary alignancies (SPM) in the phase III study of lenalidomide versus placebo maintenance therapy following autologous stem cell transplant (ASCT) for multiple myeloma (MM) CALGB (Alliance) ECOG BMTCTN. Clin Lymphoma Myeloma Leuk 13(Suppl 1):S28
80. Tricot G, Vesole DH, Jagannath S, Hilton J, Munshi N, Barlogie B (1996) Graft-versus-myeloma effect: proof of principle. Blood 87(3):1196–1198
81. Garban F, Attal M, Michallet M et al (2006) Prospective comparison of autologous stem cell transplantation followed by dose-reduced allograft (IFM99-03 trial) with tandem autologous

stem cell transplantation (IFM99-04 trial) in high-risk de novo multiple myeloma. Blood 107 (9):3474–3480

82. Bruno B, Rotta M, Patriarca F et al (2007) A comparison of allografting with autografting for newly diagnosed myeloma. N Engl J Med 356(11):1110–1120

83. Barlogie B, Jagannath S, Vesole DH et al (1997) Superiority of tandem autologous transplantation over standard therapy for previously untreated multiple myeloma. Blood 89 (3):789–793

Treatment of Relapsed/Refractory Multiple Myeloma

Paola Neri, Nizar J. Bahlis, Claudia Paba-Prada
and Paul Richardson

Abstract

Survival outcomes of patients with Multiple Myeloma (MM) have improved over the last decade due to the introduction of novel agents such as the immunomodulatory drugs thalidomide, lenalidomide (Len) and pomalidomide, and the proteasome inhibitors bortezomib (BTZ) and carfilzomib [1, 2]. However, despite these major advances, MM remains largely incurable and almost all patients relapse and require additional therapy [3]. The successful introduction of next generation novel agents including oral proteasome inhibitors, deacetylase inhibitors, and especially monoclonal antibodies as part of immunotherapy promises to further improve outcome.

Keyword

Relapsed and refractory multiple myeloma · Combination therapy · Novel agents

The terms "relapsed" and "refractory" are sometimes used interchangeably and may differ across studies, but in fact are quite distinct. In general "relapsed" refers to a disease that progresses after a period of remission. According to the International Myeloma Working Group, progressive disease is defined by at least a 25 % increase in serum or urine paraprotein from nadir (absolute increase ≥ 0.5 g/dL and ≥ 200 mg/24 h, respectively), or involved-to-uninvolved serum FLC ratio >100 mg/L. In patients with

P. Neri · N.J. Bahlis
Southern Alberta Cancer Research Institute, University of Calgary,
Calgary, AB, Canada

C. Paba-Prada · P. Richardson (✉)
Jerome Lipper Multiple Myeloma Center, Dana-Farber Cancer Institute,
Boston, MA, USA
e-mail: paul_richardson@dfci.harvard.edu

© Springer International Publishing Switzerland 2016
A.M. Roccaro and I.M. Ghobrial (eds.), *Plasma Cell Dyscrasias*,
Cancer Treatment and Research 169, DOI 10.1007/978-3-319-40320-5_10

Table 1 Definition of relapsed and refractory disease in Multiple Myeloma

Category	Definition
Relapsed myeloma	Disease that progresses after a period of remission, as defined by IMWG criteria
Relapsed and Refractory myeloma	Disease non responsive while in therapy or who progress within 60 days of last therapy
Primary refractory	Patients who never achieve at least a minimal response to therapy and are considered non-responsive
Double refractory	Patients who are relapsed and refractory to both proteasome inhibitors (PIs) and immunomodulatory drugs (IMiDs)

oligo- or nonsecretory myeloma an increase in bone marrow plasma cells (with a ≥ 10 % increase), or new bone or soft tissue lesions, or increasing size of existing bone or soft tissue lesions, or an unexplained serum calcium >11.5 mg/dL is used to define disease progression [4]. In contrast, patients with "refractory" myeloma are those with disease that has relapsed but then progresses while on therapy or who progress within 60 days of last therapy [5]. Patients who never achieve at least a minimal response are defined as "primary refractory". Patients with disease refractory to both proteasome inhibitors and immunomodulatory drugs are now defined as "double-refractory". Definitions of relapsed and refractory MM are shown in Table 1.

Treatment of relapsed and relapsed and refractory multiple myeloma (RRMM) represents a therapeutic challenge due to both disease clonal heterogeneity and intrinsic as well as acquired resistance, which is a hallmark of the disease at this stage of its evolution. It is especially challenging to achieve durable response in patients with high-risk cytogenetics such as del 17p, t(14; 16) and 1q21 amplification and in patients with extramedullary plasma cell involvement. Moreover, while now there are numerous choices for salvage therapies, the optimal timing of therapy and treatment selection at relapse can be complex. In general, patients who experience only a biochemical relapse with a 25 % increase in serum and/or urine paraprotein and are asymptomatic from their myeloma need to be carefully restaged. They can be followed closely without additional treatment if the progression appears to be biochemical only and asymptomatic, although the addition of relatively non-toxic therapy, or participation in clinical trails may be a good option in this setting. However, patients with higher risk disease and clinical progression (e.g., patient with unfavorable cytogenetics, skeletal progression, extramedullary disease, MM-related renal impairment, or aggressive disease at diagnosis) or with rapid increase in serum or urine M-protein in 2 months or less should receive treatment.

1   Treatments Options

The introduction of proteasome inhibitors (PIs) and immunomodulatory drugs (IMiDs) has dramatically increased the survival of myeloma patients. However, the outcome for patients' refractory to BTZ- and Len-based therapies is poor, with a median progression free survival (PFS) of only 5 months and an overall survival (OS) of 9 months [6]. Thus, there remains an urgent need for next generation novel drugs and newer combinations to overcome resistance to current therapies and so further improve outcome. Importantly, there are various options currently available for treatment of RRMM, making the opportunity for rational choices real.

2 Proteasome Inhibitors (PIs)

Bortezomib (BTZ) is a small molecule boronate peptide, and is a reversible, first-in class PI that targets the constitutive proteasome subunit $\beta5$ of the 26S proteasome resulting in the accumulation of misfolded proteins in the plasma cell and leads to apoptosis [7]. It was the first PI developed for treatment of MM and is a very widely used "backbone" agent, both in the upfront and relapsed/refractory setting. Two phase III trials have demonstrated its efficacy in patient with RRMM [8, 9]. In the APEX trial [8], patients treated with intravenous BTZ had significantly higher rates of overall response rate (ORR) (27 %), PFS and 1 year survival compared with high-dose Dexamethasone (Dex). Based on those results, it received FDA and EMEA full approval in 2005, subsequent to its accelerated approval for RR in 2003. In combination with dexamethasone, BTZ has demonstrated clinical benefit without affecting the safety profile and is considered as a reference regimen in the relapsed setting [10]. Based on the observed preclinical synergistic activity with other agents, various combinations have been evaluated in several phase I/II trials. BTZ was initially combined with thalidomide [11] and then with Len and dexamethasone (RVD) [12] and showed that the combination of BTZ with Dex and a third agent (specifically an IMiD) provided a response rate of 61–72 % with manageable toxicity in patients exposed to a median of 1–5 prior therapies. More recently, BTZ has been combined with alkylating agents such as cyclophosphamide [13], the third-generation IMiD pomalidomide [14], and histone deacetylase inhibitors, such as vorinostat [15] and panobinostat [16]. All these studies resulted in high ORR (55–87 %) despite prior PI/IMiD resistance, and therefore a BTZ-based triple combination can be considered a valuable option for the management of RRMM.

A summary of all BTZ-based regimens is shown in Table 2. The major toxicities of BTZ include peripheral neuropathy, thrombocytopenia, diarrhea, and a localized rash when administered subcutaneously. Of note, the MMY-3021 trial demonstrated that subcutaneous BTZ was comparable in terms of efficacy to intravenous BTZ and resulted in significantly reduced peripheral neuropathy [9].

Carfilzomib (CFZ) is a second-generation, epoxyketone, nonreversible PI, FDA approved in 2012 for the treatment of patients with RRMM who have received at least two prior therapies, including the first-generation BTZ and an IMiD. It has demonstrated single agent activity even in patients who are BTZ refractory [17]. In combination with Len and dexamethasone (Dex) CFZ demonstrated an ORR of 77 %, with an ORR of 69 % in BTZ-refractory patients and 70 % in Len-refractory patients [18]. Similar superior results with CFZ in combination with Pomalidomide (Pom) and Dex were seen in heavily pretreated patients, with a median of six lines

Table 2 Summary of key Bortezomib-based regimens in RRMM

Study	Phase	Regimen	Prior lines	PFS (months)	OS (months)
Richardson et al. [8]	III	BTZ versus Dex	2	6.2 versus 3.5	29.8 versus 23.7
Jagannath et al. [10]	II	BTZ-Dex	≥1	TTP 5.3–6.8	NR
Garderet et al. [11]	III	BTZ-TD versus TD	≥2	18.3 versus 13.6	71 % versus 65 %
Dimopoulos et al. [15]	III	BTZ + Vorinostat versus BTZ	2	7.63 versus 6.83	NR versus 28.07
Richardson et al. [16]	II	BTZ + Panobinostat	4	5.4	NR
Richardson et al. [12]	II	BTZ + Len + dex	2	9.5	30
Richardson et al. [14]	II	BTZ + Pom + dex	≥1	NR, DOR 7.4 (ORR 70 %)	NR
De Waal et al. [13]	II	BTZ + Cyclophosphamide + Prednisone	≥2	18.4	28.1

of therapies [19]. Recently, the large international phase III trial, ASPIRE, compared CFZ plus Len + Dex versus Len + Dex among relapsed patients who had received one to three prior therapies. The addition of CFZ to Len + Dex resulted in significant improvement of PFS (26.3 vs. 17.6 months) and a 31 % decrease in the relative risk of progression or death compared to Len + Dex arm [20]. Based on these results, the FDA approved the use of CFZ in combination with Len and Dex for the treatment of patients with relapsed MM who have received one to three prior lines of therapy, in July 2015. Results of the ENDEAVOUR phase 3 trial comparing the efficacy of CFZ (56 mg/m2) versus BTZ both in combination with Dex in RRMM, demonstrated the superiority of CFZ with a median PFS of 18.7 months versus 9.4 months with BTZ and Dex and ORR of 77 % versus 63 % for the CFZ and BTZ arms, respectively [21]. Phase I trials of CFZ in combination with ARRY 520 [22] and panobinostat [23] have also shown promising results.

A summary of CFZ-based regimens is shown in Table 3. It is generally well tolerated, but its use is associated with myelosuppression, fatigue, diarrhea, renal dysfunction, thrombosis and importantly cardiovascular side effects, including hypertension, stroke, myocardial ischemia, and pulmonary hypertension. Cardiotoxicity (and in particular cardiac failure) may also be exacerbated by the use of concomitant intravenous fluid hydration to reduce the risk of tumor lysis and protect renal function. Therefore patients with preexisting thrombotic risk, heart failure, or poorly controlled hypertension should be monitored closely. Neuropathy is very infrequent [24], making CFZ particularly attractive in patients with significant neuropathy, whereas other disadvantages include consecutive days of administration requiring six infusion visits in a 28-day cycle.

Ixazomib (MLN9708) is a reversible oral PI in the boronate peptide class, with superior tissue penetration and greater biological activities [25] when compared with BTZ. As a single agent in two single-arm, phase I trials, it demonstrated ORR of 15 and 27 % in 60 heavily pretreated patients with RRMM, including patients refractory to BTZ [26, 27]. In combination with Len and Dex, it has been well tolerated and has

Table 3 Summary of key Carfilzomib-based regimens

Study	Phase	Regimen	Prior lines	PFS (months)	OS (months)
Vij et al. [17]	II	CFZ 20 mg/m^2 versus 27 mg/m^2	2	8.2 versus NR	NR versus NR
Stewart et al. [20]	III	CFZ + Len + dex versus Len + dex	1–3	26.3 versus 17.6	NR
Dimopoulos et al. [21]	III	CFZ + dex versus BTZ + dex	1–3	18.7 versus 9.4	NR
Shah et al. [19]	I	CFZ + Pom + dex	≥2	7.2	20.6
Shah et al. [22]	I	CFZ + ARRY-520	4	NR	NR
Berdeja et al. [23]	I/II	CFZ + Panobinostat	≥1	3.5–18.7	NR

exhibited deeper responses as well as excellent PFS in newly diagnosed MM [28, 29]. Recent results from the Phase 3 study, TOURMALINE-MM1, showed that the addition of ixazomib to Len and Dex (IRd) in pts with RRMM significantly increased median PFS to 20.6 from 14.7 mos without a substantial increase in overall toxicity. Benefit of IRd was also noted in pts with high-risk cytogenetics, including those with del(17), in whom median PFS was similar to all IRd-treated pts indicating that ixazomib may have a favorable impact on patients with high-risk cytogentics [30]. Based on these results, in November 2015 the FDA approved the use of Ixazomib in combination with Len and Dex for the treatment of patients with relapsed MM who have received at least one prior lines of therapy. This is the first all-oral triplet regimen containing a proteasome inhibitor and an IMiD drug that may become a new standard of care in this setting. The drug is well tolerated, with a remarkably lower toxicity profile and low rate of peripheral neuropathy than other PI's. The most common side effects include fatigue, skin rash, gastrointestinal toxicity, and thrombocytopenia, but significant cardiovascular or renal toxicity is not seen.

Other next generation PIs, such as marizomib and oprozomib, are in the early stage of clinical development. A phase I trial of Marizomib in 34 RRMM, including 74 % BTZ-refractory patients, showed a PR rates of 20 % as a single agent [31]. Phase II response data for oprozomib in combination with Dex are also promising with ORR of 36 % [32]. Combination trials are currently under evaluation and show promise for marizomib and pomalidomide (Pom) in particular [33, 34]. The most common side effects of oprozomib include significant gastrointestinal toxicity such as diarrhea, nausea and vomiting, which has proven challenging. Marizomib has shown manageable CNS toxicity and fatigue but minimal neuropathy and thrombocytopenia, and no significant cardiopulmonary toxicity to date.

2.1 Immunomodulatory (IMiDs) Drugs

Thalidomide (Thal), the prototypic IMiD, was the first novel drug with known activity in the RRMM setting, with an ORR of 25 % when used as a single agent

[35] and up to 50 % when used in combination with high-dose Dex [36]. It has been effectively combined with cyclophosphamide [37], bortezomib [11], and more recently with CFZ [38]. Although now used less frequently in the management of RRMM, due to the more extensive use of next generation IMiDs, and the lack of data on its activity in Len- or Pom-refractory patients, it nonetheless remains a worldwide standard due to its accessibility, minimal myelosuppression and lack of nephrotoxicity as a combinatorial agent. Since it is almost exclusively eliminated as a hydrolysed product Thal is safe in patients with renal failure and has a role in patients with severe cytopenias in combination with steroids and BTZ, as well as other agents and in particular cytotoxic chemotherapy such as cyclophosphamide, bendamustine, liposomal doxorubicin, and melphalan. Important side effects include neuropathy, somnolence, thrombosis, and constipation.

Lenalidomide (Len) is an analog of Thal with higher potency and less toxicity [39]. Phase I and II trials demonstrated single agent activity in RRMM with PR rates of 24–29 % [40]. In 2006 it was approved by the FDA in combination with Dex for the treatment of patients with relapsed MM and at least one prior line of therapy. This approval was based on the results of two randomized, placebo-controlled phase II trials, MM009 [41] and MM010 [42] that confirmed the benefit of Len and Dex versus Dex alone in OS (38 vs. 31.6 months, respectively), although 47.6 % of patients in the Dex arm received Len-based treatment after disease progression or unblinding [43]. The combination of Len with new emerging new molecules has been extensively investigated in the last few years. It has been successfully combined with cytotoxic agents such as cyclophosphamide [44] and monoclonal antibodies such as elotuzumab [45] and daratumumab [46] as well as with PIs such as BTZ [12] and CFZ [18]. All these studies showed that the combination of Len-dex with a third agent in patients exposed to prior therapies resulted in higher ORR from 65 % to 95 % improving the outcome of RRMM patients. A summary of all Len-based regimens is shown in Table 4.

Table 4 Summary of key Lenalidomide-based regimens

Study	Phase	Regimen	Prior lines	PFS (months)	OS (months)
Weber et al. [41]	III	Len-dex versus Dex	≥2	11.1 versus 4.7	29.6 versus 20.2
Dimopoulos et al. [42]	III	Len-dex versus Dex	≥2	11.3 versus 4.7	NR versus 20.6
Richardson et al. [45]	Ib/II	Len-dex + Elotuzumab (10–20 mg/kg)	1–3	32.49 versus 25	NR
Richardson et al. [12]	II	Len-BTZ-Dex	2	9.5	30
Wang et al. [18]	II	CFZ-Len-Dex	NR	15.4	NR
Reece et al. [44]	I-II	Cyclophosphamide + Prednisone + Len	2	16.1	27.6
Plesner et al. [46]	I/II	Daratumumab + Len and Dex	≥1	72 % at 18 mo	90 % at 18 mo

In patients relapsing during Len maintenance, increasing the dose of Len to 25 mg and/or the addition of Dex may restore response in patients with low tumor burden and less aggressive disease. More commonly, the addition of a third agent is needed to induce response. Len's main toxicities include myelosuppression, fatigue, thrombosis, muscle cramps, chronic diarrhea, and possibly an increased risk of second primary malignancies. The chronic diarrhea seen may be related to bile-acid malabsorption and may respond to reduction of fat intake in the diet and treatment with bile-acid sequestrants [40, 47].

Pomalidomide (Pom) is a third-generation IMiD agent and was granted accelerated approval by the FDA in 2013 for RRMM in patients with previous use of BTZ and Len. It has similar properties to Thal and Len but is much more potent in vitro, and has proven efficacy in heavily pretreated patients, and even in those refractory to Len and BTZ, with its accelerated approval primarily based upon the favorable results of the MM-02 study [48, 49]. Furthermore, in the MM-03 trial comparing Pom-dex versus high-dose Dex in patients who had received a median of five lines of therapies, Pom-dex induced a 32 % ORR, with median PFS and OS of 4 and 13 months, respectively [50]. This randomized study resulted in the full approval of Pom-dex for RRMM in 2015. More recently, the addition of a third drug to Pom-dex has been explored in several phase I-II studies in order to improve clinical outcome. Preliminary data from phase II randomized trials showed that Pom-dex combined with alkylating agents such as Cyclophosphamide [51, 52], first- or second-generation PI BTZ [14] and with CFZ [19] or Clarithromycin [53], resulted in higher ORR from 32 % to 81 % and improved PFS from 4 to 17 months in patients with RRMM previously exposed to BTZ and Len.

A summary of the Pom-based regimens is shown in Table 5. Overall Pom is generally very well tolerated and the main side effects include myelosuppression,

Table 5 Summary of key Pomalidomide-based regimens

Study	Phase	Regimen	Prior lines	PFS (months)	OS (months)
Leleu et al. [48]	II	Pom q1-21 versus q 28 + dex	5	5.4 versus 3.7	14.9 versus 14.8
Richardson et al. [49]	II	Pom + dex versus Pom	5	4.2 versus 2.7	16.6 versus 13.6
San Miguel et al. [50]	III	Pom + dex versus Dex	5	4 versus 1.9	12.7 versus 8.1
Mark et al. [53]	II	Clarithromycin + Pom + dex	5	8.3	19.3
Richardson et al. [14]	II	Pom + BTZ + dex	≥ 1	NR, DOR 7.4	NR
Shah et al. [19]	I	CFZ + Pom + dex	≥ 2	7.2	20.6
Baz et al. [52]	II	Cyclophosphamide + Pom + Dex	3	9.5	NR
Larocca et al. [51]	II	Cyclophosphamide + Pom + Prednisone	3	10.4	NR

thrombosis, rash, and constipation. Neuropathy is rarely seen, although worsening of preexisting neuropathy has been reported but is usually mild to moderate.

2.2 Immunotherapies

Recently several immunotherapeutic approaches have been explored in patients with RRMM and have shown promising results.

Among them, monoclonal antibodies (MoAbs) have emerged as an attractive targeted strategy based on the wide range of antigens expressed on the surface of plasma cells.

Elotuzumab (Elo) is a humanized MoAb specifically targeting SLAMF7 (signaling lymphocytic activation molecule family member 7), also known as CS1, a glycoprotein highly expressed on myeloma and natural killer cells [54]. It exerts dual mechanism of action by directly activating natural killer cells and tumor cell death via antibody-dependent cellular cytotoxicity (ADCC) [57]. As a single agent, Elo has shown modest activity; however, encouraging results have been recently shown when Elo was combined with Len and Dex [55, 56]. The ELOQUENT-2 trial, a phase III randomized trial comparing the efficacy and safety of Len-Dex with or without Elo in RRMM patients has shown that the combination of Elo-Len-dex demonstrated an ORR of 79 % versus 66 % in the Len-Dex arm and resulted in an extended PFS compared with the control arm (19.4 months vs. 14.9 months, respectively), reducing the risk of progression or death by 30 %. This benefit was maintained regardless of patient age, number of prior line of therapies, previous exposure to Len or the presence of high-risk cytogenetics, such as del 17(p) or t(4;14) [58]. Based on these results, Elo was approved by FDA on November 30, 2015, for use with Len/dex in patients with RRMM and 1–3 prior therapies. A recent update of the ELOQUENT-2 trial has also shown that at 3-year follow-up, pts receiving Elo had 27 % reduction in risk of progression or death versus Len/dex alone and had median delay of 1 year in time to next treatment versus Len/dex arm [59]. In terms of the safety profile, the most common side effects were lymphocpenia, neutropenia, and fatigue. Infusion reactions to Elo occurred in 10 % or less of patients and were of mild to moderate grade only. In combination with BTZ, results of a phase II trial showed an ORR of 66 % in the Elo arm versus 63 % in patients treated with BTZ and Dex alone. Importantly, the PFS was significantly better at 9.7 months in the Elo arm versus 6.9 months in the BTZ/dex arm [60]. Infusion reactions occurred in 7 % of patients in the Elo arm and the most common side effects were thrombocytopenia and infections, with an otherwise very favorable tolerability profile.

Daratumumab (Dara) is a humanized MoAb that targets CD38-which is highly expressed in myeloma cells. It induces the killing of CD38-expressing tumor cells via ADCC, antibody-dependent phagocytosis, complement-depend cytotoxicity, and apoptosis [61]. As a single agent, in the phase II SIRIUS trial, Dara demonstrated an ORR of 29 % and a median PFS of 3.7 months in patients with RRMM, all prior exposed and refractory to BTZ and Len. The median time to response among responders was 1 month and the median duration of response was 7.4 months [63, 64]. Patients experienced modest infusion-related reactions and manageable hematological toxicity including anemia, neutropenia, and thrombocytopenia. Based on the favorable toxicity profile and efficacy, Dara was FDA approved on November 2015 for use in MM pts with ≥ 3 prior therapies. Recent results of a Phase 1/2 Study (GEN503) of Dara in combination with Len/dex showed rapid, deep, and durable responses in RRMM patients. The ORR was 81 % including 28 % VGPR and 34 % CR/sCR with median 15.6 months follow-up. At 18 months, the PFS was 72 % and the OS was 90 %. The toxicity profile was similar to that reported by studies of DARA monotherapy and no additional toxicities were observed [46]. Two phase III studies of Dara are currently ongoing, one in combination with Len and Dex versus Len and Dex (MMY3003) and one in combination with BTZ and Dex versus BTZ and Dex alone (MMY3004) with very promising early results reported in both studies. The combination of Dara with Pom and Dex is also being evaluated in ongoing Phase I trial. An early analysis has shown rapid initial responses that are deepening over time. Specifically, the ORR was 71 and 67 % in patients' double refractory to PI/IMiDs, and showed a tolerable safety profile similar to Pom/dex alone [65].

Isatuximab (SAR650984) is another MoAb that binds selectively to a unique epitope on the human CD38 receptor with strong pro-apoptotic activity in MM cells. It induces the killing of CD38-expressing plasma cells via ADCC, antibody-dependent phagocytosis and complement-depend cytotoxicity [66]. It has shown promising activity and tolerability as a single agent in a single-arm, phase I trial of patients with RRMM. The ORR was 32 % and the most side effects were GI disorders, cough, fatigue, and hematological toxicity [67]. A phase II trial and further combination strategies are current ongoing.

Indatuximab is a chimeric anti-CD138 MoAb conjugated to DM4, a maytansinoid cytotoxic agent. Preliminary results from a phase I/II trial of Indatuximab in combination with Len and dex showed an encouraging ORR of 78 %, with 10 % sCR/CR and 33 % VGPR. The most common adverse events were diarrhea, fatigue, nausea, and hypokalemia, as well as gastrointestinal toxicity [68].

Encouraging results are also emerging from the use of chimeric antigen receptor (CAR) T-cells that are engineered to target antigens expressed on MM cells leading to direct MM cells killing and T-cell immunity stimulation. Autologous transplantation followed by treatment with CAR-T cells against CD19 (CTL019) demonstrated a significant activity in a patient with refractory MM. It led to a complete response with no evidence of progression and measurable serum or urine monoclonal protein at a follow-up of 12 months [69]. Promising results are also coming from CAR-T cell therapy targeting BCMA, the B-cell maturation antigen expressed by normal and malignant plasma cells. Preliminary results of a Phase I trial of an anti-BCMA chimeric antigen receptor (CAR-BCMA) in patients with advanced MM and a median of seven prior lines of therapy, showed strong anti-MM activity at higher dose level with durable sCR achieved in two patients with a high disease burden and chemotherapy-resistant disease. Substantial but reversible toxicity was observed. These included cytopenias attributable to chemotherapy, fever, and signs of cytokine release syndrome including tachycardia and hypotension delirium, hypoxia, and coagulopathy [70]. Additional studies of other CAR-T cell therapies targeting CD38, CD138, and CS1 are currently under evaluation in clinical trials.

In addition, MoAbs generated to block the inhibitory interaction of PD-1 on T or NK cells with its ligand PD-L1 on tumor cells or tumor-promoting accessory cells have also showed remarkable responses in both solid tumors and hematologic malignancies [71]. Several studies have shown that overexpression of PD-L1 is associated with tumor invasiveness in MM cells [72] and this may be a mechanism of immune evasion. At the present, there are multiple clinical trials exploring the use of checkpoint inhibitors in patients with RRMM.

Pembrolizumab is a highly selective anti-PD-1 monoclonal antibody designed to block the interaction of PD-1 with PD-L1 and PD-L2 that has been recently evaluated in patients with RRMM in combination with IMiDs, due to their ability to enhance MM-specific cytotoxic T cells. Preliminary results of the KEYNOTE-023, a nonrandomized, open-label, dose-escalation phase I trial exploring the safety, tolerability, and efficacy of Pembrolizumab in combination with Len/dex showed promising efficacy in heavily pretreated RRMM. The ORR was 76 %, with four patients achieving a very good partial response and nine patients achieving a partial response with a duration of response of 9.7 months. Responses were observed also in patients with IMiDs-refractory and double-refractory disease [73]. The combination also had a tolerable safety profile, consistent with the individual drug profiles and no obvious additive effects. The most common adverse events were anemia, pneumonia, neutropenia, thrombocytopenia, hyperglycemia, dyspnea, and the immune-related side effects included pneumonitis, hypothyroidism, and hepatitis. Promising results are also coming from the Phase II study evaluating the safety and efficacy of Pembrolizumab with Pom + dexamethasone in RRMM. Early evidence of deep, durable responses were observed in this heavily treated population. The ORR was 59 % in all cohort of patients, and 50 % in patients' double refractory to PIs and IMiDs [74]. The combination proved tolerable with a manageable safety profile, although some evidence of an increased incidence of pneumonitis was noted. Otherwise, no overt additional toxicity was observed.

The anti-PD-1 antibody nivolumab (BMS936558), alone or in combination with the CTLA4-blocking antibody ipilimumab or the killer cell immunoglobulin-like receptor-blocking antibody lirilumab, is also under evaluation in a phase 1 clinical trial in relapsed or refractory hematologic malignancies, including MM (NCT01592370).

A summary of additional monoclonal antibodies currently in clinical development for RRMM in combination with PI or IMiD-based regimens is shown in Table 6.

Table 6 Summary of next-generation Monoclonal Antibodies under investigation in RRMM (daratumumab and elotuzumab)

MoAb	Target	Combination	Phase
Tabalumab	BAFF		II
Isatuximab	CD38	Len/dex CFZ Pom/dex	I
Indatuximab	CD138	Len/dex	I/II
Milatuzimab	CD74		I/II
MOR03087	CD38		I/II
Pidilizumab	PD-1	Len	I/II
Pembrolizumab [73, 74]	PD-1	Len/Dex Pom	I/II
Nivolumab	PD-1	Lirilumab	I
Atezolizumab	PDL-1	Len	I
Lirilumab	KIR	Elotuzumab	I
Urelumab	CD137	Elotuzumab	I

2.3 Salvage ASCT

A number of studies have examined outcomes of second ASCT for relapsed MM in patients who had ASCT at an earlier point in their disease management. Retrospective or single-center studies revealed that ASCT following high-dose therapy resulted in clinical benefit with an ORR of 65 % and prolonged control of disease with PFS and OS approaching 12 and 32 months, respectively [75–77]. However, the optimal timing of the salvage ASCT is still unclear. Recently, a phase III trial evaluating the efficacy of salvage ASCT with conventional chemotherapy (cyclophosphamide) demonstrated improvement in PFS (19 months vs. 11 months) but not OS. Patients with adverse cytogenetics had markedly poorer outcomes, suggesting that salvage ASCT may not be beneficial in this subset of patients [78]. Several studies have suggested that an interval of 18 months is at least needed, with a range of 1.5–3 years from the first ASCT to relapse to result in a second PFS of about half that time after salvage ASCT, leading many centers to consider a minimum of 18 months as a reasonable interval to recommend second ASCT in relapsed MM or RRMM patients [79–81]. With the availability of highly effective novel agents such as BTZ, Len, CFZ, and Pom in the relapsed setting, as well as the emerging role of next generation agents, the role of salvage ASCT must be weighed carefully against toxicity and activity of the more effective therapies in the salvage setting.

Overall the use of salvage ASCT may be a reasonable option to consider for young transplant eligible patients with good performance status and with prolonged response to the first ASCT (i.e., at least 18–24 months). Future prospective studies are necessary to assess the impact of salvage ASCT in the era of novel agents, as its role continues to evolve.

2.4 Allogenic Stem Cell Transplant in RRMM

The role of allogenic stem cell transplant (allo-SCT) as a salvage therapy for RRMM remains an area of debate and active research. Although a small proportion of patients may have long-term benefit, the mortality and morbidity in particular from acute/chronic graft-versus-host disease associated with allo-SCT usually outweighs the benefit [82, 83]. A retrospective case-matched analysis by the European Group for Blood and Marrow Transplantation (EBMT) compared outcomes of patients treated with allo-SCT or ASCT for RRMM. They showed inferior median survival with allo-SCT compared to ASCT (18 months vs. 34 months, respectively), mainly due to increased transplant-related mortality in allo-SCT (41 % vs. 13 %), which in turn was not compensated by the lower rate of relapse and progression [84]. Transplant-related mortality may be decreased in patients who receive a reduced-intensity or non-myeloablative conditioning allo-SCT. However, results from published studies in newly diagnosed MM patients treated with this approaches appear conflicting [85, 86].

Overall the probability of benefit from an allo-SCT in a patient with aggressive disease or in patients with high-risk RRMM remains unclear. Outside of the context of a clinical trial, the use of allo-SCT should not be routinely considered.

3 Factors Influencing Treatment Choices

With many options available there is no simple or ideal sequence of treatments that has been established. The choice is based on a series of factors summarized in Table 7 and the goal is to balance efficacy and toxicity. Those determinants include: *Disease-related factors* such as risk stratification based on chromosomal abnormalities, the presence or absence of extramedullary disease; *Regimen-related factors* such as previous drug exposure, regimen-related toxicity (such as peripheral neuropathy, myelosuppression, and other toxicities) as well as previous depth and duration of response, and finally *Patient-related factors*, such as age, frailty, renal impairment, and other comorbidities.

Table 7 Factors influencing treatment choices

Disease-related factors	High versus standard risk Presence versus absence of extramedullary disease
Regimen-related factors	Prior drug exposure: response and duration Regimen-related toxicity
Patients related factors	Age/Frailty Presence versus absence of organ function Overall goals of care

3.1 Disease-Related Factors

High-risk chromosomal abnormalities, such as deletion of 17p13 (del17p) or the presence of chromosomal translocations t(4; 14), t(14; 16), and t(14; 20) are associated with reduced response rates and shorter survival [87]. Decision-making on salvage therapy for high-risk patients is difficult due to the limited number of prospective studies available. Studies in newly diagnosed patients suggest that combinations of newer agents may partially overcome the adverse prognosis conferred by the poor-risk genetics. In a study from the IFM, it was shown that BTZ improved both the PFS and OS of patients with t(4;14) but not of patients with del(17p) [88]. Conversely, data from the HOVON-65 study indicated that patients with del(17p) in the PAD (BTZ, Adriamycin, and Dex) arm have significantly better PFS and OS when compared with the VAD arm. Better results were also achieved in patients with t(4;14) receiving PAD, though statistical significance was not reached [89]. Conflicting data merge from retrospective trials of Len and dex in pts with high-risk cytogenetics [90, 91], while Pom combination therapies have shown consistent promise. In the MM-003 study, which compared Pom in combination with low-dose Dex versus high-dose Dex, Pom and low-dose Dex was superior in terms of ORR, PFS, and OR in patients with poor-risk cytogenetics [92]. Pom therapy was also associated with longer PFS in patients with del(17p) in a prospective study from the IFM [93]. Deeper responses were observed in another combination study of Pom with BTZ and Dex in high-risk patients [94] suggesting that combinations of Pom and PI represent a valid approach for high-risk patients in particular.

As secondary genetic events are often present in the relapsed setting, patients should be evaluated at the time of relapse for the presence of del(17p) at the minimum, as well as other mutations. Patients with high-risk features should be encouraged to participate in clinical trials of novel agents, but off protocol combinations incorporating PI's, IMiDs, MoAbs, and other next generation agents are rational choices for such patients in the absence of an appropriate study.

Extramedullary disease is generally associated with poor outcome [95], and extramedullary relapses are associated with lower overall survival and increased risk of bone plasmacytomas and/or fractures [96]. At this stage, relatively few options may exist for effective disease control. Multi-agent combinations of chemotherapies incorporating novel agents have been used with some success. The most commonly used chemo-therapeutic regimen is VDT-PACE (BTZ, dex + thal with infusion of cisplatin, doxorubicin, cyclophosphamide, and etoposide), which is generally reserved as salvage therapy for aggressive MM and/or plasma cell leukemia (PCL) resistant to other therapies [97]. Although the overall response rate of approximately 50 % in this poor prognosis cohort is encouraging, these responses remain typically short and toxicity is considerable, so this regimen is used typically as a bridge to more active and durable therapies, as well as participation in clinical trials.

3.2   Regimen-Related Factors

The specific agents and drug combination regimens that patients have previously
received are important to consider when evaluating how to treat MM that has
relapsed.

Patients who have progressed on the first-generation IMiDs, PIs, double or triple
combination therapies (such as Len + Dex, BTZ + Dex, Thal + Dex, BTZ +
Thal + Dex, Cyclophosphamide + BTZ + Dex, RVD therapy) can be treated with
next generation regimens such as CFZ + Dex, Pom + Dex, Pom + Cyclo + Dex,
Pom + BTZ + Dex (PVD).

Retreatment with prior therapies can also be considered especially if the patient
has had a durable response to similar treatment previously and tolerance was
acceptable. Genetic studies have showed that MM at presentation is composed of an
array of multiple clones, each potentially associated with different clinical behavior.
The concept of clonal tides and intra-clonal heterogeneity [98, 99] becomes
extremely important when it comes to the treatment of relapsed disease. Since the
prevalence of MM clones changes over time, it is not unreasonable to retreat a
patient with a treatment that was proven to be effective in a previous disease phase
as the clone present may not have been selected for resistance to that treatment.
Data from the VISTA [100] and MM-015 [101] studies indicate that reuse of BTZ
and Len is associated with a response of 50–60 %, especially in patients who
responded to VMP or MPR, respectively.

Avoiding the agents that have resulted in significant prior regimen-related toxicity is also essential. Peripheral neuropathy is commonly observed in patients with
relapsed MM due to complication of both the disease and treatment-related toxicities. Patients previously treated with thalidomide or BTZ may have residual
peripheral neuropathy and, if significant, should be treated with other agents.
A phase III study has demonstrated that subcutaneous BTZ may be a suitable
alternative due to substantially reduced neuropathy [9]. A CFZ-based regimen is
also a potentially very valuable alternative due to its reduced incidence of peripheral
neuropathy, as long as other potential side effects such as cardiovascular risk or
renal toxicity are not a concern [24].

The duration of prior remission is also a critical consideration. A relapse within
the first 12 months should be treated differently than a relapse that occurs later in
the course of the disease. These patients should receive more intensive combinations of a PIs plus a novel IMiDs such as BTZ + Rev + Dex [12], CFZ + Rev +
Dex [20]. In summary, retreatment with agents from the initial regimen may be
considered in patients who achieved a partial response or better and a remission
lasting 12 months or longer [102, 103], and in combination. Patients who relapse
rapidly following initial treatment should ideally receive a different class of agent if
feasible, with a rational combination utilizing a PI and/or IMiD backbone, and
should also be encouraged to participate in clinical trials.

3.3   Patient-Related Factors

Patient age is a significant prognostic factor for patients with MM; specifically, patients who are ≥ 50 years of age at diagnosis have shorter survival than younger patients [104]. Since older patients usually present with multiple comorbidities and treatment-related toxicities at relapse, a geriatric assessment including the frailty indices should be performed [105]. Patients who are fit (who do not require assistance for household tasks) should receive treatments at the doses and intervals similar to the younger patients. Patients who are unfit (who can perform limited activities) should be treated with reduced doses and longer intervals. For frail patients (who need help for household tasks and personal care), supportive care with or without low doses of anti-myeloma drugs should be considered, and the involvement of internal medicine specialists to help with comorbidities is recommended.

Renal dysfunction is a common comorbidity in patient with MM and results from immunoglobulin deposition in the renal tubes that characteristically lead to kidney dysfunction. In the relapsed setting, the overproduction of the involved free light chain may lead to overt cast nephropathy, which may not be present at diagnosis. In addition 5–15 % of patients may present with "light chain escape" at relapse and may develop significant renal impairment (RI) in this setting. The presence of renal dysfunction may have an impact on treatment decisions. The Apex study [106] and the ASPIRE trial [20] have shown that the BTZ and CFZ therapies have activity in patients with renal impairment, and BTZ the drug of choice for patients on dialysis and significant renal dysfunction; BTZ can also be used without dose adjustment since BTZ has been shown to be safe in this setting. In contrast, caution with CFZ is warranted given the increased incidence of renal dysfunction seen with its use in advanced RRMM. Among IMiDs, Thal is almost exclusively eliminated as hydrolysis products and does not require dose adjustments [107], Len requires dose adjustment [108] but based upon Pom data from three pivotal trials (MM-002, MM-003, MM-010) comparable efficacy and tolerability of Pom + LoDEX in pts with or without moderate RI has been demonstrated [109]. Preliminary data from the MM-013 study also showed efficacy and safety of Pom + LoDEX in RRMM pts with moderate or severe RI, including those on dialysis [110].

Overall, patients with renal impairment should be treated with agents that are not excreted by the kidney, such as proteasome inhibitors (especially BTZ). Dose adjustments may be needed in patients with moderate or severe renal impairment who are treated with agents excreted by the kidney such as Len. Preliminary results have also shown that Pom can also be used in patients with relapsed MM and renal impairment quite safely, making it an attractive agents in this context.

4   Emerging Next Generation Novel Therapies

A range of small molecules with various mechanisms of action are currently in clinical trials in patients with RRMM; key agents are described below.

Histone Deacetylase Inhibitors (HDACi) are a new class of anticancer agents in clinical development in many malignancies including MM. HDACi target the enzyme histone deacetylase (HDAC) involved in the deacetylation of histone and non-histone cellular proteins that play important roles in epigenetic regulation of gene expression inducing death, apoptosis and cell cycle arrest in cancer cells [111]. In MM cells, HDACi inhibit cell growth and induce apoptosis as a single and are also synergistic with BTZ [112]. Clinically, the activity of HDACi is limited, but when combined with Dex or BTZ in patients with RRMM, HDACi are able to overcome BTZ resistance, due to the simultaneous targeting of the ubiquitin pro-teasome pathway by BTZ and the aggresome protein degradation pathway by HDACi. Several class-specific inhibitors or pan-deacetylase inhibitors are currently under evaluation in RRMM.

Vorinostat, a pan-HDACi, was evaluated as monotherapy in a single-arm, phase I trial of patients with advanced MM. Only modest clinical activity was observed, however the agent was well tolerated with GI disorders and fatigue being the most common adverse effects [113]. The combination of vorinostat with BTZ was eval-uated in the double blinded, phase III, VANTAGE 088 trial of early relapsed MM patients receiving one to three prior therapies. An ORR of 56 % was observed in patients receiving vorinostat in combination with BTZ, but only a modest improvement in PFS was observed, 7.6 months in the vorinostat group versus 6.8 months in the placebo arm. Adverse effects included mainly thrombocytopenia and GI toxicity, and there was a high rate of treatment discontinuation in this context [15].

In contrast, panobinostat (LBH589) is a highly potent pan-HDACi with demonstrated anti-tumor activities at low nanomolar concentration in several pre-clinical studies and so may have better tolerability. In MM, preclinical data con-firmed synergistic activity when combined with BTZ or Len [114]. Results of the phase II, PANORAMA 2, and phase III, PANORAMA 1, clinical trials showed that the addition of LBH589 to dexamethasone and BTZ induced responses in 35 % of patients with RRMM who were previously refractory to BTZ and also high risk [16, 115]. In PANORAMA 1, its addition induced an ORR of 59 % compared with 41 % in the BTZ and Dex arm, and a highly significant improvement in PFS of 10.9 months compared with 5.8 months in patients receiving BTZ and Dex alone. However, due to serious adverse effects associated with panobinostat use when combined with IV BTZ given twice a week according to the classical schedule (including severe diarrhea, fatigue and thrombocytopenia), its use needs to be closely monitored [115], and weekly BTZ appears to be better tolerated [115]. Of note, based on these results, panobinostat was recently approved in February 2015 for the treatment of relapsed MM patients who had received more than two lines of therapies, including BTZ and an IMiD. Promising results are also reported from the combination of panobinostat with Len and Dex in RRMM. Data from a recent Phase II study demonstrated that the addition of panobinostat to Len and Dex induced encouraging ORR (38 %) and a duration of response of 6 months, even in Len-ref patients with high-risk molecular findings. In contrast to PANORAMA 1, this regimen seems well tolerated with no significant GI toxicities and manageable hematologic toxicities [116]. Early phase I and II studies exploring LBH589 in combination with CFZ [23] are also ongoing.

Rocilinostat (ACY-1215) is a selective inhibitor of HDAC-6, developed to minimize the toxicities associated with the other pan-HDACi. Similar to other agents in this class, the efficacy of ACY-1215 as single agent is modest; however, it showed potent synergistic activity with PIs and IMiDs in preclinical models and early clinical results are very encouraging and support this promise [117, 118]. Specifically, results of a phase I/II trial investigating ACY-1215 in combination with BTZ and Dex in heavily pretreated patients demonstrated favorable results to date. With a median follow-up of 3 (1–18) months; ORR ($\geq$ PR) was 39 % and toxicity was manageable with diarrhea and hematologic of low grade. Responses were observed among BTZ-refractory patients [119]. Early phase I and II studies exploring ACY-1215 in combination with Len or Pom and Dex are also ongoing in patients with RRMM. Preliminary results showed encouraging tolerability and promising clinical activity [120, 121].

XPO1 inhibitors The nuclear export protein XPO1 is overexpressed in all types of hematological malignancies including MM [122, 123]. Selinexor (KPT-330) is a novel, first-in-class, slowly reversible XPO1 antagonist that forces the nuclear retention of major tumor suppressor proteins (TSPs) such as p53, IkB, FOXO, and p21 leading subsequently in cancer cell death [123]. Preclinical studies have shown that inhibitors of the nuclear export receptor XPO1, in combination with BTZ, CFZ, doxorubicin, or melphalan, synergistically induced apoptosis in MM cells in vitro and in vivo [124, 125]. In early phase I/II clinical trial, selinexor showed anti-myeloma activity as a single agents (ORR of 23 %) in heavily pretreated patients, however adverse events have been recorded, including nausea, fatigue, and anorexia that required prophylaxis with steroids, anti-nausea agents, appetite stimulants to improve tolerability [126]. Early phase I-II studies are now exploring KPT-330 in combination with CFZ in patients with RRMM. Preliminary results demonstrated encouraging activity with 75 % PR or better and no unexpected toxicities in highly refractory MM pts, including those previously refractory to CFZ [127]. In addition, a multicenter, open-label, randomized phase I-II clinical study of Selinexor (KPT-330) in combination with backbone treatments (BTZ, Len and Pom) is currently ongoing to assess its efficacy, and safety in patients with RRMM (KCP-330-017: STORM).

KSP Inhibitors ARRY-520 is a kinesin-spindle protein (KSP) inhibitor that induces cell death targeting the KSP and inhibiting spindle formation during mitosis. As a single agent ARRY-520 has modest activity, an ORR of 16 % was observed in patients' refractory to BTZ, Len, and Dex [128]. In a phase I trial, in combination with BTZ and Dex ARRY-520 was active with 31 % of PRs observed in patients with RRMM. The main toxicities were hematologic adverse events and fatigue [129]. Early phase I-II studies are now exploring ARRY-520 in combination with CFZ in patients with RRMM. Preliminary results demonstrated that the combination of ARRY-520 and CFZ was well tolerated, with limited hematological toxicities, and noticeably increased in the ORR compared to CFZ alone (30 % vs. 10 %, respectively). Responses were observed also in pts who are double refractory to IMiDs and BTZ. The ORR was 35 % in patients randomized to CFZ + ARRY-520 versus 14 % in pts treated with CFZ alone [130].

Several other small molecules as well as modified cytotoxics targeting different cell functions and pathways are still in early phases of development in MM and may represent additional treatment options for patients with RRMM in the near future.

5 Conclusion

Although MM remains an incurable disease, the improved survival rates achieved over the last decade are a reflection of more effective new therapies now available for patients both in the upfront and relapsed settings. Encouragingly, multiple treatments options are emerging for patients with RRMM. However, prospective randomized trials directly comparing the different combinations remain limited as the pace of change is proving so rapid, and thus new standards of care for the treatment of RRMM are difficult to define, although clearly three drug regimens now appear consistently superior to two drug regimens in specific settings. The choice of optimal salvage therapy and treatment sequencing therefore depends on several characteristics that relate to both disease and patient-specific features. In this context, risk stratification based on chromosomal abnormalities, age, comorbidities, and prior treatment including degree and depth of response are important determinants in choosing treatment options. In addition, a careful balance between efficacy and toxicity is required, considering that patients with advanced RRMM can be more frail and at risk of developing severe complications and end organ damage. As mentioned above, three drug therapies and in particular those combining PI's and IMiDs seem to be superior to doublet regimens for overcoming drug resistance and improve outcome in patients with RRMM. In addition, new drugs with different mechanism of actions (including immunotherapy with monoclonal antibodies as well as other novel strategies such as checkpoint and HDAC inhibition) are emerging and show promising results. Future studies also looking into the biology of MM and on other mechanisms of resistance will pave the way for further improvement in responses and especially in patients with double-refractory RRMM. In addition, the use of genomic and other molecular tools together with the validation of promising biomarkers will hopefully provide better insights into the clonal heterogeneity of MM, and so allow stratification of patients based on risk and potential therapeutic benefit in a more targeted fashion. All together, those approaches should provide a platform for a personalized approach that ultimately will further improve patient outcome.

Acknowledgments The authors gratefully acknowledge the editorial support of Michelle Maglio in the preparation of this manuscript, funded in part by the RJ Corman Multiple Myeloma Research Fund.

References

1. Kumar SK (2014) Continued improvement in survival in multiple myeloma: changes in early mortality and outcomes in older patients. Leukemia 28(5):1122–1128
2. Kumar SK, Rajkumar SV, Dispenzieri A et al (2008) Improved survival in multiple myeloma and the impact of novel therapies. Blood 111(5):2516–2520
3. Palumbo A, Anderson K (2011) Multiple myeloma. N Engl J Med 364(11):1046–1060
4. Rajkumar SV, Harousseau JL, Durie B et al (2011) Consensus recommendations for the uniform reporting of clinical trials: report of the international myeloma workshop consensus panel 1. Blood 117(18):4691–4695
5. Richardson PG, Barlogie B, Berenson J et al (2003) A phase 2 study of bortezomib in relapsed, refractory myeloma. N Engl J Med 348(26):2609–2617
6. Kumar SK, Lee JH, Lahuerta JJ et al (2012) Risk of progression and survival in multiple myeloma relapsing after therapy with IMiDs and bortezomib: a multicenter international myeloma working group study. Leukemia 26(1):149–157
7. Obeng EA, Carlson LM, Gutman DM, Harrington WJ Jr, Lee KP, Boise LH (2006) Proteasome inhibitors induce a terminal unfolded protein response in multiple myeloma cells. Blood 107(12):4907–4916
8. Richardson PG, Sonneveld P, Schuster MW et al (2005) Bortezomib or high-dose dexamethasone for relapsed multiple myeloma. N Engl J Med 352(24):2487–2498
9. Moreau P, Pylypenko H, Grosicki S et al (2011) Subcutaneous versus intravenous administration of bortezomib in patients with relapsed multiple myeloma: a randomised, phase 3, non-inferiority study. Lancet Oncol 12(5):431–440
10. Jagannath S, Richardson PG, Barlogie B et al (2006) Bortezomib in combination with dexamethasone for the treatment of patients with relapsed and/or refractory multiple myeloma with less than optimal response to bortezomib alone. Haematologica 91(7):929–934
11. Garderet L, Iacobelli S, Moreau P et al (2012) Superiority of the triple combination of bortezomib-thalidomide-dexamethasone over the dual combination of thalidomide-dexamethasone in patients with multiple myeloma progressing or relapsing after autologous transplantation: the MMVAR/IFM 2005-04 Randomized Phase III Trial from the Chronic Leukemia Working Party of the European Group for Blood and Marrow Transplantation. J Clin Oncol 30(20):2475–2482
12. Richardson PG, Xie W, Jagannath S et al (2014) A phase 2 trial of lenalidomide, bortezomib, and dexamethasone in patients with relapsed and relapsed/refractory myeloma. Blood 123 (10):1461–1469
13. de Waal EG, de Munck L, Hoogendoorn M et al (2015) Combination therapy with bortezomib, continuous low-dose cyclophosphamide and dexamethasone followed by one year of maintenance treatment for relapsed multiple myeloma patients. Br J Haematol 171 (5):720–725
14. Richardson PG, Hofmeister C, Raje NS et al (2015) A phase 1, multicenter study of pomalidomide, bortezomib, and low-dose dexamethasone in patients with proteasome inhibitor exposed and lenalidomide-refractory myeloma (Trial MM-005). Blood 126 (23):3036
15. Dimopoulos M, Siegel DS, Lonial S et al (2013) Vorinostat or placebo in combination with bortezomib in patients with multiple myeloma (VANTAGE 088): a multicentre, randomised, double-blind study. Lancet Oncol 14(11):1129–1140

16. Richardson PG, Schlossman RL, Alsina M et al (2013) PANORAMA 2: panobinostat in combination with bortezomib and dexamethasone in patients with relapsed and bortezomib-refractory myeloma. Blood 122(14):2331–2337

17. Vij R, Siegel DS, Jagannath S et al (2012) An open-label, single-arm, phase 2 study of single-agent carfilzomib in patients with relapsed and/or refractory multiple myeloma who have been previously treated with bortezomib. Br J Haematol 158(6):739–748

18. Wang M, Martin T, Bensinger W et al (2013) Phase 2 dose-expansion study (PX-171-006) of carfilzomib, lenalidomide, and low-dose dexamethasone in relapsed or progressive multiple myeloma. Blood 122(18):3122–3128

19. Shah JJ, Stadtmauer EA, Abonour R et al (2015) Carfilzomib, pomalidomide, and dexamethasone for relapsed or refractory myeloma. Blood 126(20):2284–2290

20. Stewart AK, Rajkumar SV, Dimopoulos MA et al (2015) Carfilzomib, lenalidomide, and dexamethasone for relapsed multiple myeloma. N Engl J Med 372(2):142–152

21. Dimopoulos MA, Moreau P, Palumbo A et al (2015) Carfilzomib and dexamethasone versus bortezomib and dexamethasone for patients with relapsed or refractory multiple myeloma (ENDEAVOR): a randomised, phase 3, open-label, multicentre study. Lancet Oncol

22. Shah JJ, Feng L, Thomas SK et al (2015) Phase 1 study of the novel kinesin spindle protein inhibitor filanesib + carfilzomib in patients with relapsed and/or refractory multiple myeloma (RRMM). Blood 126(23):376

23. Berdeja JG, Gregory TB, Faber EA et al (2015) A Phase I/II study of the combination of panobinostat (PAN) and Carfilzomib (CFZ) in patients (pts) with relapsed or relapsed/refractory multiple myeloma (MM): comparison of two expansion cohorts. Blood 126(23):1825

24. Siegel D, Martin T, Nooka A et al (2013) Integrated safety profile of single-agent carfilzomib: experience from 526 patients enrolled in 4 phase II clinical studies. Haematologica 98(11):1753–1761

25. Chauhan D, Tian Z, Zhou B et al (2011) In vitro and in vivo selective antitumor activity of a novel orally bioavailable proteasome inhibitor MLN9708 against multiple myeloma cells. Clin Cancer Res 17(16):5311–5321

26. Kumar SK, Bensinger WI, Zimmerman TM et al (2014) Phase 1 study of weekly dosing with the investigational oral proteasome inhibitor ixazomib in relapsed/refractory multiple myeloma. Blood 124(7):1047–1055

27. Richardson PG, Baz R, Wang M et al (2014) Phase 1 study of twice-weekly ixazomib, an oral proteasome inhibitor, in relapsed/refractory multiple myeloma patients. Blood 124 (7):1038–1046

28. Kumar SK, Berdeja JG, Niesvizky R et al (2014) Safety and tolerability of ixazomib, an oral proteasome inhibitor, in combination with lenalidomide and dexamethasone in patients with previously untreated multiple myeloma: an open-label phase 1/2 study. Lancet Oncol 15 (13):1503–1512

29. Richardson PG, Hofmeister CC, Rosenbaum CA et al (2013) Twice-weekly oral MLN9708 (Ixazomib Citrate), an investigational proteasome inhibitor, in combination with lenalidomide (Len) and dexamethasone (Dex) in patients (Pts) with newly diagnosed multiple myeloma (MM): final phase 1 results and phase 2 data. proceedings of the American society of hematology meeting; Dec 7–10; New Orleans, LA. Blood 122(21) [abstract 535]

30. Moreau P, Masszi T, Grzasko N et al (2015) Ixazomib, an Investigational Oral Proteasome Inhibitor (PI), in Combination with Lenalidomide and Dexamethasone (IRd), Significantly Extends Progression-Free Survival (PFS) for Patients (Pts) with Relapsed and/or Refractory Multiple Myeloma (RRMM): the P. Blood 126(23):727

31. Richardson PG, Spencer A, Cannell P et al (2011) Phase 1 clinical evaluation of twice-weekly marizomib (NPI-0052), a novel proteasome inhibitor, in patients with relapsed/refractory multiple myeloma (MM). Blood 118(21):302

32. Kaufman JL, Siegel DS, Vij R et al (2013) Clinical profile of single-agent modified-release oprozomib tablets in patients (Pts) with hematologic malignancies: updated results from a multicenter, open-label, dose escalation phase 1b/2 study. Blood 122(21):3184

33. Das DS, Ray A, Song Y et al (2015) Synergistic anti-myeloma activity of the proteasome inhibitor marizomib and the IMiD(®) immunomodulatory drug pomalidomide. Br J Haematol 171(5):798–812

34. Spencer A, Laubach JP, Zonder JA et al (2015) Phase 1, multicenter, open-label, combination study (NPI-0052-107; NCT02103335) of pomalidomide (POM), marizomib (MRZ, NPI-0052), and low-dose dexamethasone (LD-DEX) in patients with relapsed and refractory multiple myeloma. proceedings of the American society of hematology meeting; Dec 5–8; Orlando, FL. Blood 126(23):[poster 4220]

35. Singhal S, Mehta J, Desikan R et al (1999) Antitumor activity of thalidomide in refractory multiple myeloma. N Engl J Med 341(21):1565–1571

36. Dimopoulos MA, Zervas K, Kouvatseas G et al (2001) Thalidomide and dexamethasone combination for refractory multiple myeloma. Ann Oncol 12(7):991–995

37. Dimopoulos MA, Hamilos G, Zomas A et al (2004) Pulsed cyclophosphamide, thalidomide and dexamethasone: an oral regimen for previously treated patients with multiple myeloma. Hematol J 5(2):112–117

38. Sonneveld P, Asselbergs E, Zweegman S et al (2015) Phase 2 study of carfilzomib, thalidomide, and dexamethasone as induction/consolidation therapy for newly diagnosed multiple myeloma. Blood 125(3):449–456

39. Zou Y, Sheng Z, Niu S, Wang H, Yu J, Xu J (2013) Lenalidomide versus thalidomide based regimens as first-line therapy for patients with multiple myeloma. Leuk Lymphoma 54 (10):2219–2225

40. Richardson P, Jagannath S, Hussein M et al (2009) Safety and efficacy of single-agent lenalidomide in patients with relapsed and refractory multiple myeloma. Blood 114(4):772–778

41. Weber DM, Chen C, Niesvizky R et al (2007) Lenalidomide plus dexamethasone for relapsed multiple myeloma in North America. N Engl J Med 357(21):2133–2142

42. Dimopoulos M, Spencer A, Attal M et al (2007) Lenalidomide plus dexamethasone for relapsed or refractory multiple myeloma. N Engl J Med 357(21):2123–2132

43. Dimopoulos MA, Chen C, Spencer A et al (2009) Long-term follow-up on overall survival from the MM-009 and MM-010 phase III trials of lenalidomide plus dexamethasone in patients with relapsed or refractory multiple myeloma. Leukemia 23(11):2147–2152

44. Reece DE, Masih-Khan E, Atenafu EG et al (2015) Phase I-II trial of oral cyclophosphamide, prednisone and lenalidomide for the treatment of patients with relapsed and refractory multiple myeloma. Br J Haematol 168(1):46–54

45. Richardson PG, Jagannath S, Moreau P et al (2015) Elotuzumab in combination with lenalidomide and dexamethasone in patients with relapsed multiple myeloma: final phase 2 results from the randomised, open-label, phase 1b-2 dose-escalation study. Lancet Haematol 2(12):e516–527

46. Plesner T, Arkenau H-T, Gimsing P et al (2015) Daratumumab in combination with lenalidomide and dexamethasone in patients with relapsed or relapsed and refractory multiple myeloma: updated results of a phase 1/2 study (GEN503). Blood 126(23):507

47. Pawlyn C, Khan MS, Muls A et al (2014) Lenalidomide-induced diarrhea in patients with myeloma is caused by bile acid malabsorption that responds to treatment. Blood 124 (15):2467–2468

48. Leleu X, Attal M, Arnulf B et al (2013) Pomalidomide plus low-dose dexamethasone is active and well tolerated in bortezomib and lenalidomide-refractory multiple myeloma: Intergroupe Francophone du Myelome 2009-02. Blood 121(11):1968–1975

49. Richardson PG, Siegel DS, Vij R et al (2014) Pomalidomide alone or in combination with low-dose dexamethasone in relapsed and refractory multiple myeloma: a randomized phase 2 study. Blood 123(12):1826–1832

50. San Miguel J, Weisel K, Moreau P et al (2013) Pomalidomide plus low-dose dexamethasone versus high-dose dexamethasone alone for patients with relapsed and refractory multiple myeloma (MM-003): a randomised, open-label, phase 3 trial. Lancet Oncol 14(11):1055–1066

51. Larocca A, Montefusco V, Bringhen S et al (2013) Pomalidomide, cyclophosphamide, and prednisone for relapsed/refractory multiple myeloma: a multicenter phase 1/2 open-label study. Blood 122(16):2799–2806

52. Baz R, Martin TG, Alsina M, Shain KH et al (2013) Pomalidomide (Pom) Dexamethasone (D) with or without oral weekly Cyclophosphamide (Cy) for lenalidomide refractory multiple myeloma (LRMM): a multicenter randomized phase II trial. Blood 122(21):3200

53. Mark TM, Boyer A, Yadlapati S et al (2015) Clapd (Clarithromycin, Pomalidomide, Dexamethasone) therapy in relapsed or refractory multiple myeloma overcomes negative prognostic impact of adverse cytogenetics and prior resistance to lenalidomide and bortezomib. Blood 126(23):4232

54. Hsi ED, Steinle R, Balasa B et al (2008) CS1, a potential new therapeutic antibody target for the treatment of multiple myeloma. Clin Cancer Res 14(9):2775–2784

55. Lonial S, Vij R, Harousseau JL et al (2012) Elotuzumab in combination with lenalidomide and low-dose dexamethasone in relapsed or refractory multiple myeloma. J Clin Oncol 30 (16):1953–1959

56. Richardson PG, Jagannath S, Moreau P et al (2015) Elotuzumab in combination with lenalidomide and dexamethasone in patients with relapsed multiple myeloma: final phase 2 results from the randomised, open-label, phase 1b-2 dose-escalation study. Lancet Haematol 2(12):e516–527

57. Collins SM, Bakan CE, Swartzel GD et al (2013) Elotuzumab directly enhances NK cell cytotoxicity against myeloma via CS1 ligation: evidence for augmented NK cell function complementing ADCC. Cancer Immunol Immunother 62(12):1841–1849

58. Lonial S, Dimopoulos M, Palumbo A et al (2015) Elotuzumab Therapy for Relapsed or Refractory Multiple Myeloma. N Engl J Med 373(7):621–631

59. Dimopoulos MA, Lonial S, White D et al (2015) Eloquent-2 Update: a phase 3, randomized, open-label study of elotuzumab in combination with lenalidomide/dexamethasone in patients with relapsed/refractory multiple myeloma—3-year safety and efficacy follow-up. Blood 126 (23):28

60. Palumbo A, Offidani M, Pégourie B et al (2015) Elotuzumab plus bortezomib and dexamethasone versus bortezomib and dexamethasone in patients with relapsed/refractory multiple myeloma: 2-year follow-up. Blood 126(23):510

61. de Weers M, Tai YT, van der Veer MS et al (2011) Daratumumab, a novel therapeutic human CD38 monoclonal antibody, induces killing of multiple myeloma and other hematological tumors. J Immunol 186(3):1840–1848

62. Lokhorst HM, Plesner T, Laubach JP et al (2015) Targeting CD38 with daratumumab monotherapy in multiple myeloma. N Engl J Med 373(13):1207–1219

63. Lonial S, Weiss BM, Usmani SZ et al (2015) Phase II study of daratumumab (DARA) monotherapy in patients with >= 3 lines of prior therapy or double refractory multiple myeloma (MM): 54767414MMY2002 (Sirius). ASCO Meeting Abstracts 33(18_suppl): LBA8512

64. Lonial S, Weiss BM, Usmani SZ et al (2016) Daratumumab monotherapy in patients with treatment-refractory multiple myeloma (SIRIUS): an open-label, randomised, phase 2 trial. Lancet. 2016 Jan 6. pii: S0140–6736(15)01120-4. doi:10.1016/S0140-6736(15)01120-4. [Epub ahead of print]

65. Chari A, Lonial S, Suvannasankha A et al (2015) Open-label, multicenter, phase 1b study of daratumumab in combination with pomalidomide and dexamethasone in patients with at least 2 lines of prior therapy and relapsed or relapsed and refractory multiple myeloma. Blood 126 (23):508

66. Deckert J, Wetzel MC, Bartle LM et al (2014) SAR650984, a novel humanized CD38-targeting antibody, demonstrates potent antitumor activity in models of multiple myeloma and other CD38 + hematologic malignancies. Clin Cancer Res 20(17):4574–4583

67. Martin T, Richter J, Vij R et al (2015) A dose finding phase II trial of Isatuximab (SAR650984, Anti-CD38 mAb) as a single agent in relapsed/refractory multiple myeloma. Blood 126(23):509

68. Kelly KR, Chanan-Khan A, Heffner LT et al (2014) Indatuximab Ravtansine (BT062) in combination with lenalidomide and low-dose dexamethasone in patients with relapsed and/or refractory multiple myeloma: clinical activity in patients already exposed to lenalidomide and bortezomib. Blood 124(21):4736

69. Garfall AL, Maus MV, Hwang WT et al (2015) Chimeric antigen receptor T cells against CD19 for multiple myeloma. N Engl J Med 373(11):1040–1047

70. Ali SA, Shi V, Wang M et al (2015) Remissions of multiple myeloma during a first-in-humans clinical trial of T cells expressing an anti-B-cell maturation antigen chimeric antigen receptor. Blood 126(23):LBA-1-LBA

71. Pardoll DM (2012) The blockade of immune checkpoints in cancer immunotherapy. Nat Rev Cancer 12(4):252–264

72. Paiva B, Azpilikueta A, Puig N et al (2015) PD-L1/PD-1 presence in the tumor microenvironment and activity of PD-1 blockade in multiple myeloma. Leukemia 29 (10):2110–2113

73. San Miguel J, Mateos M-V, Shah JJ et al (2015) Pembrolizumab in Combination with Lenalidomide and low-dose dexamethasone for relapsed/refractory multiple myeloma (RRMM): keynote-023. Blood 126(23):505

74. Badros AZ, Kocoglu MH, Ma N et al (2015) A phase II study of anti PD-1 antibody pembrolizumab, pomalidomide and dexamethasone in patients with relapsed/refractory multiple myeloma (RRMM). Blood 126(23):506

75. Atanackovic D, Schilling G (2013) Second autologous transplant as salvage therapy in multiple myeloma. Br J Haematol 163(5):565–572

76. Morris C, Iacobelli S, Brand R et al (2004) Benefit and timing of second transplantations in multiple myeloma: clinical findings and methodological limitations in a European group for blood and marrow transplantation registry study. J Clin Oncol 22(9):1674–1681

77. Sellner L, Heiss C, Benner A et al (2013) Autologous retransplantation for patients with recurrent multiple myeloma: a single-center experience with 200 patients. Cancer 119 (13):2438–2446

78. Cook G, Williams C, Brown JM et al (2014) High-dose chemotherapy plus autologous stem-cell transplantation as consolidation therapy in patients with relapsed multiple myeloma after previous autologous stem-cell transplantation (NCRI Myeloma X Relapse [Intensive trial]): a randomised, open-label, phase 3 trial. Lancet Oncol 15(8):874–885

79. Gonsalves WI, Gertz MA, Lacy MQ ct al (2013) Second auto-SCT for treatment of relapsed multiple myeloma. Bone Marrow Transplant 48(4):568–573

80. Lemieux E, Hulin C, Caillot D et al (2013) Autologous stem cell transplantation: an effective salvage therapy in multiple myeloma. Biol Blood Marrow Trans 19(3):445–449

81. Olin RL, Vogl DT, Porter DL et al (2009) Second auto-SCT is safe and effective salvage therapy for relapsed multiple myeloma. Bone Marrow Trans 43(5):417–422

82. Kroger N, Perez-Simon JA, Myint H et al (2004) Relapse to prior autograft and chronic graft-versus-host disease are the strongest prognostic factors for outcome of melphalan/fludarabine-based dose-reduced allogeneic stem cell transplantation in patients with multiple myeloma. Biol Blood Marrow Trans 10(10):698–708

83. Freytes CO, Vesole DH, LeRademacher J et al (2014) Second transplants for multiple myeloma relapsing after a previous autotransplant-reduced-intensity allogeneic vs autologous transplantation. Bone Marrow Trans 49(3):416–421

84. Bjorkstrand BB, Ljungman P, Svensson H et al (1996) Allogeneic bone marrow transplantation versus autologous stem cell transplantation in multiple myeloma: a retrospective case-matched study from the European group for blood and marrow transplantation. Blood 88(12):4711–4718

85. Moreau P, Garban F, Attal M et al (2008) Long-term follow-up results of IFM99-03 and IFM99-04 trials comparing nonmyeloablative allotransplantation with autologous transplantation in high-risk de novo multiple myeloma. Blood 112(9):3914–3915

86. Rosinol L, Perez-Simon JA, Sureda A et al (2008) A prospective PETHEMA study of tandem autologous transplantation versus autograft followed by reduced-intensity conditioning allogeneic transplantation in newly diagnosed multiple myeloma. Blood 112 (9):3591–3593

87. Avet-Loiseau H, Attal M, Moreau P et al (2007) Genetic abnormalities and survival in multiple myeloma: the experience of the Intergroupe Francophone du Myelome. Blood 109 (8):3489–3495

88. Avet-Loiseau H, Leleu X, Roussel M et al (2010) Bortezomib plus dexamethasone induction improves outcome of patients with t(4;14) myeloma but not outcome of patients with del (17p). J Clin Oncol 28(30):4630–4634

89. Sonneveld P, Schmidt-Wolf IG, van der Holt B et al (2012) Bortezomib induction and maintenance treatment in patients with newly diagnosed multiple myeloma: results of the randomized phase III HOVON-65/ GMMG-HD4 trial. J Clin Oncol 30(24):2946–2955

90. Reece D, Song KW, Fu T et al (2009) Influence of cytogenetics in patients with relapsed or refractory multiple myeloma treated with lenalidomide plus dexamethasone: adverse effect of deletion 17p13. Blood 114(3):522–525

91. Avet-Loiseau H, Soulier J, Fermand JP et al (2010) Impact of high-risk cytogenetics and prior therapy on outcomes in patients with advanced relapsed or refractory multiple myeloma treated with lenalidomide plus dexamethasone. Leukemia 24(3):623–628

92. Dimopoulos MA, Weisel KC, Song KW et al (2015) Cytogenetics and long-term survival of patients with refractory or relapsed and refractory multiple myeloma treated with pomalidomide and low-dose dexamethasone. Haematologica 100(10):1327–1333

93. Leleu X, Karlin L, Macro M et al (2015) Pomalidomide plus low-dose dexamethasone in multiple myeloma with deletion 17p and/or translocation (4;14): IFM 2010-02 trial results. Blood 125(9):1411–1417

94. Richardson PG, Siegel D, Baz R et al (2013) Phase 1 study of pomalidomide MTD, safety, and efficacy in patients with refractory multiple myeloma who have received lenalidomide and bortezomib. Blood 121(11):1961–1967

95. Oriol A (2011) Multiple myeloma with extramedullary disease. Adv Ther 28(Suppl 7):1–6

96. Papanikolaou X, Repousis P, Tzenou T et al (2013) Incidence, clinical features, laboratory findings and outcome of patients with multiple myeloma presenting with extramedullary relapse. Leuk Lymphoma 54(7):1459–1464

97. Gerrie AS, Mikhael JR, Cheng L et al (2013) D(T)PACE as salvage therapy for aggressive or refractory multiple myeloma. Br J Haematol 161(6):802–810

98. Egan JB, Shi CX, Tembe W et al (2012) Whole-genome sequencing of multiple myeloma from diagnosis to plasma cell leukemia reveals genomic initiating events, evolution, and clonal tides. Blood 120(5):1060–1066

99. Keats JJ, Chesi M, Egan JB et al (2012) Clonal competition with alternating dominance in multiple myeloma. Blood 120(5):1067–1076

100. Mateos MV, Richardson PG, Schlag R et al (2010) Bortezomib plus melphalan and prednisone compared with melphalan and prednisone in previously untreated multiple myeloma: updated follow-up and impact of subsequent therapy in the phase III VISTA trial. J Clin Oncol 28(13):2259–2266

101. Dimopoulos MA, Petrucci MT, Foa R et al (2015) Impact of maintenance therapy on subsequent treatment in patients with newly diagnosed multiple myeloma: use of "progression-free survival 2" as a clinical trial end-point. Haematologica 100(8):e328–330

102. Conner TM, Doan QD, Walters IB, LeBlanc AL, Beveridge RA (2008) An observational, retrospective analysis of retreatment with bortezomib for multiple myeloma. Clin Lymphoma Myeloma 8(3):140–145

103. Madan S, Lacy MQ, Dispenzieri A et al (2011) Efficacy of retreatment with immunomodulatory drugs (IMiDs) in patients receiving IMiDs for initial therapy of newly diagnosed multiple myeloma. Blood 118(7):1763–1765

104. Ludwig H, Durie BG, Bolejack V et al (2008) Myeloma in patients younger than age 50 years presents with more favorable features and shows better survival: an analysis of 10 549 patients from the international myeloma working group. Blood 111(8):4039–4047

105. Palumbo A, Bringhen S, Mateos MV et al (2015) Geriatric assessment predicts survival and toxicities in elderly myeloma patients: an international myeloma working group report. Blood 125(13):2068–2074

106. San-Miguel JF, Richardson PG, Sonneveld P et al (2008) Efficacy and safety of bortezomib in patients with renal impairment: results from the APEX phase 3 study. Leukemia 22 (4):842–849

107. Eriksson T, Hoglund P, Turesson I et al (2003) Pharmacokinetics of thalidomide in patients with impaired renal function and while on and off dialysis. J Pharm Pharmacol 55(12):1701–1706

108. Dimopoulos M, Alegre A, Stadtmauer EA et al (2010) The efficacy and safety of lenalidomide plus dexamethasone in relapsed and/or refractory multiple myeloma patients with impaired renal function. Cancer 116(16):3807–3814

109. Siegel DS, Weisel KC, Dimopoulos MA et al (2015) Analysis of pomalidomide plus low-dose dexamethasone in patients with relapsed/refractory multiple myeloma with vs without moderate renal impairment. Blood 126(23):3031

110. Ramasamy K, Dimopoulos MA, van de Donk NWCJ et al (2015) Safety of treatment (Tx) with pomalidomide (POM) and low-dose dexamethasone (LoDEX) in patients (Pts) with relapsed or refractory multiple myeloma (RRMM) and renal impairment (RI), including those on dialysis. Blood 126(23):374

111. Jones PA, Baylin SB (2007) The epigenomics of cancer. Cell 128(4):683–692

112. Hideshima T, Richardson PG, Anderson KC (2011) Mechanism of action of proteasome inhibitors and deacetylase inhibitors and the biological basis of synergy in multiple myeloma. Mol Cancer Ther 10(11):2034–2042

113. Richardson P, Mitsiades C, Colson K et al (2008) Phase I trial of oral vorinostat (suberoylanilide hydroxamic acid, SAHA) in patients with advanced multiple myeloma. Leuk Lymphoma 49(3):502–507

114. Ocio EM, Vilanova D, Atadja P et al (2010) In vitro and in vivo rationale for the triple combination of panobinostat (LBH589) and dexamethasone with either bortezomib or lenalidomide in multiple myeloma. Haematologica 95(5):794–803

115. San-Miguel JF, Hungria VT, Yoon SS et al (2014) Panobinostat plus bortezomib and dexamethasone versus placebo plus bortezomib and dexamethasone in patients with relapsed or relapsed and refractory multiple myeloma: a multicentre, randomised, double-blind phase 3 trial. Lancet Oncol 15(11):1195–1206

116. Chari A, Cho HJ, Leng S et al (2015) A phase II study of panobinostat with lenalidomide and weekly dexamethasone in myeloma. Blood 126(23):4226

117. Santo L, Hideshima T, Kung AL et al (2012) Preclinical activity, pharmacodynamic, and pharmacokinetic properties of a selective HDAC6 inhibitor, ACY-1215, in combination with bortezomib in multiple myeloma. Blood 119(11):2579–2589

118. Mishima Y, Santo L, Eda H et al (2015) Ricolinostat (ACY-1215) induced inhibition of aggresome formation accelerates carfilzomib-induced multiple myeloma cell death. Br J Haematol 169(3):423–434

119. Vogl DT, Raje NS, Jagannath S et al (2015) Ricolinostat (ACY-1215), the first selective HDAC6 inhibitor, in combination with bortezomib and dexamethasone in patients with relapsed or relapsed-and-refractory multiple myeloma: phase 1b results (ACY-100 Study). Blood 126(23):1827

120. Yee AJ, Bensinger W, Voorhees PM et al (2015) Ricolinostat (ACY-1215), the first selective HDAC6 inhibitor, in combonation with lenalidomide and dexamethasone in patients with relapsed and relapsed-and-refractory multiple myeloma: phase 1b results (ACE-MM-101 Study). Blood 126(23):3055

121. Raje NS, Bensinger W, Cole CE et al (2015) Ricolinostat (ACY-1215), the first selective HDAC6 inhibitor, combines safely with pomalidomide and dexamethasone and shows promosing early results in relapsed-and-refractory myeloma (ACE-MM-102 Study). Blood 126(23):4228

122. Kojima K, Kornblau SM, Ruvolo V et al (2013) Prognostic impact and targeting of CRM1 in acute myeloid leukemia. Blood 121(20):4166–4174

123. Tai YT, Landesman Y, Acharya C et al (2014) CRM1 inhibition induces tumor cell cytotoxicity and impairs osteoclastogenesis in multiple myeloma: molecular mechanisms and therapeutic implications. Leukemia 28(1):155–165

124. Turner JG, Dawson J, Emmons MF et al (2013) CRM1 inhibition sensitizes drug resistant human myeloma cells to topoisomerase II and proteasome inhibitors both in vitro and ex vivo. J Cancer 4(8):614–625

125. Rosebeck S, Alonge MM, Kandarpa M et al (2016) Synergistic myeloma cell death via novel intracellular activation of caspase-10-dependent apoptosis by Carfilzomib and Selinexor. Mol Cancer Ther 15(1):60–71

126. Chen C, Garzon R, Gutierrez M et al (2015) Safety, efficacy, and determination of the recommended phase 2 dose for the oral selective inhibitor of nuclear export (SINE) selinexor (KPT-330). Blood 126(23):258

127. Jakubowiak A, Jasielec J, Rosenbaum CA et al (2015) Phase 1 MMRC trial of selinexor, carfilzomib (CFZ), and dexamethasone (DEX) in relapsed and relapsed/refractory multiple myeloma (RRMM). Blood 126(23):4223

128. Shah JJ, Zonder J, Bensinger WI et al (2013) Prolonged survival and improved response rates with ARRY-520 in relapsed/refractory multiple myeloma (RRMM) patients with low α-1 acid glycoprotein (AAG) levels: results from a phase 2 study. Blood 122(21):285

129. Htut M, Zonder J, Fay JW et al (2013) A phase 1 study of ARRY-520 with bortezomib (BTZ) and dexamethasone (dex) in relapsed or refractory multiple myeloma (RRMM). Blood 122(21):1938

130. Zonder JA, Usmani S, Scott EC et al (2015) phase 2 study of carfilzomib (CFZ) with or without filanesib (FIL) in patients with advanced multiple myeloma (MM). Blood 126(23):728

Treatment of MM: Upcoming Novel Therapies

Sagar Lonial

Abstract

Treatment for myeloma has dramatically changed over the past decade, as has overall survival, due in large part to the development of new targeted agents. While proteasome inhibitors and immunomodulatory agents have contributed to improved outcomes, additional new options remain an unmet medical need. Classes of emerging agents include those targeting epigenetics, such as histone deacetylase inhibitors, monoclonal antibodies, and other emerging targets, such as kinesin spindle protein (KSP) inhibitors, cyclin dependent kinase (CDK) inhibitors, and nuclear protein export inhibitors. Future treatment approaches will need to identify how and when to incorporate these treatment options to optimally treat patients with relapsed or refractory myeloma.

Keywords

Multiple myeloma · New drugs · Proteasome inihibitor · Monoclonal antibodies

1 Introduction

Treatment choices for myeloma patients at each phase of their disease have become a complex decision-making process, due to a deeper understanding of plasma cell biology [1]. This has resulted in more therapeutic options for patients at each stage of treatment. Treatment of patients with relapsed or refractory multiple myeloma presents a special therapeutic challenge, due to the heterogeneity of disease at

S. Lonial (✉)
Department of Hematology and Medical Oncology, Emory University School of Medicine, 1365 Clifton Rd, Building C, Room 4004, Atlanta, GA 30322, USA
e-mail: sloni01@emory.edu

© Springer International Publishing Switzerland 2016
A.M. Roccaro and I.M. Ghobrial (eds.), *Plasma Cell Dyscrasias*,
Cancer Treatment and Research 169, DOI 10.1007/978-3-319-40320-5_11

Table 1 New drugs in Development for Myeloma

New targets in myeloma	Phase of development
Oral proteasome inhibitors	
MLN9708 Ixazomib	Phase III
ONX0912 Oprozomib	Phase II
HDAC inhibitors	
Panobinostat	Phase III
ACY1215 Rocilinostat	Phase II
Monoclonal antibodies	
Elotuzumab	Phase III
Daratumumab	Phase III
SAR650984	Phase III
Other	
Array 520 Filanesib	Phase II
Dinaciclib	Phase II
Selinexor	Phase II

relapse and the absence of biomarker-based recommendations regarding the choice of salvage therapies [2]. With recognition of clonal heterogeneity and genomic instability in plasma cell disorders, the identification of new targets and agents has become critical. Several new agents and targets are currently under development and show considerable promise. The next-generation proteasome inhibitors (ixazomib and oprozomib), and other molecularly targeted therapies directed at specific cell signaling pathways (including histone deacetylase inhibitors) are currently in development. Even newer approaches such as monoclonal antibodies targeting SLAMF7, CD38, CD138, and others have also demonstrated promising anti-myeloma activity (Table 1). Incorporation of these new agents into the treatment paradigm as well as establishment of biomarkers to identify optimal patients for these new targets remains a major focus of research and clinical investigation.

2 Newer Proteasome Inhibitors

2.1 Ixazomib

Ixazomib (MLN9708) is a reversible oral boronate peptide, a next-generation proteasome inhibitor that is in phase III clinical development. While structurally similar to bortezomib, ixazomib is pharmacokinetically and pharmacodynamically different from bortezomib [3]. Weekly and twice-weekly schedules of ixazomib have been evaluated among relapsed and refractory myeloma patients, and clinical data suggest that weekly dosing is effective and associated with less toxicity compared with twice a week dosing. One study administered ixazomib on a twice-weekly schedule similar to bortezomib (days 1, 4, 8, 11) of a 21-day cycle [4]. The second study administered ixazomib once weekly for 3 out of 4 weeks (days 1, 8, 15) of a 28-day cycle. The drug was well tolerated with lower rates of PN than were seen with botezomib either through the SQ or IV route [5]. In combination with lenalidomide and dexamethasone, twice-weekly dosing of ixazomib was also well tolerated, with similar efficacy to weekly dosing in combination with lenalidomide and dexamethasone [6]. Based upon a lower rate of gastrointestinal and skin toxicity for the weekly dosing, most studies are moving toward weekly dosing both as a single agent or in combination studies. These results are encouraging for the possibility of a highly efficacious, oral triplet-regimen in the induction therapy for those newly diagnosed or relapsed MM [7].

2.2 Oprozomib

Oprozomib (ONX0912) is an oral abbreviated derivative of the irreversible proteasome inhibitor carfilzomib. Similar to bortezomib, it predominantly inhibits chymotryptic-like activity of $\beta 5$ subunit of the proteasome. Among the 30 RRMM patients and 12 WM patients treated on twice-weekly (2/7) schedule or 5 days every 2 weeks (5/14) schedule. 2 DLTs both occurring on 5/14 schedule were seen (renal failure and tumor lysis syndrome). Currently, dose formulation changes and dose ramp up studies are in progress. Preliminary data suggest that oprozomib monotherapy has promising activity, but additional studies are in progress to optimize drug delivery and dose in myeloma as well as other diseases [8].

3 HDAC Inhibitors

Histone deacetylase inhibitors (HDACi) prevent deacetylation, which is a process involved in the epigenetic regulation of gene expression promoting cell proliferation and cell death [9]. In myeloma cells, HDACi's inhibit cell growth and induce apoptosis as a single agent, but are also synergistic with proteasome inhibitors and immunomodulatory agents [10]. Clinically, the activity of HDACi's as single agents are limited [11], but when combined bortezomib in relapsed or refractory myeloma patients, HDACi's are able to overcome bortezomib resistance. This is also the case when combined with carfilzomib [12]. This is likely a result of simultaneous inhibition both the proteasome (bortezomib) and the aggresome/autophagy (HDACi) systems through combination therapy. Additional preclinical work is emerging that also suggests synergy when HDAC inhibitors are combined with immunomodulatory agents [13]. Several class–specific inhibitors or as pan-deacetylase inhibitors [14] are under evaluation (Table 2).

Table 2 HDAC inhibitors in Myeloma

Treatment	N	Trial	Overall response (%)
Panobinostat	38	Monotherapy	2.6
Panobinostat + Bz	55	Bz Refractory	34
Panobinostat + BZ	387	Bz Sensitive	60.7
ACY1215 + Bz	48	Refractory Ds	39
ACY 1215 + Len	31	Refractory D	55
ACY 1215 + Pom	28	Refractory D	29

3.1 Panobinostat

Phase 1 studies evaluating panobinostat and bortezomib in relapsed or refractory myeloma patients identified panobinostat 20 mg given days 1–14 and BTZ 1.3 mg/m^{2}days 1,4,8,11 every 21 days as the MTD [15]. In the expansion phase of the same study, a majority of patients responded to therapy (ORR 73.3 %) however, $\geq$ G3 thrombocytopenia was higher at 89 %. In the subsequent phase 2 trial, PANORAMA-2 evaluating the combination of panobinostat with bortezomib and dexamethasone among patients who were refractory to bortezomib at study entry, the ORR was 34.5 %, with a median PFS of 5.4 months. It should be noted that the overall response rate was higher among patients who were refractory as defined by progression within 60 days of stopping treatment as compared with the patients who progressed on therapy. Toxicity included $\geq$ G3 thrombocytopenia and diarrhea rates of 60 and 20 %, respectively [16]. This trial was followed by the large randomized phase 3 PANORAMA-1 trial that randomized 768 patients to receive panobinostat with bortezomib and dexamethasone versus bortezomib and dexamethasone alone in an early relapsed disease setting. Panobinostat 20 mg PO or placebo was given 3 times/week on days 1–14 was given in combination with twice-weekly VD in treatment phase I (TP1) for cycles 1–8. In TP2 (cycles 9-12), patients would receive weekly VD. The median PFS was 12 vs. 8.1 months favoring the panobinostat group ($p < 0.0001$ with a HR 0.63) [17]. Among patients able to complete TP2 in the panobinostat arm, the response rates were higher and had longer median PFS [18]. The rates of grade 3/4 AEs in TP1 versus TP2 were: diarrhea (25.5 % vs. 8.8 %), thrombocytopenia (47.1 % vs. 5.9 %), and fatigue (14.7 % vs. 2.0 %) supporting once weekly administration of bortezomib when used in combination with panobinostat and dexamethasone in the maintenance setting. Additionally, it suggests that toxicity is not cumulative, but rather dose and dose density related [18, 19]. Additional subgroup analyses were performed and demonstrated that among patients who had received >2 prior lines and were exposed to bortezomib and lenalidomide, the difference in PFS was more significant (12.5 months for panobinostat bortezomib/dexamethasone treated patients vs. 4.7 months for bortezomib/dexamethasone alone) further supporting the ability of the HDACi to overcome intrinsic or acquired proteasome inhibitor and/or immunomodulatory agent resistance (Table 2).

Table 3 Monoclonal antibodies in Myelomax

Treatment	N	Overall response (%)
Daratumumab	106	29
Daratumumab + Len	32	87
SAR690854	13	31
SAR690854 + Len	31	58
Elotuzumab + Len	321	79

Based upon encouraging data utilizing HDAC inhibitors on relapsed myeloma as part of a combination strategy, other more selective HDAC inhibitors are in development. Additional phase I and II data in combination with proteasome inhibitors and IMIDS are currently ongoing, and will provide what is hoped to be additional safety and efficacy data for this new and important class of agents [20, 21].

4 Rocilinostat (ACY 1215)

Rocilinostat is a selective HDAC6 inhibitor that has been studied in preclinical models and synergizes with bortezomib and with the IMIDs [22]. Early clinical trials did not demonstrate single agent activity, similar to what has been demonstrated with other agents in this class, however, the toxicology profile did suggest much less diarrhea and nausea. Early phase trials combining this agent with bortezomib supported the ability of this agent to potentially overcome bortezomib resistance. Additional preclinical work suggested impressive synergy when combined with pomalidomide, and early clinical trial data support the preclinical observation as well. Trials are currently ongoing to determine the optimal formulation and combination partner.

5 Monoclonal Antibodies

Monoclonal antibodies represents and important target for a number of different reasons. Their activity allows one to target the tumor cell in a method that may be in part independent of intracellular signaling mechanisms, which in cancer can be a major source of drug resistance. Additionally, they can represent a unique target on cancer cells, or at least a target that may have a much more limited effect when compared with targeting a specific kinase or DNA damage response. Potential antibody targets in myeloma include the use of agents that target CD38, SLAMF7 (Formerly known as CS1), CD138, as well as other microenvironmental targets such as BAFF or cytokines including IL6 [23] (Table 3).

5.1 Elotuzumab

Elotuzumab is a humanized monoclonal antibody that targets the cell surface glycoprotein CS1 (SLAMF7). Elotuzumab mediates ADCC in myeloma cell lines and myeloma cells, from patients with MM resistant or refractory to conventional therapies and bortezomib [24]. Elotuzumab as a single agent demonstrated no objective responses, but in a phase1 study, in combination with standard dose and schedule lenalidomide dexamethasone, objective responses were observed in 23/28 treated patients (82 %) [25]. Dose limiting toxicities were not noted up to a dose of 20 mg/kg, leading to a phase 2 extension phase where the response rates for elotuzumab doses of 10 mg/kg versus 20 mg/kg were 92 % versus 76 % and median progression free survival was 33 versus 26 months, respectively [26]. Data combining bortezomib and dex with elotuzumab were presented in a randomized phase 2 study from Jakubowiak et al. and demonstrate an improvement in PFS with suggestions in OS improvements, though the study was too small to be powered for that endpoint [27]. Recently, data from the randomized phase III trial, Eloquent 2 (Elo/len/dex vs. Len/dex), were published demonstrating an improvement in progression free survival favoring the group that received elotuzumab [28]. Additional analyses showed that patient with high risk genetics, specifically del 17p, appeared to benefit from treatment with elotuzumab as did patient older than age 65. An interesting subset analysis tested the PFS by response and treatment group. This demonstrated that among patients who achieved a PR or >VGPR, the PFS was improved if they received elotuzumab as compared with those who did not. This suggests that the immune mechanism of activity is important not only for inducing a response, in maintaining the response over a longer time. There are additional studies evaluating the impact of elotuzumab among other patients populations including the ELOQUENT 1 trial comparing the efficacy and the safety of lenalidomide and dexamethasone with or without 10-mg/kg elotuzumab in patients with newly diagnosed myeloma.

5.2 Daratumumab

Daratumumab is a humanized anti-CD38 antibody that not only directly targets tumor cells but also effectively mediates killing of CD38-expressing plasma cells via antibody-dependent cell-mediated cytotoxicity (ADCC), antibody-dependent cellular phagocytosis (ADCP), complement-dependent cytotoxicity (CDC), and apoptosis. In a phase 1 dose escalation study, heavily pretreated relapsed and refractory myeloma patients were treated with single agent daratumumab with doses ranging from 0.005 to 24.0 mg/kg. Marked reduction in paraprotein and bone marrow plasma cells were observed at doses ≥ 4 mg/kg. Overall, 42 % of this heavily pretreated population of patients achieved $\geq$ PR at doses ≥ 4 mg/kg [29, 30]. The combination of lenalidomide and daratumumab demonstrated enhanced NK-mediated cytotoxicity in vitro using ADCC assays [31]. Based on this rationale, a phase 1/2 study of daratumumab in combination with lenalidomide and oral dexamethasone in the relapsed and refractory myeloma patients was initiated with primary objective of establishing the safety profile. Daratumumab dosing ranged from 2 to 16 mg/kg weekly for 8 weeks, twice a month for 16 weeks, and once a month until disease progression. Among 20 patients reported, preliminary safety data show a manageable safety profile in line with what has previously been reported for lenalidomide. The high overall response rate of 75 % with this combination is encouraging [32]. More recently, a large phase II study was presented that utilized 16 mg/kg of Daratumumab as a single among a group of patients with refractory MM [33]. This trial enrolled 106 patients with IMID and PI resistant myeloma, and these patients had received a median of five prior lines of treatment. The overall response rate for this group was 29 %, with three patients achieving a sCR, and an additional 10 patients achieving a VGPR. The median duration of response was 7.4 months, and the median overall survival was 65 % at 12 months. This data clearly identifies daratumumab as having a major benefit among patients with refractory MM, sets the stage for accelerated approval and for combination therapy in earlier lines of treatment.

5.3   SAR650984

SAR650984 is another humanized anti-CD38 antibody with strong proapoptotic activity independent of cross-linking agents. Killing is mediated by ADCC, ADCP, and CDC [34]. In a phase, 1 dose escalation trial SAR is administered as a single agent IV infusion every week (QW) or every 2 weeks (Q2W) to adult patients with selected CD38 + hematological malignancies with doses ranging from 0.0001 mg/kg Q2W to 10 mg/kg QW. MTD has not been reached and DLTs were limited to G2 infusion reactions. Among the six MM patients treated at the 10 mg/kg Q2W dose, three patients had PR, and two had SD [35]. Additional studies combining with proteasome inhibitors and with lenalidomide have demonstrated encouraging activity as well, supporting the notion that monoclonal antibodies can be safely combined with the two most active classes of anti-myeloma agents with no concerns. As with elotuzumab and daratumomab, the IMID combination appears to be particularly promising.

5.3.1   Kinesin Spindle Protein

The use of anti-mitotics in myeloma has been hindered by significant toxicity and questionable activity. Anti-mitotics were widely used in myeloma as part of the VAD (vincristine, doxorubicin, and dexamethasone) combination that was a standard of care prior to the introduction of PIs and ImIDs. However, the role of vincristine in this combination was brought into question. Toxicity of anti-microtubule agents is due to inhibition of non-mitotic actions of microtubules in post-mitotic cells. Therefore, anti-mitotics that do not function through inhibition of microtubules are desirable for therapy as they should have an enhanced therapeutic index. One such agent that has been developed to function in this fashion is ARRY-520. ARRY-520 is an inhibitor of kinesin spindle protein (KSP). KSP is essential for spindle assembly and equal segregation of sister chromatids; therefore, inhibition of KSP results in metaphase arrest but does not alter non-mitotic effects of microtubules. A recent study demonstrated that ARRY-520 induces mitotic arrest and apoptosis in human myeloma cell lines. Mitotic arrest and cell death correlated with loss of Mcl-1, an anti-apoptotic protein that is essential for myeloma cell survival. Consistent with this model, silencing of the Mcl-1 inhibitor, Noxa, also results in ARRY-520 resistance while silencing of Mcl-1 sensitizes cells. Clinical trials with ARRY-520 are underway in myeloma and recently presented data from a phase II study suggests activity in patients that are refractory to bortezomib and ImIDs. A phase I study of the combination of ARRY-520 and carfilzomib, and a combination with bortezomib are underway.

5.3.2 Cyclin Dependant Kinase

It is well known that dysregulation of cyclin dependent kinases represent a common pathogenic mechanism for several subsets of myeloma. Several groups have reported that targeting of specific CDKs can induce myeloma cell death, but often these agents induce significant myelosuppression or other adverse events limiting their long-term use. Additionally, identification of the specific genetic subset of myeloma patients who may gain the greatest benefit from CDK inhibition has not been clearly reported from preclinical models. Kumar and colleagues reported a clinical trial testing the CDK 1, 2, 5, and 9 inhibitor dinaciclib among a group of refractory myeloma and demonstrated single agent activity of around 20 % [36]. These patients had received a median of five prior lines of therapy, and were heavily refractory based upon prior therapy. A second clinical trial from Niesvizky et al. tested the CDK 4/6 inhibitor palbociclib in combination with bortezomib in a heavily refractory myeloma patient population as well, and demonstrated a combination overall response rate of 20 % [37]. Both of these agents had significant preclinical rationale supporting their use, yet neither demonstrated overwhelming single agent activity suggesting that the impact of CDK inhibition may be most important among smaller subsets of patients who harbor specific translocations that may render their survival more sensitive to CDK inhibtion. Currently, which genetic mutations sensitize to CDK inhibition remains unclear.

5.3.3 Targeting Nuclear Export Signals

Cargo transported from the nucleus to the cytoplasm is exported through the nuclear pore complex (NPC) and while small proteins can pass freely through the NPC, larger ones must be assisted by a transport receptor. Transport receptors belong to the karyopherin-β family of proteins including chromosome maintenance protein-1 (CRM1)/exportin-1 (XPO1). CRM1 recognizes a leucine-rich export signal in the cargo protein and when complexed, will export proteins into the cytoplasm. CRM1 has been shown to be overexpressed in many tumors. Interestingly many of the cargo proteins exported by CRM1 are tumor-suppressor proteins and can contribute to tumorigenesis through the export of proteins including p53 and pRb. Moreover, CRM1 was identified as a promising target in myeloma cells via an RNAi screen of 6,722 druggable targets. CRM1 ranked in the top 50 targets in this screen [38].

Together these findings point to the promise of targeting CRM1 as a therapeutic strategy in cancer, especially myeloma. Early studies focused on the use of leptomycin B, which inhibits CRM1 through covalent modification of the reactive site on cysteine residue(528). While active in preclinical models, leptomycin B was shown to be too toxic for clinical use in a phase I study. A new series of CRM1 inhibitors referred to as selective inhibitors of nuclear export (SINE) has been developed and has shown promise in preclinical models, including in myeloma. KPT-330 an orally available SINE is in phase I and II trials in both solid tumors and hematologic malignancies. Preliminary data in myeloma suggests single agent activity, and larger phase II studies are currently ongoing.

6 Conclusions

The use of currently available agents has dramatically changed the outcome for patients with relapsed myeloma. Sequencing versus combination therapy in the relapsed setting now becomes the focus for future investigation. Studies such as the ASPIRE trial demonstrate significant benefit for combining new agents, and supports the idea that patients treated aggressively in early relapse can enjoy long periods of progression free survival. Expanding this concept with the use of antibodies suggests that not only can patient achieve durable remissions, but that the tolerance of these long term treatments may be improved over currently available agents. As such, emerging concepts and targets suggests that ultimately we will need more personalized approaches to therapy as we seek to sort out what agents to use at which times.

References

1. Lonial S, Mitsiades CS, Richardson PG (2011) Treatment options for relapsed and refractory multiple myeloma. Clin Cancer Res Official J Am Assoc Cancer Res 17(6):1264–1277
2. Nooka AK, Kastritis E, Dimopoulos MA, Lonial S (2015) Treatment options for relapsed and refractory multiple myeloma. Blood 125(20):3085–3099
3. Chauhan D, Tian Z, Zhou B et al (2011) In vitro and in vivo selective antitumor activity of a novel orally bioavailable proteasome inhibitor MLN9708 against multiple myeloma cells. Clin Cancer Res 17(16):5311–5321
4. Richardson PG, Baz R, Wang M et al (2014) Phase 1 study of twice-weekly ixazomib, an oral proteasome inhibitor, in relapsed/refractory multiple myeloma patients. Blood 124(7):1038–1046
5. Kumar SK, Bensinger WI, Zimmerman TM et al (2014) Phase 1 study of weekly dosing with the investigational oral proteasome inhibitor ixazomib in relapsed/refractory multiple myeloma. Blood 124(7):1047–1055
6. Kumar SK, Berdeja JG, Niesvizky R et al (2014) Safety and tolerability of ixazomib, an oral proteasome inhibitor, in combination with lenalidomide and dexamethasone in patients with previously untreated multiple myeloma: an open-label phase 1/2 study. Lancet Oncol 15 (13):1503–1512
7. Richardson P, Rosenbaum CA, Htut M et al (2013) Twice-weekly oral MLN9708 (Ixazomib Citrate), An investigational proteasome inhibitor, in combination with Lenalidomide (Len) and

dexamethasone (Dex) in patients (Pts) with newly diagnosed multiple myeloma (MM): final phase 1 results and phase 2 data. Blood 122(21):535

8. Ghobrial I, Kaufman JL, Siegel DS et al (2013) Clinical profile of single-agent modified-release oprozomib tablets in patients (Pts) with hematologic malignancies: updated results from a multicenter, open-label, dose escalation phase 1b/2 study. ASH Annula Meeting Abstracts. 2013-11-15 00:00:00 2013;122(21):3184

9. Kaufman JL, Fabre C, Lonial S, Richardson PG (2013) Histone deacetylase inhibitors in multiple myeloma: rationale and evidence for their use in combination therapy. Clin Lymphoma Myeloma Leuk 13(4):370–376

10. Richardson PG, Wolf J, Jakubowiak A et al (2011) Perifosine plus bortezomib and dexamethasone in patients with relapsed/refractory multiple myeloma previously treated with bortezomib: results of a multicenter phase I/II trial. Clin Cancer Res Official J Am Assoc Cancer Res 29(32):4243–4249

11. Wolf JL, Siegel D, Goldschmidt H et al (2012) Phase II trial of the pan-deacetylase inhibitor panobinostat as a single agent in advanced relapsed/refractory multiple myeloma. Leukemia Lymphoma 53(9):1820–1823

12. Berdeja JG, Hart LL, Mace JR et al (2015) Phase I/II study of the combination of panobinostat and carfilzomib in patients with relapsed/refractory multiple myeloma. Haematologica 100 (5):670–676

13. Hideshima T, Cottini F, Ohguchi H et al (2015) Rational combination treatment with histone deacetylase inhibitors and immunomodulatory drugs in multiple myeloma. Blood Cancer J 5: e312

14. Qian DZ, Kato Y, Shabbeer S et al (2006) Targeting tumor angiogenesis with histone deacetylase inhibitors: the hydroxamic acid derivative LBH589. Clin Cancer Res 12 (2):634–642

15. San-Miguel JF, Richardson PG, Günther A et al (2013) Phase Ib study of panobinostat and bortezomib in relapsed or relapsed and refractory multiple myeloma. J Clin Oncol October 10, 2013 2013;31(29):3696–3703

16. Richardson PG, Schlossman RL, Alsina M et al (2013) PANORAMA 2: panobinostat in combination with bortezomib and dexamethasone in patients with relapsed and bortezomib-refractory myeloma. Blood 122(14):2331–2337

17. Richardson PG, Hungria VTM, Yoon S-S et al (2014) Panorama 1: a randomized, double-blind, phase 3 study of panobinostat or placebo plus bortezomib and dexamethasone in relapsed or relapsed and refractory multiple myeloma. ASCO Meeting Abstracts 32 (15_suppl):8510

18. San Miguel J, Hungria VT, Yoon S-S et al (2014) Efficacy and safety based on duration of treatment of panobinostat plus bortezomib and dexamethasone in patients with relapsed or relapsed and refractory multiple myeloma in the phase 3 panorama 1 study. Blood. 2014-12-06 00:00:00 2014;124(21):4742

19. Richardson PG, Hungria VTM, Yoon S-S et al (2014) Characterization of the incidence and management of gastrointestinal toxicity in the phase 3 panorama 1 study of panobinostat plus bortezomib and dexamethasone versus placebo plus bortezomib and dexamethasone in patients with relapsed or relapsed and ref.... Blood. 2014-12-06 00:00:00 2014;124(21):2120

20. Raje N, Vogl DT, Hari PN et al (2013) ACY-1215, a selective histone deacetylase (HDAC) 6 inhibitor: interim results of combination therapy with bortezomib in patients with multiple myeloma (MM). Blood 122(21):759

21. Yee A, Vorhees P, Bensinger WI et al (2013) ACY-1215, a selective histone deacetylase (HDAC) 6 inhibitor, in combination with lenalidomide and dexamethasone (dex), is well tolerated without dose limiting toxicity (DLT) in patients (Pts) with multiple myeloma (MM) at doses demonstrating biologic ac.... Blood 122(21):3190

22. Santo L, Hideshima T, Kung AL et al (2012) Preclinical activity, pharmacodynamic, and pharmacokinetic properties of a selective HDAC6 inhibitor, ACY-1215, in combination with bortezomib in multiple myeloma. Blood 119(11):2579–2589

23. Lonial S, Durie B, Palumbo A, Miguel JS (2015) Monoclonal antibodies in the treatment of multiple myeloma: current status and future perspectives. Leukemia

24. Hsi ED, Steinle R, Balasa B et al (2008) CS1 A potential new therapeutic antibody target for the treatment of multiple myeloma. Clin Cancer Res 14(9):2775–2784

25. Lonial S, Vij R, Harousseau JL et al (2012) Elotuzumab in combination with lenalidomide and low-dose dexamethasone in relapsed or refractory multiple myeloma. J Clin Oncol Official J Am Soc Clin Oncol 30(16):1953–1959

26. Richardson PG, Jagannath S, Moreau P et al (2012) A Phase 2 study of elotuzumab (Elo) in combination with lenalidomide and low-dose dexamethasone (Ld) in patients (pts) with relapsed/refractory multiple myeloma (R/R MM): updated results. Blood 120(21):202

27. Jakubowiak A, Offidani M, Pegourie B et al (2015) A randomized phase II study of bortezomib (Btz)/dexamethasone (dex) with or without elotuzumab (Elo) in patients (pts) with relapsed/refractory multiple myeloma (RRMM). Paper presented at: ASCO; June 2015; Chicago, Ill

28. Lonial S, Dimopoulos M, Palumbo A et al (2015) Elotuzumab therapy for relapsed or refractory multiple myeloma. New Engl J Med 373(7):621–631

29. Plesner T, Lokhorst H, Gimsing P, Nahi H, Lisby S, Richardson PG. (2012) Daratumumab, a CD38 monoclonal antibody in patients with multiple myeloma - data from a dose-escalation phase I/II study. ASH Annual Meeting Abstracts 120(21):73

30. Lokhorst HM, Plesner T, Gimsing P et al (2013) Phase I/II dose-escalation study of daratumumab in patients with relapsed or refractory multiple myeloma. ASCO Meeting Abstracts; 31(15_suppl):8512

31. Nijhof IS, Noort WA, Lammerts van Bueren J et al (2013) CD38-targeted immunochemotherapy of multiple myeloma: preclinical evidence for its combinatorial use in lenalidomide and bortezomib refractory/intolerant MM patients. 2013;122(21):277

32. Plesner T, Arkenau T, Lokhorst H et al (2013) Preliminary safety and efficacy data of daratumumab in combination with lenalidomide and dexamethasone in relapsed or refractory multiple myeloma 122(21):1986

33. Lonial S, Weiss B, Usmani S et al (2015) Phase II study of daratumumab (DARA) monotherapy in patients with ≥ 3 lines of prior therapy or double refractory multiple myeloma (MM): 54767414MMY2002 (Sirius). Paper presented at: ASCO; June 2015; Chicago,Ill

34. Deckert J, Wetzel MC, Bartle LM et al (2014) SAR650984, a novel humanized cd38-targeting antibody, demonstrates potent antitumor activity in models of multiple myeloma and other cd38 + hematologic malignancies. Clin Cancer Res Official J Am Assoc Cancer Res 20 (17):4574–4583

35. Martin TG III, Strickland SA, Glenn M, Zheng W, Daskalakis N, Mikhael JR (2013) SAR650984, a CD38 monoclonal antibody in patients with selected CD38 + hematological malignancies- data from a dose escalation phase I study. ASH Annu Meet Abs 122(21):284

36. Kumar SK, LaPlant B, Chng WJ et al (2015) Dinaciclib, a novel CDK inhibitor, demonstrates encouraging single-agent activity in patients with relapsed multiple myeloma. Blood 125 (3):443–448

37. Niesvizky R, Badros AZ, Costa LJ et al (2015) Phase 1/2 study of CDK4/6 inhibitor palbociclib (PD-0332991) with bortezomib and dexamethasone in relapsed/refractory multiple myeloma. Leukemia Lymphoma 1–21

38. Schmidt J, Braggio E, Kortuem KM et al (2013) Genome-wide studies in multiple myeloma identify XPO1/CRM1 as a critical target validated using the selective nuclear export inhibitor KPT-276. Leukemia 27(12):2357–2365

Role of the Immune Response in Disease Progression and Therapy in Multiple Myeloma

Susan J. Lee and Ivan Borrello

Abstract

Multiple myeloma (MM) is a hematologic cancer derived from malignant plasma cells within the bone marrow. Unlike most solid tumors, which originate from epithelial cells, the myeloma tumor is a plasma cell derived from the lymphoid cell lineage originating from a post-germinal B-cell. As such, the MM plasma cell represents an integral component of the immune system in terms of both antibody production and antigen presentation, albeit not efficiently. This fundamental difference has significant implications when one considers the implications of immunotherapy. In the case of lymphoid malignancies such as myeloma, immune-based strategies must take into consideration this important difference, potentially necessitating immunotherapy targeted toward MM to be altered from that targeted at solid tumors. Typically, the immune system "surveys" cells within our body and is able to recognize and attack cancerous cells that may arise. However, some cancer cells are able to evade immune surveillance and continue to flourish, causing disease. The major mechanism leading to an effective tumor-specific response is one that enables effective antigen processing and presentation with subsequent T-cell activation, expansion, and effective trafficking to the tumor site. Plasma cells employ several mechanisms to escape immune surveillance which include altered interactions with T-cells, DCs, bone marrow stromal cells (BMSC's), and natural killer cells (NK Cells) that can be mediated by immunosuppressive cells such as and myeloid-derived suppressor cells (MDSC's) and cytokines such as IL-10, TGFβ, and IL-6 as well as down-regulation of the antigen processing machinery. Many therapies have been developed to reestablish a functional immune system in MM patients. These include adoptive T-cell therapies to deliver more tumor-specific

S.J. Lee · I. Borrello (✉)
Sidney Kimmel Comprehensive Cancer Center, Johns Hopkins University,
Baltimore, MD 21205, USA
e-mail: iborrell@jhmi.edu

© Springer International Publishing Switzerland 2016
A.M. Roccaro and I.M. Ghobrial (eds.), *Plasma Cell Dyscrasias*,
Cancer Treatment and Research 169, DOI 10.1007/978-3-319-40320-5_12

T-cells, vaccines to increase the tumor-specific precursor frequency of the endogenous T-cell population, immunomodulatory agents (IMiDs) such as thalidomide and lenalidomide to enhance global endogenous immunity, immunostimulatory cytokines, and antibodies to specifically target tumor-specific cell-surface proteins or cytokines. This review will dissect these various approaches currently being explored in MM as well as highlight some future directions for myeloma-specific immune-based strategies.

Keyword

Myeloma · Immunotherapy · T-cells · Cytokines

1 Interactions with Bone Marrow Stromal Cells (BMSC)

As with most tumors, interactions with the surrounding microenvironment are critical to their survival [1–3]. BMSC interactions with plasma cells are a key factor for the survival of MM tumor cells. Adhesion of MM cells to BMSC's stimulates the production of various anti-apoptotic and cell cycle activating proteins [4, 5]. A major factor contributing to plasma cell survival through BMSC interaction is IL-6, which has a wide range of functions that serve to increase MM proliferation and survival [4] as well as IL-1β which is largely responsible for the production of IL-6 in BMSC's.

IL-6 induces MM proliferation by activating the Ras/Raf/MEK/ERK pathway as well as by blocking p21 and p27, which inhibit CDK. IL-6 also initiates a pro-survival cascade in MM cells though the MAPK/JAK/STAT3 pathway by activating Mcl1, Bcl-xL, and cMyc as well as down-regulating Bim [4].

The Wnt pathway has been found to be aberrantly expressed in myeloma and is responsible for cell proliferation, differentiation, and apoptosis. Dickkopf 1 (Dkk1) inhibits Wnt signaling and plays a role in osteolytic bone disease. Dkk1 inhibition with a neutralizing antibody has been shown to increase osteoblast activity, reduce osteoclast activation, and restore bone mineral density. Additionally, it reduces IL-6 levels and adhesion of MM cells to BMSC's [6].

CCL25 and its receptor CCR9 can increase MM survival in a stroma-dependent interaction [5]. CCL25 is secreted by MM tumor cells and is proposed to be a chemo-attractant for mesenchymal stem cells (MSCs), promoting the survival MM tumor. Detectable CCL25 expression was found in 5 of 6 MM cell lines and 11 of 14 primary MM tumor cells by Western blot. When mice were co-injected with MM and mesenchymal stem cells (MSC's), more than twice as many MM cells were observed in the femur compared to injecting MM cells alone. Additionally, an in vitro transwell system showed that MSCs had elevated levels of IL-6, VEGF, IL-10, IGF-1, and DKK1 after 48 h of coculture with MM cells, and MM cells showed both increased levels of pAKT, pERK, Cyclin D2, CDK4, and Bcl-xL as well as decreased levels of Caspase-3 and PARP after 24 h of coculture with MSC's.

1.1   CD4/CD8 T-Cells

Extensive evidence exists to suggest that disease progression in MM is associated with a loss of tumor-specific immunity [7]. suggesting that immune surveillance may play a role in the prevention of MM disease progression. In MM patients demonstrating long-term survival (MM-LTS), clonally expanded T-cell populations have a much higher proliferative capacity than in non-LTS-MM patients. Interestingly however, no significant differences in IFNγ production were observed between T-cells from LTS versus non-LTS patients. Additionally, MM patients have fewer TH17 cells than LTS-MM patients by both absolute number and percentage of total T-cells. The Treg/Th17 ratio was also higher in MM patients compared to MM-LTS patients, with the ratio in MM-LTS rivaling that of healthy donors [8].

1.2   Th17

Th17 cells are pro-inflammatory T-cells that may aid in mounting T-cell responses against tumor. Conversely, Tregs have been shown to suppress immune responses, including those mounted by Th17 cells. In MM, the balance between immunosuppressive Tregs and pro-inflammatory Th17 cells is thought to play an important role in mediating an effective immune response. Patients with MM show increased levels of Th17 cells in the peripheral blood (PB) compared to healthy donors. Additionally higher PB Th17 levels (3.7 % vs. 5.14 %; $p = 0.019$) correlate with more advanced clinical disease (Stage I/II vs. stage III, respectively) [9].

When the ratio of Treg:Th17 in PB was examined, patients with a Treg/Th17 ratio greater than 2SD above the mean had significantly reduced OS ($p = 0.025$) [10]. Of note in this study, patients with high Treg/Th17 ratios all had normal Treg levels, indicating that a decrease in the number of Th17 cells in PB is the driving force in increased disease burden, contradicting the previously discussed data.

While these data look at Th17 cells in the peripheral blood, MM is a disease that originates in the bone marrow (BM) which provides the rationale for examining immune responses in that compartment. IL-6 plays a role in both Th17 and Treg cells promoting Th17 differentiation while suppressing Treg production [11, 12]. Furthermore, cytokines such as IL-6, TGFβ and IL-1b that skew CD4 cells toward a TH17 phenotype are largely found in the BM of MM patients, but not in the PB or in BM or healthy donors [13].

1.3   Regulatory T-Cells

Regulatory T-cells (Tregs) are CD4+ T-cells that express high levels of CD25 as well as FoxP3, CTLA-4, and GITR. Tregs secrete the inhibitory cytokines, IL-10 and TGFβ, suppress immune function, and prevent autoimmunity by killing T-cells via granzyme and perforin. IL-10 is required for the suppressive function of Tregs in vivo [14] as well as for transplant immunity [15]. TGFβ is both secreted and expressed on the surface of Tregs. Transmembrane TGFβ is important for inhibition of NK activation via NKG2D [16], while secreted TGFβ is necessary for T-cell suppression [17–19]. Tregs suppress the immune system but the full effect this has on an immune-derived malignancy such as MM remains to be fully elucidated.

Peripheral blood (PB) Tregs are elevated in MM patients compared to healthy volunteers [20, 21]. Additionally, it was observed that both naïve and activated Tregs were elevated ($p = 0.015$ and $p = 0.036$, respectively). However, no differences were seen in PB Tregs between healthy volunteers and MGUS, SMM, or patients in remission. BM Tregs were elevated in relapse patients compared to healthy volunteers ($p = 0.035$), however, no differences were seen between any other groups of patients. Furthermore, Treg function was similar in MM and healthy patients [20].

In contrast to the above-mentioned data, patients with MGUS and MM have significantly reduced numbers of Tregs compared to healthy donors [22]. This shows that Tregs in MGUS and MM patients are significantly less functional and ineffectively suppress T-cells, which could ultimately result in greater numbers of hyperactivated T-cells.

When $CD4^+/CD25^+$ cells from the PB are compared to that of the BM, MM patients were found to have significantly more $FoxP3^+$ cells in the PB compared to BM (52.2 % versus 2.2 %). Additionally, these $FoxP3^+/CD4^+/CD25^+$ cells from the PB had the ability to suppress T-cell proliferation by greater than 90 %, whereas those from the BM demonstrated no suppressive capabilities. These data indicate that $FoxP3^+/CD4^+/CD25^+$ cells in the PB and BM of MM patients are functionally distinct cell types [13].

CD8+ Tregs have been identified as well [23, 24] and while they also express FoxP3, CTLA4, and GITR, their mechanism of action does not involve TGFβ or IL-10, but rather TNFα and CCL4, causing cells to become cytostatic. CD8+ Tregs in both PB and BM are elevated in patients with MM compared to healthy donors. Multiple studies have demonstrated that tumor-induced CD4+ iTregs are created in a contact-dependent manner by MM tumor cells and express higher levels of FoxP3, PD-1 and GITR than nTregs [23, 25]. Additionally, proliferation of MM induced CD4+ iTregs is mediated by ICOS/ICOS-L interactions and not by the standard IL-10 or TGFβ interactions [25].

Tregs have multifaceted interactions and functions with T-cells in the myeloma setting. Tregs cannot simply be grouped together as having a single mechanism of action or effect on T-cells or the myeloma environment. There are clear differences in both phenotype and function of Tregs, which must be taken into consideration and studied, to better understand their role in Myeloma.

2   NK Cells

Natural killer (NK) cells are cytotoxic lymphocytes that do not express CD3, defined by the expression of CD56 in humans and function as cytotoxic cells in a non-HLA-restricted manner. Immunophenotyping was done on MM patients following HSCT. They found that at 1 month post-transplant, NK levels were predictive of PFS. Patients with NK counts below 100 cells/uL had an average PFS of 2.2 months compared to 11.6 months for patients with NK counts above 100 cells/uL. However, this was not predictive of OS or time to next treatment [26].

NK cells from healthy donors do not express PD-1, however, NK cells from MM patients do. This phenotypic difference indicates that there is potentially a functional change occurring in NK cells in response to the MM tumor helping to create an immunosuppressive environment for the tumor to thrive [27].

NK cells also express a variety of surface receptors, including NKG2D, that can be used to recognize tumor cells, or cells that are in a state of stress expressing ligands such as MICA, MICB, and ULBP1-6. The NKG2D receptor, also expressed on CD4 and CD8 cells, has been shown to be critical for the recognition and lysis of MM cells [28]. Additionally, MICA expression on plasma cells and shedding of MICA (sMICA) correlates with MM progression. MGUS patients express high levels of MICA on their plasma cells compared to normal donors, and MM patients express intermediate MICA levels but high sMICA levels. MGUS patients also have high levels of anti-MICA antibodies whereas MM patients do not [29]. The presence of anti-MICA antibodies ameliorates the suppressive effects of MICA on NKG2D, whereas the loss of these antibodies contributes to MM disease progression. Therefore, the use of anti-MICA antibodies may prove to be a viable therapeutic in MM.

3   DC's

Dendritic cells (DCs) are one of the most effective antigen presenting cells (APCs) for stimulating naïve T-cells. However, MM patients have not only fewer DC cells and precursors compared to healthy donors [30, 31], but also have impaired DC function. Peripheral blood DCs (PBDCs) from MM patients have decreased expression of HLA-DR, CD40, and CD80 and are nonfunctional. This effect is mediated by IL-6. Conversely, CD14+ derived DCs (Mo-DCs) are fully functional in both normal in MM patients [31]. This observation brings into question the use of PBDCs for therapeutic use in MM, discussed later.

4   MDSC's

Myeloid-derived suppressor cells (MDSC's) are immunosuppressive cells of the myeloid lineage. They suppress the function of T-cells mainly via up-regulation of iNOS, ROS, and Arg-1. Two subsets of MDSC's have been described, polymorphonuclear MDSCs (PMN-MDSCs) and monocytic MDSCs (M-MDSCs). PMN-MDSCs are Ly6Clo/Ly6G+ and use ROS to mediate T-cell suppression, while M-MDSC are Ly6Chi/Ly6G− and have increased levels of NO, but not ROS [32]. Significant MDSC accumulation is observed in BM and PB of MM patients compared to healthy donors [32, 33], and the majority of MDSC's in the BM are PMN-MDSC's. Additionally, the frequency of MDSCs increases with disease progression (newly diagnosed < relapsed < relapsed/refractory) with significantly different ($p < 0.025$) frequencies between healthy donors and relapsed/refractory patients [33].

In a murine model in which MDSCs are unable to accumulate in tumor-bearing mice (S100A9 model), reduced tumor growth is observed, accompanied by an accumulation of antigen-specific CD8+ T-cells in the spleen and BM. Either adoptive transfer of MDSCs or anti-CD8 mAb negate this effect. Interestingly, there is no correlation between disease extent and MDSC levels in this murine model [32].

PDE5 inhibition is an approach to inhibiting MDSC function. PDE5 inhibition increases proliferation and infiltration of T-cells in the myeloma tumor environment that can render adoptive T-cell therapy more effective [34]. In fact, in one case study, PDE5 inhibition regenerated tumor-specific T-cell function in a patient with end-stage MM [35].

5   Therapies

5.1   Autologous Stem Cell Transplant

Autologous stem cell transplantation (ASCT) is largely considered frontline therapy for myeloma patients under the age of 65. The primary goal of ASCT is a platform to deliver high dose chemotherapy with stem cell rescue. However, there is an increasing appreciation of the role myeloablative chemotherapy can play as a platform for immunotherapy. Specifically, through its myeloablation, it can: (1) provide effective lymphodepletion to enhance homeostatic lymphocytic proliferation following adoptive T-cell transfer; (2) abolish the intrinsic tolerogenic mechanisms that usually serve to impair the generation of effective antitumor immunity; and (3) potentially augment the efficacy of tumor-specific vaccines by enabling such vaccine to effectively skew the developing T-cell repertoire toward greater tumor recognition [36, 37].

5.2   Allogeneic Bone Marrow Transplant (BMT)

Allogeneic SCT (allo-SCT) using HLA-identical (or haploidentical) donor cells has also been used to treat MM. However, graft versus host disease (GVHD) remains a sizeable obstacle with a significant morbidity and mortality. Patients who receive allo-SCT upfront as opposed to upon relapse or progressive disease show an increase in 2-year progression free survival (PFS) (63 % vs. 25 %) and overall survival (OS) (81 % vs. 52 %) [38]. However, myeloablative allo-SCT has historically been associated with an unacceptably high transplant-related mortality of >40 % [39–41]. In conclusion, the high graft v myeloma effect of allogeneic transplants must be balanced with the significant mortality. An approach to reduce such toxicity includes the use of post-transplant cyclophosphamide which has dramatically reduced the incidence of GVHD, minimized the use of immunosuppression in HLA-identical transplants and opened this modality as a therapeutic option even to HLA-mismatched donors thus dramatically increasing donor availability [42].

6 Adoptive T-Cell Therapy

Adoptive T-cell therapy activates and expands tumor-specific T-cells ex vivo to reverse T-cell tolerance and increase their numbers. One advantage of adoptive T-cell therapy is the quantity of T-cells that can be generated and infused into patients. Evidence from several studies has shown the extent to which T-cells can rapidly and efficiently eradicate rather large tumor burdens. A limitation of this approach has been the expense and manufacturing needs required to implement such an approach.

7 Marrow-Infiltrating Lymphocytes

Marrow-infiltrating lymphocytes (MILs) are bone marrow-derived T-cells expanded ex vivo using CD3/CD28 beads in the presence of all cells from the bone marrow, including the tumor cells. The rationale for the development of this approach was to utilize an endogenous T-cell population obtained from the tumor microenvironment. However, in addition to it being the site of disease in hematologic malignancies such as myeloma, the bone marrow also has several unique immunologic properties. It is also a reservoir for central memory T-cells, which are the most efficient at maintaining long-term immunity [43, 44]. Furthermore, MILs possess many other important and unique properties essential to effective adoptive T-cell therapy: they are present in all patients; they can traffic to the bone marrow upon reinfusion; and can kill tumor and persist over time [45]. This has led to the development of clinical trials showing the ability of MILs to impart a measurable myeloma-specific response that correlates with clinical outcomes in patients.

8 CARs

Chimeric antigen receptors (CARs) are T-cells with genetically modified transmembrane proteins that confer target specificity. CARs posses an antigen-specific extracellular domain as well as an intracellular domain that transduces an activation signal. While first generation CARs targeted CD19 and were stimulated via a CD3ζ, second generation CARs have co-stimulatory molecules, such as CD28 or 41BB in addition to CD3ζ and third generation CARs have multiple intracellular signaling domains. A group at Ohio State has developed a second generation CAR using NK cells that target CS-1/SLAM7, a surface protein highly expressed in MM cells. These SLAM7 CAR NK cells demonstrate increased cytotoxicity via cell lysis of tumor cell lines, and increased specificity for myeloma tumor compared to mock-transduced or empty vector NK cells. Promising results were seen in both in vitro models as well as in mouse models [46]. Mice with IM9 MM tumor showed a significant reduction in tumor burden and increased survival when treated with SLAM7 CAR NK cells as compared to mock-transduced NK cells and untreated controls ($p < 0.05$ and <0.01, respectively) [46].

Another CAR NK cell (NK-92MI) has been developed targeting CD138 with encouraging preclinical activity. These CD138 CARs show increased cytotoxicity and antitumor activity in both in vitro and xenograft studies [47]. Both IFNγ and granzymeB were significantly increased in the NK-92MI cells compared to mock transfected cells in response to CD138+ tumor cell lines as well as primary patient tumor cells, demonstrating tumor-specific cytotoxicity. Furthermore, the cytotoxicity of the NK-92MI cells was maintained even after irradiation with 10 Gy. This finding has important implications in ameliorating the risk of unrestrained proliferation after transplant of the transplanted cells.

Non-antigen-specific CARs may also prove to be effective in MM. NKG2D is a receptor expressed on some CD8+ T-Cells, γδT-cells, and NK cells. It facilitates cell lysis in a non-MHC restricted and TCR-independent manner and has multiple ligands, several of which are selectively expressed in MM tumor cells. Enriching for NGK2D+CD3+CD8+ T-cells increases autologous myeloma cell lysis and demonstrates a role for NKG2D in killing autologous myeloma tumor [28, 48]. Therefore, creating a CAR targeting NKG2D or other non-antigen-specific molecules may prove to be an effective means of targeting the MM tumor as well.

9   Vaccines

Cancer vaccines aim to prime an endogenous T-cell response to tumor-specific antigens. Approaches used are highly variable but all seek to achieve this goal.

10   DC Vaccines

Dendritic cell (DCs) vaccines aim to elicit antitumor responses by overcoming the immunosuppressive environment created by the tumor. Several approaches have been applied to DC vaccines to ultimately generate measurable tumor-specific T-cell responses. One historical approach used idiotype-pulsed (Id-pulsed) DCs [49–53]. However, a potential drawback in using Id as a tumor target in myeloma is that it is largely a secreted protein potentially more likely to induce tolerance but incapable of effectively mounting a tumor-specific immune response that could result in tumor cell killing.

Tumor lysate-pulsed DCs is another approach that has been used in MM. In the 5TGM1 myeloma mouse model, DCs pulsed with tumor lysate have a much more potent antitumor response than Id-pulsed DCs [54]. This data suggests that tumor lysates serve as better tumor antigens than Id. Considering that the whole tumor cell likely possesses multiple tumor antigens that include, but are not limited to Id, these findings are not unexpected. A potential risk in using whole tumor lysates, however, is that antigens expressed on normal cells may also be expressed in the tumor, presented by the DC and recognized by T-cells as a foreign antigen, mounting a non-tumor-specific response.

Creating DC/tumor fusions is another means of creating at DC-based vaccine. This approach attempts to combine the entire antigenic repertoire of autologous tumors with efficient antigen presentation of a DC to maximize the immune response that can be generated by such an approach. In a clinical trial with patients who had undergone ASCT and had a minimum of 20 % plasma cells in the BM, 36 patients received a DC/tumor fusion vaccine and 12 of these patients also received GM-CSF. 78 % of patients achieved a CR or VGPR (47 % and 31 %, respectively) and at a median follow-up time of 45.6 months, the 2-year PFS was 57 % [55].

10.1 Tumor Associated Antigen Vaccines

MM lacks many defined tumor-specific antigens making it difficult to specifically target the tumor using an antigen-specific approach. One study used the RHAMM-R3 peptide (CD168) as a vaccine to treat MM. RHAMM is expressed in 100 % of MM tumor cells, but is not expressed in PBMCs or healthy donor CD34+ BMSCs. Following treatment with R3, 2 of 4 (50 %) of patients had reduced plasma cells and β2-microglobulin in the BM as well as a reduction of free light chains in the serum and/or urine [56]. Additionally, in 4/9 (44 %) of patients, a CD8+ RHAMM-R3-specific T-cell response was observed. Of these 4 patients showing an immunological response, one had decreased blasts in the BM and another had a reduction of free light chains. However, the other two patients showed no clinical changes [57].

Wilms tumor gene (WT-1) is a universal tumor antigen that is processed by MM cells and expressed in the context of HLA class 1. WT-1 is recognized by cytotoxic CD8+ T-cells, that are able to efficiently kill MM tumor cells via perforin-mediated cytotoxicity and WT-1-specific CTLs are found in MM patients [58]. Based on this preclinical data, a patient was given WT-1 vaccine. In this case report, the percentage of MM cells in the BM decreased from 85 to 25 % and the M-protein levels decreased from 3.6 to 0.6 g/day [59] making a strong case for further studies using a WT-1 vaccine.

While vaccines against tumor antigens is a promising means of eliciting a tumor-specific immune response, finding MM-specific antigens has proven to be a major obstacle.

10.2 Whole Cell Vaccines

Allogeneic vaccines can be used to target MM via shared tumor antigens between the MM tumor and the cells used in the vaccine. In one study, a combination of MM tumor cell lines (H929 and U266) and a GM-CSF-producing cell line (K562/GM) are irradiated and combined to form a vaccine. Patients received 3 monthly vaccinations and a booster vaccination at 6 months. All patients were previously on a Len-containing regimen, which was continued as a single agent in addition to the vaccine. Additionally, these patients needed to be in one of three categories to receive vaccine: (1) in a stable nCR for at least 4 months, (2) converting from IFE negative to positive, or (3) show signs of early relapse from nCR to an M-spike <0.3 g/dL. Twelve patients were vaccinated and 16 were observed without vaccination. PFS was significantly improved for patients who received the vaccine compared to those who did not and the overall CR rate for patients receiving vaccine was 64 %. Of the 4 patients receiving vaccine in category 1, 3 achieved a true CR and one achieved an nCR. All 3 patients in category 2 achieved true CRs. In category 3, 1 patient achieved a CR, 1 SD and 3 PD. Additionally, patients achieving a CR had more central memory CD8 T-cells at baseline in the BM and blood, more phenotypically active CD8 in the BM and had more tumor-specific IFNγ production. This study demonstrates that in the MRD setting, the combination of an allogenic vaccine with Len has significant clinical benefit compared to Len alone [60].

Allogeneic vaccines are an off-the-shelf product. Since it is made using cell lines and not primary cells, there is a theoretically unlimited supply available for treating patients.

---

11 Antibodies

Using monoclonal antibodies (mAbs) to specifically target proteins expressed on tumor cells is a desirable treatment approach for many cancers, including MM, since it is a universally applicable, highly specific form of therapy available to all patients. Several mAbs have been developed to target the MM tumor based on cell-surface expression of proteins as well as secreted survival factors. Rituximab, targets CD20 and it's primary use is in non-Hodgkin lymphomas, but has been used in myeloma as well. Rituximab targets CD20, which is differentially expressed on MM plasma cells. Less than one third of MM tumor cells express CD20, as mature plasma cells tend to lose CD20 expression. However, patients who do have CD20-expressing MM tend to have more aggressive disease and lower overall survival [61]. Furthermore, there are data suggesting that CD20 is expressed on what may be precursor myeloma cells [62], providing suitable rationales for targeting CD20 in myeloma. In one study, out of 19 MM patients treated, 6 (32 %) had a clinical response to Rituximab therapy (1 PR, 5 SD), and all 6 of these patients had CD20+ BMPCs (Bone Marrow Plasma Cells) [63]. Another study in relapsed/refractory MM showed that no patients achieved an objective response.

22 % of patients (2 of 9) had SD at 6 months while the rest (88 %) had progressive disease [64]. A subsequent study selected only for patients with CD20+ MM and showed that 7 % of patients (1 of 14) had a minor response while 36 % (5 of 14) had stable disease yielding a clinical response rate of 43 % [65].

CD38 is expressed in many heme malignancies including MM and may have a pro-survival role [66]. CD38 ligation to CD31 activates NFκB, leading to cytokine secretion and proliferation of T-cells. Several CD38 mAbs have been created, including daratumumab (DARA) and SAR650984. DARA is an IgG1 k antibody that has therapeutic efficacy in MM patients, especially in combination with IMiDs and/or proteasome inhibitors [67]. Several mechanisms have been proposed for DARA, including Ab-dependent cellular cytotoxicity (ADCC), complement-dependent cytotoxicity (CDC) [68], Fc receptor-mediated crosslinking [69] and antibody-vdependent cellular phagocytosis (ADCP) [70]. Promising preliminary clinical results have been seen with DARA. When treated with 4, 8, or 16 mg/kg DARA, patients showed 80–100 % reduction of bone marrow plasma cells [71]. Additionally, in combination with lenalidomide and dexamethasone, 8/11 patients achieved a PR or better while the remaining 3 patients achieved MR (2) and SD (1) [72].

SAR650984 is a newer IgG1 antiCD38 mAb that also has ADCC, CDC, and ADCP activity against MM tumor cell lines and cytotoxicity of both MM cell lines and primary patient tumor. Additionally, SAR650984 drastically decreased tumor volume in xenograft studies of MOLP-8 and H929 cells compared to bortezomib [73]. However, SAR650984 has not yet entered the clinic.

CD56, also known as neural cell adhesion molecule (N-CAM) is not expressed by benign plasma cells, but is highly expressed in MM cells [74]. Lorvotuzumab mertansine (LM) is an antibody-drug conjugate that targets MM cells via high affinity CD56 mAb and is conjugated to the drug Maytansine, which inhibits tubulin. As a single agent in heavily pretreated patients with CD56+ MM, 16.2 % had objective responses (OR) and 40.5 % had SD for greater than 3 months, including those with ORs [75]. LM in combination with Lenalidomide and Dex-amethasone shows greater clinical benefit with a 56.4 % OR and 66.1 % CR rate in relapsed/refractory MM [76].

CS1 (CRACC, SLAMF7) is a glycoprotein highly expressed on the surface of plasma cells. It is a member of the CD2 receptor family and contains an immunoreceptor tyrosine-based switch motif (ITSM) that is involved in lymphocyte activation [77]. Elotuzumab targets CS1 and is currently entering phase III clinical trials. Data from phase I trials show that elotuzumab alone yielded no objective responses (≥PR), while 26.5 % of patients had stable disease after about two months and the rest had progressive disease [78]. When combined with bortezomib, 48 % of patients had an objective responses and a median time to progression (TTP) of 9.5 months [79]. When elotuzumab is combined with lenalidomide and low-dose dexamethasone, objective responses were seen in 82 % of patients with a median TTP not reached after 16.4 months [80]. Preliminary data from a phase II study with elotuzumab combined with lenalidomide and dexamethasone show an overall ORR of 84 %, with a 92 % ORR in the cohort receiving 10 mg/kg elo-tuzumab and 76 % in those receiving 20 mg/kg. Patients receiving 10 mg/kg had not reached PFS at 20.8 months while PFS was 18.6 months for those receiving 20 mg/kg. While elotuzumab may not work well as a single agent, in combination with lenalidomide and dexamethasone elotuzumab appears to be a promising new therapeutic for MM.

CD40 is a member of the TNF-receptor family. It is required for B-cell activation and differentiation and is more highly expressed in patients with B-cell malignancies, such as MM. Dacetuzumab, a CD40 mAb, has not shown promising results in a phase 1 trial as a single agent; no patients achieved an OR and 20 % achieved SD [81]. Lucatumumab, another CD40 mAb, has completed a phase 1 study in which 33 patients were evaluated. One patient achieved a PR while 12 (43 %) had SD as a best response [82]. Neither Lucatumumab nor Dacetuzumab show promising clinical results as a single agent, however, like many therapeutics they warrant further investigation in combination with other therapies, but no data has been published to date.

IL-6 is not expressed on the surface of MM cells, however, it is an important factor in their proliferation. Siltuximab is an anti-IL-6 mAb that so far has shown minimal clinical benefit. In a Phase I trial, 13 MM patients were treated and 2 (15 %) had a CR [83]. In a Phase II trial and RRMM, initially 14 patients received siltuximab alone, 10 whom later received dexamethasone. 39 additional patients were then treated with a combination of siltuximab and dexamethasone with a response rate of 23 % (17 % CR and 6 % PR). No responses were seen with siltuximab alone [84]. Another phase II trial evaluated bortezomib, melphalan and prednisone therapy with or without siltuximab (VMP versus S + VMP) in newly diagnosed transplant eligible patients. ORR was only 8 % higher in S + VMP than VMP alone (88 % versus 80 %, respectively) whereas ≥VGPR was 20 % higher in S + VMP than VMP (71 % vs. 51 %). Finally, median PFS as well as 1 year OS were equivalent in both groups showing definitively that siltuximab has no additional benefit to VMP therapy in MM [85].

12 Checkpoint Blockade

The role of PD-1 is to maintain T-cell homeostasis by limiting the proliferation and activation of T-cells. However, many tumors usurp this mechanism and over-express PD-L1, engaging PD-1 on T-cells and generating tumor-specific T-cell tolerance [86–89]. Therapy targeted at blocking programmed death-1 (PD-1) and its ligand (PD-L1) transformed the field of immunotherapy in immunogenic solid tumors, such as renal cell carcinoma and melanoma [90, 91] and more recently Hodgkin's lymphoma [92]. More recently, inhibition of PD-1 and PD-L1 has also been shown to work in non-immunogenic solid tumors such as lung, ovarian, and breast cancers [91, 93]. These findings have opened the door to studying PD-1 and PD-L1 in a wide variety of tumor types. There are four PD-1 mAbs (Nivolumab, Pidilizumab, Pembrolizumab, and MK-3475) and four PD-L1 mAbs (BMS-936559, MSB0010718C, MEDI4736, and MDPL3280A) currently in clinical trials. Despite the significant efficacy in certain malignancies, the overall efficacy of single agent PD-1 blockade in relapsed MM is negligible [94].

Syngeneic mice lacking PD-1 completely suppress MM tumor (J558L) formation whereas mice expressing PD-1 form rapidly growing tumor demonstrating a clear role of PD-1 and its interaction with PD-L1 in MM [89]. More recently, data shows that treatment with a PD-L1 mAb in combination with lymphodepletion with irradiation eliminate MM in a murine 5T33 model, again highlighting the importance of the PD-1/PD-L1 axis in MM [95].

CTLA4 is an inhibitory molecule expressed on T-cells that binds to CD80 and competes with CD28, a co-stimulatory molecule that also binds CD80, but with lower affinity. CTLA4 has been shown to maintain control to T-cell proliferation [96] as well as being critical for proper function of Tregs [97, 98]. 70 % of MM patients have increased CTLA4 expression and may be associated with an accumulation of immunosuppressive Tregs in the bone marrow microenvironment [99]. Blocking CTLA4 has proven to be an effective therapeutic strategy in patients with metastatic melanoma [100], opening the doors for its use in other malignancies, including MM.

13　IMiDs

Immunomodulatory drugs (IMiDs), such as thalidomide, lenalidomide, and pomalidomide, are often used as both frontline and maintenance therapy for MM. Beneficial clinical outcomes are seen with the use of IMiDs, and while many studies have given insights into how these drugs work, their exact mechanism of action is only recently being understood.

IMiDs have been shown to increase the proliferation and function of T-cells. Greater lytic capacity as well as higher percentages of polyfunctional T-cells (T-cells secreting multiple cytokines) was observed in MM patients receiving IMiDs following ASCT, due at least in part to decreased Tregs and increased DC function [101]. Furthermore, the immunomodulatory properties of lenalidomide (Len) was confirmed by demonstration about its ability to enhance both infectious vaccines [102] as well as possibly tumor vaccines [60]. The induction of Rho GTPases with pomalidomide (Pom) may contribute to improving immune synapses in T-cells [103]. IMiDs effects on DCs could also play a role in the enhanced T-cell functionality. DCs treated with lenalidomide or pomalidomide have enhanced endocytic ability as well as an increased levels of CD86, MHC I, and MHC II on the DC cell surface [104]. Additionally, DCs that have been pretreated with Len or Pom show significantly enhanced cross-priming of CD8+ T-cells and priming of CD4+ T-cells. Additionally, these CD8+ T-cells are more cytotoxic, exhibiting increased levels of both IFNγ and perforin.

However, other studies suggest that IMiDs may prove to be harmful to immune surveillance long-term for myeloma patients. Clave et al., observed that 6 months post ASCT, terminally differentiated CD8 T-cells are reduced in the presence of Len.

Pro-inflammatory cytokines such as TNFα were also reduced in the blood of patients receiving Len after ASCT. Furthermore, Len also significantly increased the NK cell activity as well as the percentage of Treg cells 18 months post ASCT [105, 106].

14   Summary

There are many promising immunotherapeutic treatments available for the Multiple myeloma, however, we have not yet been able to cure this disease by enabling the immune system to fight off the cancer completely. The immune system is an intricate network of cells and signaling molecules with multifaceted microenvironments creating a complex system for targeted therapies. However, as we learn more about the immune system and how it interacts with the tumor, we can continue to create more potent and targeted therapies.

References

1. Alifano M et al (2014) Systemic inflammation, nutritional status and tumor immune microenvironment determine outcome of resected non-small cell lung cancer. PLoS ONE 9: e106914–11
2. Song G et al (2014) Effects of tumor microenvironment heterogeneity on nanoparticle disposition and efficacy in breast cancer tumor models. Clin Cancer Res 20:6083–6095
3. Kumar V, Gabrilovich DI (2014) Hypoxia-inducible factors in regulation of immune responses in tumour microenvironment. Immunology 143:512–519
4. Manier S, Sacco A, Leleu X, Ghobrial IM, Roccaro AM (2012) Bone marrow microenvironment in multiple myeloma progression. J Biomed Biotechnol 2012:1–5
5. Xu S et al (2012) Bone marrow-derived mesenchymal stromal cells are attracted by multiple myeloma cell-produced chemokine CCL25 and favor myeloma cell growth in vitro and in vivo. Stem Cells 30:266–279
6. Fulciniti M et al (2009) Anti-DKK1 mAb (BHQ880) as a potential therapeutic agent for multiple myeloma. Blood 114:371–379
7. Spisek R et al (2007) Frequent and specific immunity to the embryonal stem cell-associated antigen SOX2 in patients with monoclonal gammopathy. J Exp Med 204:831–840
8. Bryant C et al (2013) Long-term survival in multiple myeloma is associated with a distinct immunological profile, which includes proliferative cytotoxic T-cell clones and a favourable Treg/Th17 balance. Blood Cancer J 3:e148
9. Shen CJ, Yuan ZH, Liu YX, Hu GY (2012) Increased numbers of T helper 17 cells and the correlation with clinicopathological characteristics in multiple myeloma. J Int Med Res 40:556–564
10. Favaloro J et al (2014) Myeloid derived suppressor cells are numerically, functionally and phenotypically different in patients with multiple myeloma. Leuk Lymphoma 55:2893–2900
11. Zhou L et al (2007) IL-6 programs TH-17 cell differentiation by promoting sequential engagement of the IL-21 and IL-23 pathways. Nat Immunol 8:967–974
12. Lichtenstein A, Berenson J, Norman D, Chang M-P, Charlie A (1989) Production of cytokines by bone marrow cells obtained from patients with multiple myeloma. Blood 74:1266–1273
13. Noonan K et al (2010) A novel role of IL-17-producing lymphocytes in mediating lytic bone disease in multiple myeloma. Blood 116:3554–3563

14. Asseman C, Mauze S, Leach MW, Coffman RL, Powrie F (1999) An essential role for interleukin 10 in the function of regulatory T cells that inhibit intestinal inflammation. J Exp Med 190:995–1004

15. Kingsley CI, Karim M, Bushell AR, Wood KJ (2002) CD25+CD4+ regulatory T cells prevent graft rejection: CTLA-4- and IL-10-dependent immunoregulation of alloresponses. J Immunol 168:1080–1086

16. Ghiringhelli F (2005) CD4+CD25+ regulatory T cells inhibit natural killer cell functions in a transforming growth factor-dependent manner. J Exp Med 202:1075–1085

17. Strauss L et al (2007) A unique subset of CD4+CD25highFoxp3+ T cells secreting interleukin-10 and transforming growth factor-beta1 mediates suppression in the tumor microenvironment. Clin Cancer Res 13:4345–4354

18. Fahlen L (2005) T cells that cannot respond to TGF- escape control by CD4+CD25+ regulatory T cells. J Exp Med 201:737–746

19. Shull MM et al (1992) Targeted disruption of the mouse transforming growth factor-beta 1 gene results in multifocal inflammatory disease. Nature 359:693–699

20. Muthu Raja KR et al (2012) Increased T regulatory cells are associated with adverse clinical features and predict progression in multiple myeloma. PLoS ONE 7:e47077–11

21. Giannopoulos K, Kaminska W, Hus I, Dmoszynska A (2012) The frequency of T regulatory cells modulates the survival of multiple myeloma patients: detailed characterisation of immune status in multiple myeloma. Br J Cancer 106:546–552

22. Prabhala RH (2006) Dysfunctional T regulatory cells in multiple myeloma. Blood 107:301–304

23. Muthu Raja KR et al (2012) Functionally suppressive CD8 T regulatory cells are increased in patients with multiple myeloma: a cause for immune impairment. PLoS ONE 7:e49446–10

24. Ablamunits V, Bisikirska B, Herold KC (2010) Acquisition of regulatory function by human CD8(+) T cells treated with anti-CD3 antibody requires TNF. Eur J Immunol 40:2891–2901

25. Feyler S et al (2012) Tumour cell generation of inducible regulatory T-cells in multiple myeloma is contact-dependent and antigen-presenting cell-independent. PLoS ONE 7:e35981–10

26. Rueff J, Medinger M, Heim D, Passweg J, Stern M (2014) Lymphocyte subset recovery and outcome after autologous hematopoietic stem cell transplantation for plasma cell myeloma. Biol Blood Marrow Transplant 20:896–899

27. Benson DM et al (2010) The PD-1/PD-L1 axis modulates the natural killer cell versus multiple myeloma effect: a therapeutic target for CT-011, a novel monoclonal anti-PD-1 antibody. Blood 116:2286–2294

28. Talebian L et al (2014) The natural killer-activating receptor, NKG2D, on CD3+CD8+ T cells plays a critical role in identifying and killing autologous myeloma cells. Transfusion 54:1515–1521

29. Jinushi M et al (2008) MHC class I chain-related protein A antibodies and shedding are associated with the progression of multiple myeloma. Proc Natl Acad Sci 105:1285–1290

30. Pasiarski M, Grywalska E, Kosmaczewska A, Gozdz S, Rolinski J (2013) The frequency of myeloid and lymphoid dendritic cells in multiple myeloma patients is inversely correlated with disease progression. Potepy Hig Med Dosw 67:1–7

31. Ratta M et al (2002) Dendritic cells are functionally defective in multiple myeloma: the role of interleukin-6. Blood 100:230–237

32. Ramachandran IR et al (2013) Myeloid-derived suppressor cells regulate growth of multiple myeloma by inhibiting T cells in bone marrow. J Immunol 190:3815–3823

33. Görgün GT et al (2013) Tumor-promoting immune-suppressive myeloid-derived suppressor cells in the multiple myeloma microenvironment in humans. Blood 121:2975–2987

34. Serafini P et al (2006) Phosphodiesterase-5 inhibition augments endogenous antitumor immunity by reducing myeloid-derived suppressor cell function. J Exp Med 203:2691–2702

35. Noonan KA, Ghosh N, Rudraraju L, Bui M, Borrello I (2014) Targeting immune suppression with PDE5 inhibition in end-stage multiple myeloma. Cancer Immunol Res 2:725–731

36. Borrello I et al (2000) Sustaining the graft-versus-tumor effect through posttransplant immunization with granulocyte-macrophage colony-stimulating factor (GM-CSF)–producing tumor vaccines. Blood 95:3011–3019

37. Gorin NC (2000) New developments in the therapy of acute myelocytic leukemia. Hematology 2000:69–89

38. Gerull S et al (2013) Allo-SCT for multiple myeloma in the era of novel agents: a retrospective study on behalf of Swiss Blood SCT. Bone Marrow Transplant 48:408–413

39. Bjorkstrand BB et al (1996) Allogeneic bone marrow transplantation versus autologous stem cell transplantation in multiple myeloma: a retrospective case-matched study from the European Group for Blood and Marrow Transplantation. Blood 88:4711–4718

40. Gahrton G et al (1999) Syngeneic transplantation in multiple myeloma—a case-matched comparison with autologous and allogeneic transplantation. Bone Marrow Transplant 24:741–745

41. Barlogie B (2006) Standard chemotherapy compared with high-dose chemoradiotherapy for multiple myeloma: final results of phase III US intergroup trial S9321. J Clin Oncol 24:929–936

42. Kanakry CG et al (2014) Single-agent GVHD prophylaxis with posttransplantation cyclophosphamide after myeloablative, HLA-matched BMT for AML, ALL, and MDS. Blood 124:3817–3827

43. Mazo IB et al (2005) Bone marrow is a major reservoir and site of recruitment for central memory CD8+ T cells. Immunity 22:259–270

44. Di Rosa F, Pabst R (2005) The bone marrow: a nest for migratory memory T cells. Trends Immunol 26:360–366

45. Noonan K et al (2005) Activated marrow-infiltrating lymphocytes effectively target plasma cells and their clonogenic precursors. Cancer Res 65:2026–2034

46. Chu J et al (2014) CS1-specific chimeric antigen receptor (CAR)-engineered natural killer cells enhance in vitro and in vivo antitumor activity against human multiple myeloma. Leukemia 28:917–927

47. Jiang H et al (2014) Transfection of chimeric anti-CD138 gene enhances natural killer cell activation and killing of multiple myeloma cells. Mol Oncol 8:297–310

48. Meehan KR et al (2013) Adoptive cellular therapy using cells enriched for NKG2D+CD3 +CD8+ T cells after autologous transplantation for myeloma. Biol Blood Marrow Transplant 19:129–137

49. Curti A et al (2007) Phase I/II clinical trial of sequential subcutaneous and intravenous delivery of dendritic cell vaccination for refractory multiple myeloma using patient-specific tumour idiotype protein or idiotype (VDJ)-derived class I-restricted peptides. Br J Haematol 139:415–424

50. Reichardt VL et al (1999) Idiotype vaccination using dendritic cells after autologous peripheral blood stem cell transplantation for multiple myeloma—a feasibility study. Blood 93:2411–2419

51. Lim SH, Bailey-Wood R (1999) Idiotypic protein-pulsed dendritic cell vaccination in multiple myeloma. Int J Cancer 83:215–222

52. Yi Q, Desikan R, Barlogie B, Munshi N (2002) Optimizing dendritic cell-based immunotherapy in multiple myeloma. Br J Haematol 117:297–305

53. Rollig C et al (2011) Induction of cellular immune responses in patients with stage-I multiple myeloma after vaccination with autologous idiotype-pulsed dendritic cells. J Immunother 34:100–106

54. Hong S et al (2012) Optimizing dendritic cell vaccine for immunotherapy in multiple myeloma: tumour lysates are more potent tumour antigens than idiotype protein to promote anti-tumour immunity. Clin Exp Immunol 170:167–177

55. Rosenblatt J et al (2013) Vaccination with dendritic cell/tumor fusions following autologous stem cell transplant induces immunologic and clinical responses in multiple myeloma patients. Clin Cancer Res 19:3640–3648

56. Schmitt M et al (2007) RHAMM-R3 peptide vaccination in patients with acute myeloid leukemia, myelodysplastic syndrome, and multiple myeloma elicits immunologic and clinical responses. Blood 111:1357–1365

57. Greiner J et al (2010) High-dose RHAMM-R3 peptide vaccination for patients with acute myeloid leukemia, myelodysplastic syndrome and multiple myeloma. Haematologica 95:1191–1197

58. Azuma T (2004) Myeloma cells are highly sensitive to the granule exocytosis pathway mediated by WT1-specific cytotoxic T lymphocytes. Clin Cancer Res 10:7402–7412

59. Tsuboi A et al (2007) Wilms tumor gene WT1 peptide-based immunotherapy induced a minimal response in a patient with advanced therapy-resistant multiple myeloma. Int J Hematol 86:414–417

60. Noonan K et al (2014) Lenalidomide immunomodulation with an allogeneic myeloma GVAX in a near complete remission induces durable clinical remissions. Blood 124:2137

61. Miguel JFS et al (1990) Immunophenotypic heterogeneity of multiple myeloma: influence on the biology and clinical course of the disease. Br J Haematol 77:185–190

62. Matsui W et al (2004) Characterization of clonogenic multiple myeloma cells. Blood 103:2332–2336

63. Treon SP et al (2002) CD20-directed serotherapy in patients with multiple myeloma: biologic considerations and therapeutic applications. J Immunother 25:72–81

64. Zojer N, Kirchbacher K, Vesely M, Hübl W, Ludwig H (2006) Rituximab treatment provides no clinical benefit in patients with pretreated advanced multiple myeloma. Leuk Lymphoma 47:1103–1109

65. Moreau P et al (2007) Rituximab in CD20 positive multiple myeloma. Leukemia 1–2. doi:10.1038/sj.leu.2404558

66. Deaglio S (2006) In-tandem insight from basic science combined with clinical research: CD38 as both marker and key component of the pathogenetic network underlying chronic lymphocytic leukemia. Blood 108:1135–1144

67. van der Veer MS et al (2011) The therapeutic human CD38 antibody daratumumab improves the anti-myeloma effect of newly emerging multi-drug therapies. Blood Cancer J 1:e41–e43

68. de Weers M et al (2011) Daratumumab, a novel therapeutic human CD38 monoclonal antibody, induces killing of multiple myeloma and other hematological tumors. J Immunol 186:1840–1848

69. Jansen JHM et al (2012) Daratumumab, a human CD38 antibody induces apoptosis of myeloma tumor cells via Fc receptor-mediated crosslinking. Blood 120:2974

70. Overdijk MB et al (2012) Phagocytosis is a mechanism of action for daratumumab. Blood 120:4054

71. Plesner T et al (2012) Daratumumab, a CD38 monoclonal antibody in patients with multiple myeloma—data from a dose-escalation phase I/II study. Blood 120:73

72. Plesner T et al (2013) Preliminary safety and efficacy data of daratumumab in combination with lenalidomide and dexamethasone in relapsed or refractory multiple myeloma. Blood 122:1986

73. Deckert J et al (2014) SAR650984, a novel humanized CD38-targeting antibody, demonstrates potent antitumor activity in models of multiple myeloma and other CD38+ hematologic malignancies. Clin Cancer Res 20:4574–4583

74. Harada H et al (1993) Phenotypic difference of normal plasma cells from mature myeloma cells. Blood 81:2658–2663

75. Chanan-Khan A et al (2010) Efficacy analysis from phase I study of Lorvotuzumab mertansine(IMGN901), used as monotherapy, in patients with heavily pre-treated CD56-positive multiple myeloma—a preliminary efficacy analysis. Blood 116:1962

76. Berdeja JG et al (2012) Phase i study of Lorvotuzumab mertansine (LM, IMGN901) in combination with Lenalidomide (Len) and Dexamethasone (Dex) in patients with CD56-positive relapsed or relapsed/refractory multiple myeloma (MM). Blood 120:4048

77. Kumaresan PR, Lai WC, Chuang SS, Bennett M, Mathew PA (2002) CS1, a novel member of the CD2 family, is homophilic and regulates NK cell function. Mol Immunol 39:1–8
78. Zonder JA et al (2012) A phase 1, multicenter, open-label, dose escalation study of elotuzumab in patients with advanced multiple myeloma. Blood 120:552–559
79. Jakubowiak AJ et al (2012) Phase I trial of anti-CS1 monoclonal antibody elotuzumab in combination with bortezomib in the treatment of relapsed/refractory multiple myeloma. J Clin Oncol 30:1960–1965
80. Lonial S et al (2012) Elotuzumab in combination with lenalidomide and low-dose dexamethasone in relapsed or refractory multiple myeloma. J Clin Oncol 30:1953–1959
81. Hussein M et al (2010) A phase I multidose study of dacetuzumab (SGN-40; humanized anti-CD40 monoclonal antibody) in patients with multiple myeloma. Haematologica 95: 845–848
82. Bensinger W et al (2012) A phase 1 study of lucatumumab, a fully human anti-CD40 antagonist monoclonal antibody administered intravenously to patients with relapsed or refractory multiple myeloma. Br J Haematol 159:58–66
83. Kurzrock R et al (2013) A phase I, open-label study of siltuximab, an anti-IL-6 monoclonal antibody, in patients with B-cell non-Hodgkin lymphoma, multiple myeloma, or Castleman disease. Clin Cancer Res 19:3659–3670
84. Voorhees PM et al (2013) A phase 2 multicentre study of siltuximab, an anti-interleukin-6 monoclonal antibody, in patients with relapsed or refractory multiple myeloma. Br J Haematol 161:357–366
85. San-Miguel J et al (2014) Phase 2 randomized study of bortezomib-melphalan-prednisone with or without siltuximab (anti-IL-6) in multiple myeloma. Blood 123:4136–4142
86. Chapon M et al (2011) Progressive Upregulation of PD-1 in Primary and Metastatic Melanomas Associated with Blunted TCR Signaling in Infiltrating T Lymphocytes. Journal of Investigative Dermatology 131:1300–1307
87. Topalian SL, Drake CG, Pardoll DM (2012) Targeting the PD-1/B7-H1(PD-L1) pathway to activate anti-tumor immunity. Curr Opin Immunol 24:207–212
88. Yao S, Chen L (2013) Adaptive resistance: a tumor strategy to evade immune attack. Eur J Immunol 43:576–579
89. Iwai Y et al (2002) Involvement of PD-L1 on tumor cells in the escape from host immune system and tumor immunotherapy by PD-L1 blockade. Proc Natl Acad Sci 99:12293–12297
90. Topalian SL et al (2014) Survival, durable tumor remission, and long-term safety in patients with advanced melanoma receiving Nivolumab. J Clin Oncol 32:1020–1030
91. Brahmer JR et al (2012) Safety and activity of anti–PD-L1 antibody in patients with advanced cancer. N Engl J Med 366:2455–2465
92. Ansell SM et al (2015) PD-1 blockade with Nivolumab in relapsed or refractory Hodgkin's lymphoma. N Engl J Med 372:311–319
93. Creelan BC (2014) Update on immune checkpoint inhibitors in lung cancer. Cancer Control 21:1–10
94. Lesokhin AM et al (2014) Preliminary results of a phase I study of Nivolumab (BMS-936558) in patients with relapsed or refractory lymphoid malignancies. Blood 124:291–291
95. Kearl TJ, Jing W, Gershan JA, Johnson BD (2013) Programmed death receptor-1/programmed death receptor ligand-1 blockade after transient lymphodepletion to treat myeloma. J Immunol 190:5620–5628
96 Schneider H et al (2006) Reversal of the TCR stop Signal by CTLA-4. Sci 313(5795):1972–5
97. Schmidt EM et al (2008) CTLA-4 controls regulatory T cell peripheral homeostasis and is required for suppression of pancreatic islet autoimmunity. J Immunol 182:274–282
98. Friedline RH et al (2009) CD4+ regulatory T cells require CTLA-4 for the maintenance of systemic tolerance. J Exp Med 206:421–434

99. Braga WMT, Vettore AL, Carvalho AC, Atanackovic D, Colleoni GWB (2011) Overexpression of *CTLA-4* in the bone marrow of patients with multiple myeloma as a sign of local accumulation of immunosuppressive Tregs—perspectives for novel treatment strategies. Blood 118:1829

100. Hodi FS et al (2010) Improved survival with ipilimumab in patients with metastatic melanoma. N Engl J Med 363:711–723

101. De Keersmaecker B et al (2014) Immunomodulatory drugs improve the immune environment for dendritic cell-based immunotherapy in multiple myeloma patients after autologous stem cell transplantation. Cancer Immunol Immunother 63:1023–1036

102. Noonan K et al (2012) Lenalidomide-induced immunomodulation in multiple myeloma: impact on vaccines and antitumor responses. Clin Cancer Res 18:1426–1434

103. Xu Y et al (2009) Immunomodulatory drugs reorganize cytoskeleton by modulating Rho GTPases. Blood 114:338–345

104. Henry JY et al (2013) Enhanced cross-priming of naive CD8+ T cells by dendritic cells treated by the IMiDs ®immunomodulatory compounds lenalidomide and pomalidomide. Immunology 139:377–385

105. Clave E et al (2014) Lenalidomide consolidation and maintenance therapy after autologous stem cell transplant for multiple myeloma induces persistent changes in T-cell homeostasis. Leuk Lymphoma 55:1788–1795

106. Hayashi T et al (2005) Molecular mechanisms whereby immunomodulatory drugs activate natural killer cells: clinical application. Br J Haematol 128:192–203

Transplantation for Multiple Myeloma

Yogesh S. Jethava and Frits van Rhee

Abstract

Multiple myeloma is a disorder characterized by accumulation of malignant plasma cells in the bone marrow, hypercalcemia, monoclonal protein, and end organ damage. Recently newer generation proteosome inhibitors, monoclonal antibodies and novel agents have been approved by FDA, which is undoubtedly increasing life expectancy of the patients. However, hematopoietic stem cell transplantation still remains the cornerstone of the treatment. In this chapter, we are discussing the autologous stem cell transplant, allogeneic stem cell transplant and total therapy trials with outcomes.

Keyword

Myeloma · Stem cell transplant · Tandem transplants · Clinical trials with transplant

1   Introduction

A Surveillance Epidemiology and End Results (SEER) data indicate that the number of new cases of multiple myeloma (MM) was 6.3 per 100,000 men and women per year. Multiple myeloma is the most common indication for autologous stem cell transplantation (AT). AT is still considered the standard of care for multiple myeloma (MM) patients. In the USA, eligibility for hemopoetic stem cell

Y.S. Jethava (✉) · F. van Rhee
Stem Cell and Allogeneic Transplant, Department of Hematology/Oncology,
University of Arkansas for Medical Sciences, Little Rock, AR, USA
e-mail: YSJethava@uams.edu

© Springer International Publishing Switzerland 2016
A.M. Roccaro and I.M. Ghobrial (eds.), *Plasma Cell Dyscrasias*,
Cancer Treatment and Research 169, DOI 10.1007/978-3-319-40320-5_13

transplant (HSCT) is principally determined by biological fitness rather than age while in Europe, patients are often considered who are 65 years or younger. New chemotherapeutic agents (e.g., bortezomib, thalidomide, lenalidomide) are being incorporated into treatment paradigm for multiple myeloma as a result, outcomes with AT have been improving. Recent studies with long-term follow-up suggest that cure is now feasible for subsets of patients.

2 Advances in Disease Biology and Risk-Adapted Treatment

Several algorithms for the management of myeloma have been suggested. Most of these incorporate cytogenetics and standard prognostic factors such as serum albumin and beta 2 microglobulin [1].

The cytogenetic-based risk stratification model is demonstrated in Table 1.

Apart from the cytogenetic-based risk model, gene expression profiling offers more robust way of risk stratification of MM [2]. So far, GEP is available in large institutions and the disadvantages of GEP include sample attrition (especially in multicenter trials), expense, requirement for stringent quality control, and sample turnaround time, which limits application. The introduction of a "myeloma PCR kit" has negated these issues and is enabling genetic stratification based on biologic disease risk. Based on RT-PCR data of 70 genes, MM patients are divided into standard risk and high-risk groups. High-risk patients do poorly with all current approaches and should be entered into clinical trials exploring novel therapies and combination of novel drugs. It is conceivable that standard or low-risk patients in the elderly population would be amenable to therapeutic approaches aimed at providing long-term disease control.

In subsequent sections we will discuss

- Early versus late transplant in MM
- Single autologous transplant
- Tandem autologous transplants
- Evidence related to allogeneic transplant

Table 1 Risk stratification of myeloma based on cytogenetics

High risk	Intermediate risk	Low risk
17p13 deletion t (14;16) t (14;20) LDH ≥ 2 times institutional upper limit of normal Features of primary plasma cell leukemia High-risk gene expression profiling signature	t (4;14) Deletion 13 or hypodiploidy by conventional karyotyping	Trisomies (hyperdiploidy) t (11;14) t (6;14)

Table 2 Studies of early autologous transplantation

Trial	Induction	Randomization	Results
Gay et al. N = 402 [6]	Lenalidomide + Dexamethasone	Arm A-MPR Arm B-tandem AT with melphalan 200 mg/m^2	Follow up 45 months from the diagnosis. PFS for AT superior. 38 versus 26 months ($p < 0.0001$)
Italian group N = 389 [7]	RD	Arm A = CRD Arm B = AT with mel 200 Second randomization = lenalidomide + prednisone versus lenalidomide maintenance	PFS at 2 years = mel arm 72 % and 61 % for CRD arm. ($p < 0.001$)

3   Early Versus Late Transplant in the Era of Novel Agents

Novel agents have resulted in increased response rates especially with the triplet therapy. This has raised the question whether AT should be considered early or reserved for relapse. There are not many studies, comparing up-front AT versus salvage AT. There has been one phase 3 study, reported more than 10 years ago, which examined up-front autologous HSCT compared with rescue autologous HSCT at disease progression/relapse and found no difference in the two approaches [3]. Early reports from two phase 3 trials examining chemotherapy versus up-front tandem autologous HSCT have shown an improved PFS without a difference in OS [4, 5]. Table 2 summarizes studies of early autologous transplantation versus standard chemotherapy. Recent genomic studies have shown that MM patients have significant clonal heterogeneity. Hence one could argue that, in younger patients, AT should be applied to maximize cytoreduction followed by consolidation and maintenance therapy with an objective to eliminate myeloma completely or minimize the myeloma burden to prevent the emergence of treatment-refractory clones. Further, the novel therapies carry the risk of generating drug-refractory disease, which may prove difficult to control even with a melphalan-based AT. At present it is difficult to identify patients with genomically unstable disease and therefore with with aggressive subclones and those who do not harbor more aggressive subclones, allowing for more expectant management. It is also important to realize that there is an increased tendency in the field to treat patients, who are not transplanted up-front, until progression prolonging the exposure to drugs and their potential toxicities. A large randomized study US/French study enrolling 1000 patients is currently in progress comparing the outcomes of patients receiving up-front AT and AT at relapse This study will elucidate more information on the timing of AT transplantation strategy. At present, we recommend up-front AT for the transplant eligible patients.

4   Single Autologous Transplant Versus Standard Chemotherapy

Melphalan (MEL) was first introduced in 1962 for the therapy of myeloma [4, 5]. McElwain and Powles first reported the efficacy of high-dose MEL in inducing complete biochemical and bone marrow responses in three of nine patients [8, 9]. Barlogie et al. reported that the prolonged myelosuppression due high-dose MEL therapy could be considerably shortened by infusing autologous bone marrow cells [10]. Several prospective, randomized studies in newly diagnosed patients have addressed whether high-dose Mel is superior to standard chemotherapy (Table 3). These include studies conducted by the Intergroupe Francais de Myélome (IFM), the Medical Research Council of the United Kingdom (MRC), the Group Myelome-Autogreffe (MAG), the Programa para el Estudio de la Terapéutica en Hematopatía Maligna (PETHEMA), and the US Intergroup Trial S9321 [11–13]. Collectively, the evidence of both retrospective and prospective studies indicates

Table 3 Randomized trials of standard chemotherapy compared to high-dose Mel treatment

Author	Group	N	Age (years)	Median Follow-up (month)	TRM (%)	CR%(STD vs. HDT)	Median EFS (month)	Median OS (month)	Conclusion
Attal et al. [14]	IFM 90	200	≤65	37 STD, 41 AT	5 versus 7	5 versus 22	18 versus 22	44 versus 57	Benefit in EFS and OS
Child et al. [15]	MRC7	401	≤64	32 STD 40AT		8 versus 44	20 versus 32	42 versus 54	Benefit in EFS and OS
Blade et al. [12]	PETHEMA	164	≤65	56	3.6 versus 3.7	11 versus 30	33 versus 42	66 versus 61	No benefit
Palumbo [16]	M97G	194	50–70'	39 STD 41 AT	0 versus 2.1	6 versus 25	16 versus 28	43 versus NR	Benefit in EFS and OS
Fermand et al. [11]	MAG	190	55–65	120	2.1 versus 5.3	4 versus 6	19 versus 25	48 versus 48	Benefit in EFS, but not OS
Segeren et al. [8]	HOVON	261	<65	33	1.3 versus 5.2	13 versus 29	21 versus 22	50 versus 47	No benefit in EFS or OS
Barlogieet al. [13]	USIG	516	<70	76	0.4 versus 3.4	15 versus 17	22 versus 25	54 versus 62	No benefit in EFS or OS

that high dose treatment (HDT) confers a survival benefit in younger patients (<60 years of age).

In IFM90 study involving patients younger than 65 years of age, HDT arm had shown higher CR and VGPR rates (38 vs 14 % respectively) [14]. The 5-year OS and EFS rates in the HDT arm were superior (52 vs. 12 %; $p = 0.03$ and 28 vs. 10 %; $p = 0.01$) and the best results were seen in patients <60 years with 5-year OS of 70 %. In MRCVII study of 407 patients <65 years, CR rates of 44 versus 8 % ($p < 0.001$) were reported. HDT with MEL 200 mg/m^2 not only increased median survival by almost 1 year (54.1 vs. 42.3 months) but also significantly improved time to progression in this trial.

Few trials such as MAG, PETHEMA, and the US Intergroup studies did not show a definite benefit in terms of OS for MEL-based HDT. This can be explained by several factors. In the US Intergroup Trial, CR rates were similar (17 vs. 15 %) between high-dose MEL arm and standard chemotherapy arm however the conditioning used was reduced dose of Mel 140 mg/m^2 and 8 Gy of total body irradiation (TBI). The dose if MEL is certainly inferior to MEL 200 mg/m^2 which was used in historical and randomized trials. Also in this trial, the large percentage of patients in the standard chemotherapy arm crossed over to MEL arm, making it difficult to interpret OS [17–19].

The MAG study compared VMCP chemotherapy and high-dose treatment, comprising MEL 200 or MEL140 mg/m2 with busulfan 16 mg/kg in patients between 55 and 65 years old. There was a trend to better EFS in the high-dose arm at a median follow-up at 10 years but the OS survival was identical at 48 months in both the arms. However, it is important to note that 22 % of patients in the STD arm received salvage HDT, which may have contributed to equalizing OS in both the arms in this trial.

In the PETHEMA study, randomization to high-dose chemotherapy or standard chemotherapy was not performed at diagnosis. Also, the therapy delivered in the standard arm, comprised of 12 cycles of VBMP/VBAD, which is considerably heavy and it mitigated any survival benefit conferred by HDT [20].

In general, most investigators would agree that single MEL-based high-dose treatment is superior to standard chemotherapy in patients less than 65 years [19].

5 Tandem Autologous Transplant

The role of tandem autologous transplants is explored in various total therapy trials and European trials.

5.1 Total Therapies

Total Therapy I, trial intended to increase the frequency and duration of complete response, thus extending OS [9]. The concept was inspired by the St Jude's Children's Hospital Total Therapy (TT) programs for acute leukemia which have

Total Therapy Trials 1 and 2

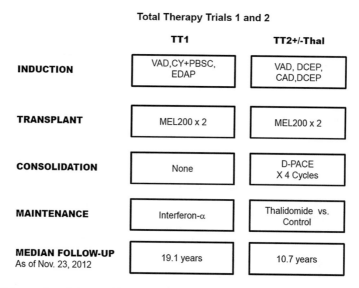

Fig. 1 Schema of total therapy 1(TT1) and total therapy 2(TT2) trials

made unprecedented progress in curing children with both acute lymphoblastic and myeloid leukemias. It was recognized in adult acute leukemia that cures were only obtained when a CR rate of $\geq$40 % was accomplished. A single MEL 200 AT resulted in a CR rate of usually no more than 20 % [10, 21, 22]. Thus, using CR as a substitute for survival, the underlying hypothesis was that a more marked increase in CR rate, from less than 5 % with standard MEL-prednisone (MP) to 40 % would produce significant prolongation of EFS and OS, and perhaps attain cure [5]. These observations led to initiation of Total Therapy Trials in MM.

The schema for TT1, TT2, and TT3 trials is already published (Figs. 1 and 2). The results of TT4, TT5, and TT6 trials are still awaited. The long-term results of TT1, which enrolled 231 patients, were published and the median follow-up was an unprecedented 12 years [23]. At 10 and 15 years, respectively, 33 and 17 % of patients are alive; 15 and 7 % are event free; and 18 and 12 % of those achieving CR remain in uninterrupted remission.

The successor Phase III trial, TT2 with 668 enrollees, delivered more intense treatment by intensifying remission induction, by adding consolidation chemotherapy post-tandem AT, and by providing high-dose pulsed dexametasone during maintenance with INF-α [24]. In addition, patients were randomized to receive thalidomide from the outset until disease progression or adverse events.

The thalidomide group had significantly higher CR rates and 5-year EFS compared to the control group (62 vs. 43 %, and 56 vs. 44 %, respectively). However, the 5-year OS was approximately 65 % in both arms of the study, which could be explained by worse post-relapse survival in the thalidomide arm, suggesting that continuous exposure to thalidomide may promote drug resistance.

Total Therapy Trials 3A and 3B

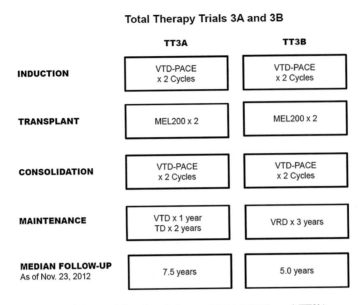

Fig. 2 Schema of total therapy 3A and total therapy 3B trial (TT3a and TT3b)

EFS and OS were adversely influenced by calcium (CA), elevated LDH and albumin <3.5 g/dl.

The non-thalidomide arms in TT2 and TT1 were recently compared in order to examine the potential benefit conferred by dose-intensified induction chemotherapy and post-tandem AT consolidation chemotherapy applied in TT2 without having thalidomide as a confounding variable [25]. The CR rates in both trials were similar at 41 and 43 %. However, the 5-year estimates of continuous CR (45 vs. 32 %), and 5-year EFS (43 vs. 28 %) were significantly superior in TT2, with a trend to improved OS (62 vs. 57 %). Patients who achieved CR in the first year and had tandem AT within 1 year also had superior OS.

The treatment-related mortality was similar in both trials at approximately 7 %. These data indicate that, overall, TT2 without thalidomide was superior to TT1. Since CA is an important prognostic factor, the outcome was examined in both trials in patients with good-risk (normal CA) and high-risk features (abnormal CA). TT2 especially benefited the two-thirds of good-risk patient who entered CR more frequently and had a longer duration of CR with superior EFS and OS. Thaldomide conferred benefit to patients with a standard risk GEP and abnormal metaphase cytogenetics; a surprising finding, which has not been satisfactorily explained. The TT3 trial combined bortezomib with DTPACE portion as induction and consolidation. The initial results of TT3 trial are, respectively, with an unprecedented 80 % of patients remaining in CR at 2 years with a treatment-related mortality of only 5 %.

These TT trials demonstrated that it is feasible in myeloma to achieve a long-term survival of >30 % at 10 years with tandem transplants with high-dose MEL. This also sets a new yardstick against which recently developed newer drugs should be tested.

5.2 European Randomized Studies

In the IFM 94 study, French intergroup compared single transplant with MEL 140 with tandem transplants. In tandem transplant arm comprised of conditioning with MEL 140 and MEL 140/TBI with the first and second transplant, respectively [26]. A superior 7-year probability of EFS and OS in the tandem AT arm (20 vs. 10 % and 42 vs. 21 %, respectively) was observed.

In Bologna, 96 studies showed that tandem AT significantly increased the probability to achieve CR from 33 to 47 % and extended the 5-year EFS from 29 to 17 % [27]. Tandem AT prolonged EFS by approximately 1 year and was related to a higher CR rate. Twenty percent of patients who failed to achieve (n)CR post after the first transplant did so after the second transplant. Patients who were sensitive to conventional chemotherapy with VAD achieved a CR rate of 73 % with double AT, versus 52 % in the single AT group. Conversely, the CR rates in the single and tandem AT arms were similar in patients' refractory to VAD, suggesting that resistance to conventional chemotherapy was difficult to overcome even by double AT. There was no benefit in terms of OS, which was similar after single and double AT (46 vs. 43 %). The 2-year OS from relapse in the single transplant arm was longer than in the second transplant arm (62 vs. 51 %), which can be explained by the sequential application of salvage therapies. Approximately one-third of the patients received a second, unplanned AT, obscuring the survival benefit conferred by a second planned procedure. In addition, half were treated with novel agents such as thalidomide and bortezomib, which may have the potential to reverse resistance to HDT.

The French MAG 95 used a two × two design in 230 patients younger than 56 years to study the effects of both tandem AT and purging of the autograft using CD34+ selection. Tandem AT using unselected CD34+ cells resulted in improved OS compared to single AT. CD34+ cell selection did not confer survival benefit and was associated with an increased risk of infectious complications [28].

Table 4 summarizes the studies of tandem transplants in MM patients.

We recommend that tandem transplant should not be done outside the context of clinical trials. The studies show that tandem AT is well tolerated by younger patients with good performance status. It has acceptable treatment-related morbidity and mortality. Patients who appear to benefit most from a second AT procedure are those who are not in (n)CR after the first AT. Patients with aggressive disease, e.g., abnormal CA, do not seem to do better with tandem AT.

Table 4 Randomized trials of single versus double AT

Group	N	Age	Median Follow-up (Mo)	Regimen	CR% (single vs. double)	Median EFS (mo) (single vs. double)	Median OS (single vs. double)	Conclusion
IFM 94 [25]	339	60	75	MEL 140 + TBI and MEL 140	42 versus 50	25 versus 30	48 versus 58	OS/EFS better in double AT
MAG 95 [27]	227	55	53	MEL 140 + CCNU/VP 16/Cy/TBI versus MEL 140 → MEL 140 + TBI	39 versus 37	31 versus 33	49 versus 73	No diff in EFS. OS is better with double AT
Bologna 96 [29]	228	60	55	MEL 200 → MEL 120 + BU 12	35 versus 48	25 versus 35	59 versus 73	OS/EFS better in double AT
GMMG HD2 [30]	210	65	NR	MEL 200 → MEL 200	Not available	23 versus 29	No difference	EFS better with double AT

6 Autologous Stem Cell Transplant

6.1 Collection and Processing of Stem Cells

Alkylating agents such as melphalan and the immunomodulatory lenalidomide can impair the collection of hemopoeitic stem cells (HSC). Melphalan is best completely avoided, whilst lenalidomide exposure should be limited to four cycles prior to collection. HSC are typically collected by apheresis from the peripheral blood after stimulation with granulocyte colony-stimulating factor (G-CSF). Peripheral blood progenitor cells (PBPCs) are preferable to bone marrow cells for transplantation due to quicker engraftment and a potential for less contamination of the infused cells with tumor cells. G-CSF alone and G-CSF plus cyclophosphamide are the most common regimens used for stem cell mobilization [31–33]. The usual dose of G-CSF is 10 mcg/kg per day subcutaneous. Cyclophosphamide is usually administered at a dose of 1.5–3 g/m^2 intravenous for 1 or 2 days. The choice between the two methods is mainly dependent on institutional preference and experience. There are no randomized trials comparing the two approaches. Some institutions use G-CSF plus cyclophosphamide as their standard. G-CSF plus cyclophosphamide has the advantage of providing much higher PBPCs than G-CSF alone, but also carries the risk of longer time to start collection and the risk of neutropenia. Plerixafor is a chemokine receptor type 4 inhibitor (CXCR4) and it impairs the binding of hematopoietic stem cells within the bone marrow microenvironment [34]. Plerixafor is by some, primarily reserved for patients who fail stem cell collection with either G-CSF or G-CSF plus cyclophosphamide, while some use pleraxifor up-front usually together with G-CSF [35, 36]. Once the mobilization regimen is initiated, patients are monitored by peripheral blood CD34 counts. Apheresis is started when the peripheral CD34+ counts reach 20 CD34 cells/microL. Apheresis is performed with a goal of collecting between at least minimum 3×10^6 CD34+ to 6×10^6 CD34+ cells/kg. A minimum of 2×106 CD34+ cells/kg is considered essential for one transplant. We routinely collect >20 × 106 CD34+ cells/kg. Infusion of a larger number of stem cells will hasten recovery, minimize blood product use, and reduce area of CRP under the curve, the latter being a surrogate marker for infectious complication. This leaves ample cells for use as salvage transplant or for reestablishing hematopoiesis if multiple lines of salvage therapy have exhausted hematopoiesis. In general, enough PBPCs are harvested for two transplantations. PBPCs are cryopreserved in 5 % dimethylsulfoxide to be thawed at the bedside at the time of infusion [16].

6.2 Preparatory Regimen

The standard conditioning regimen used for AT in multiple myeloma is melphalan at a dose of 200 mg/m^2, with dose reductions based on age and renal function.

The use of this dose is primarily based upon two randomized trials that have compared melphalan 200 mg/m^2 with a lower dose of melphalan in conditioning for HCT. The French cooperative study compared melphalan 140 mg/m^2 plus 8 Gy total body irradiation versus Melphalan 200 mg/m^2 in 282 newly diagnosed patients. Patients randomly assigned to melphalan 200 mg/m^2 had faster hematologic recovery, less mucositis, less transfusion requirements and, shorter hospitalizations. In this study, survival at 45 months was significantly better in patients receiving melphalan 200 mg/m^2 (66 versus 46 %).The Italian study comparing melphalan 200 mg/m^2 with melphalan 100 mg/m^2 as preparative regimens for HCT in 298 newly diagnosed symptomatic patients <65 years of age [37], patients who received melphalan 200 m/m^2 had significantly longer median progression-free survival (31.4 versus 26.2 months) and a trend towards improved projected overall survival at 5 years (62 versus 48 %). Higher percentage of gastrointestinal toxicity (11 versus 1 %), mucositis (17 versus 3 %), need for intravenous broad-spectrum antibiotics (41 versus 29 %), and need for platelet transfusions (56 versus 38 %) was noted in melphalan 200 mg/m^2 group. In two other randomized studies, the use of more intensive preparative regimens, such as thiotepa, busulfan, and cyclophosphamide [38] or high-dose idarubicin, cyclophosphamide, and melphalan [39] did not result in better outcomes than melphalan at a dose of 200 mg/m^2. Dose adjustments for melphalan for obese patients can lead to a lower dose of melphalan when calculated per kg and could potentially lead to under treatment.

6.3   Special Circumstances

(a) **Patients with renal insufficiency**—Randomized trials that have shown benefit with HCT compared with chemotherapy have mainly studied patients with serum creatinine <2.0 mg/dL. The data for melphalan use in patients with serum creatinine >2.0 mg/dL comes from a retrospective review of 81 patients with MM and renal failure (plasma creatinine >2 mg/dL) who underwent autologous HCT [40]. Sixty patients who received melphalan 200 mg/m^2, excessive toxicity was noted in patients than the subsequent 21 patients who received melphalan 140 mg/m^2. The patients who received melphalan 200 mg/m^2 had significantly higher rates of severe pulmonary toxicity (57 versus 17 %) and mucositis (93 versus 67 %). In the patients with creatinine >2.0 mg/dl, the treatment-related mortality, event-free, and overall survival were not significantly different between melphalan 200 mg/m^2 and melphalan 140 mg/m^2.

(b) **Older adults**—In order to reduce toxicity in patients over 65 years of age, various strategies are studied. For example, once two sequential courses of an intermediate dose of melphalan (100 mg/m^2) followed by hematopoietic stem cell rescue (MEL100) has been studied as an alternative to high-dose melphalan 200 mg/m2. In a multicenter trial of 194, in the subgroup of 80 patients aged 65–70, higher rates of near complete plus partial remissions (47 versus 16 %), longer median event-free survival (28 versus 16 months), and overall survival (58 versus

37 months) were observed in patients receiving melphalan 100 mg/m^2. However, higher short-term toxicity (e.g., mucositis, fever, need for red cell, or platelet transfusions) was noted. The French Intergroupe Francophone du Myelome (IFM) group reported on 447 previously untreated patients with myeloma patients aged 65–75 years who received melphalan, prednisone, and thalidomide (MPT) or melphalan and prednisone alone (MP) or tandem autologous HCT using MEL100 [41]. There was no difference in median overall survival between the MP and transplant arms. This study suggests that an intermediate dose of melphalan may not be the optimal conditioning regimen. At present, we use melphalan 200 mg/m^2 as standard conditioning regimen for HCT myeloma patients and reduce the dose to 140 mg/m^2 in patients with renal impairment or those over the age of 65.

6.4 Care During Transplantation

Autologous hematopoietic cell transplantation (HCT) has been performed in both the inpatient and outpatient settings. Approximately 24 h after completion of the preparative chemotherapy, peripheral blood progenitor cells (PBPCs) are reinfused. A period of pancytopenia follows. Red blood cell and platelet transfusions are administered as necessary while hematopoietic colony-stimulating factors (i.e., G-CSF) are used to speed neutrophil engraftment. Neutrophil engraftment usually occurs by day 10–11 and platelet counts are expected to recover to greater than 20,000 by day 16 [42]. Red blood cell transfusion requirements during autologous HCT are usually minimal. HCT without transfusion support, although not ideal has recently been reported in a series of 50 Jehova's witnesses with acceptable toxicity [43]. At our institution, approximately 80–90 % of patients undergo autologous transplantation entirely as an outpatient, with daily monitoring until full engraftment has occurred [44]. Patients who undergo HCT are at risk for bacterial, viral, and fungal infections, the time course of which varies in the post-transplant period, according to the degree of immune deficiency and cytopenia induced by the transplantation procedure. Approximately 40 % of patients with multiple myeloma undergoing autologous HCT will experience febrile neutropenia [45]. As a result, prophylactic therapies to prevent infection including antiviral and antifungal drugs are recommended during the period of increased risk. In addition, all markers of potential infection must be investigated thoroughly.

6.5 Maintenance After AT

The absence of a plateau on survival curves post HDT and AT with ongoing relapses justifies the exploration of maintenance strategies with the prolongation of response duration as the goal. In addition, AT may result in a very low tumor burden, which may be susceptible to long-term suppression by drugs or immunomodulatory agents. A number of agents have been or are being explored for maintenance, including interferon alpha (IFN-α), corticosteroids, biphosphonates, thalidomide, lenalidomide, bortezomib, and combinations of these drugs. Several studies show that consolidation and maintenance post AT can further reduce tumor burden and improve outcome.

IFN was one of the first drugs to be studied as maintenance post AT. It yielded a small benefit in a meta-analysis from the European Group for Blood and Marrow Transplantation (EBMT) [46]. The study by Australian myeloma group (with a median follow-up 5.4 years), thalidomide administered in combination with prednisolone for 1 year was found to significantly prolong PFS and OS compared with prednisolone alone: 5-year PFS was 27 % for Thal/Pred versus 15 % for Pred, $P = 0.005$; 5-year OS was 66 versus 47 %, respectively, $P = 0.007$) [47]. Minimum thalidomide exposure required was at least 8 months to gain a PFS and OS advantage and there was no difference between the two arms regarding overall response rate to salvage therapy or post relapse. This suggested that acquired resistance in this study was not an important issue for thalidomide-treated patients.

In the meta-analysis of five trials involving patients, Morgan et al. found a significant late OS benefit for thalidomide ($P < 0.001$, 7-year difference hazard ratio (HR) = 12.3; 95 % confidence interval, 5.5–19.0). Similarly, Lenalidomide has been investigated in the post-transplant setting in three large studies. In the study conducted by the IFM group, patients were randomized to lenalidomide maintenance until progression or no maintenance following a single or tandem ASCT step and two cycles of lenalidomide consolidation in both arms [48]. The lenalidomide was stopped at a median of 2 years (range 1–3 years) due to concerns regarding second primary malignancies. With a median follow-up of 67 months from randomization, the PFS for patients who had received lenalidomide maintenance was significantly longer than for those who had not received any maintenance therapy (46 versus 24 months, $P < 0.001$) [49]. Although OS did not achieve statistical significance in two arms (82 versus 81 months, respectively, $P = 0.8$), the second PFS and survival after the first progression were shorter in the lenalidomide maintenance arm. In addition, the cumulative incidence of second primary malignancy was significantly higher with lenalidomide. When examining cytogenetic risk, progression was superior for the lenalidomide arm for patients with or without 13q deletion and without t(4;14) or 17p deletion, but did not reach significance for patients with either t(4;14) or 17p deletion. The CALGB conducted a large placebo-controlled randomized study of lenalidomide maintenance following ASCT [50]. In this study, lenalidomide was administered until disease progression. 86 of 128 eligible patients received lenalidomide maintenance. At a median follow-up of 34 months, 37 % who received lenalidomide maintenance and 58 % who received placebo had disease progression or had died. The median time to progression was 46 months in the lenalidomide group and 27 months in the placebo group ($P < 0.001$). The median OS in both arms had not been reached, with 85 % of the lenalidomide-arm patients and 77 % of the placebo-arm patients who were alive at the time of the analysis having died ($P < 0.03$). The rate of second primary malignancy appeared to plateau at 2 years post SCT. This study was updated in 2013. At median follow-up of 48 months, the intent-to-treat analysis demonstrated that the OS was 80 % for the lenalidomide arm and 70 % for the placebo group ($P = 0.008$) with a continued PFS advantage in the lenalidomide arm. In the study by GIMEMA group, at a median follow-up of 51.2 months, the median PFS was superior with lenalidomide maintenance (PFS: 41.9 months for lenalidomide versus 21.6 months for placebo, $P < 0.0001$), but 3-year OS was not significantly prolonged (3-year OS: 88.0 % versus 79.2 %, respectively, $P = 0.14$).

Bortezomib maintenance therapy has been investigated in two phase 3 studies, the HOVON and GMMG studies. A landmark analysis from the start of maintenance showed that OS was superior for patients on the bortezomib arm, while PFS was comparable. The limitation of these studies was that, while the results of these trials confirmed the important role of bortezomib-containing regimen in the treatment of newly diagnosed MM, the design of the trials made it difficult to interpret the role of bortezomib maintenance difficult as it was not possible to delineate the individual contributions of induction versus the maintenance treatment as part of this design. Furthermore, the OS benefit was seen only for patients with del17p cytogenetic abnormalities and those who presented in renal failure. In a large randomized phase 3 study conducted by the Spanish myeloma group, the combination of bortezomib and thalidomide was compared to thalidomide and to Interferon as maintenance therapy and a significant benefit in PFS was found for the VT combination with a median follow-up of 34.9 months [15].

7   Importance of MRD

7.1   Is Complete Remission (CR) Important?

In the context of AT trials for myeloma, disappearance of the M-protein is generally thought to play a pivotal role in predicting superior survival [9, 14, 18, 47, 49, 51]. However, several observations have challenged the notion that a CR is an absolute requirement for prolongation of survival in myeloma. The Mayo Clinic has reported that patients who underwent AT have similar PFS and OS irrespective of whether they achieved CR [52]. Patients with CA in TT2 had similar CR rates of 40 % compared to those without CA, yet their median survival was significantly shorter post high-dose MEL therapy. A similar observation applied to the thalidomide arm in TT2 where a higher CR rate and EFS did not translate into superior survival. The median time to CR in TT2 was 12 months despite the application of an intensive therapeutic program [24] In addition, the disappearance of MRI-defined focal lesions (FL), which are potential sites for surviving resistant myeloma cells, lags 2 years behind the disappearance of M-protein from blood and urine [53]. Paradoxically more aggressive disease features such as CA, elevated LDH, and IgA isotype are predictors of CR [25]. We have recently reported that high serum free light chain levels at diagnosis and a rapid reduction after induction therapy are predictive for achieving CR [54]. These parameters reflect more proliferative myeloma which, on the one hand, is inherently more sensitive to combination chemotherapy, and on the other is linked to shorter EFS and OS due to rapid myeloma regrowth when tumor reduction is insufficient.

Conversely, patients with myeloma evolving from monoclonal gammopathy of unknown significance (MGUS) or with smoldering myeloma have significantly lower CR rates, yet equal EFS and OS compared to patients with de novo myeloma. The lower CR rate in these patients is likely to be due to a lower proliferative rate, reflecting more indolent disease, which is less susceptible to eradication by both standard- and high-dose chemotherapy. Interestingly, these patients also have fewer MRI-defined FL. Patients with MGUS-like myeloma have favorable clinical characteristics, with lower CR rates yet superior survival compared to patients with non-MGUS-like myeloma. Attainment of CR in myeloma is often a gradual and cumulative process. It appears, therefore, that achieving a CR is only critical for prolonging survival in a truly high-risk group of myeloma that thus far can only be captured by gene expression profiling [55]. These data also suggest that the use of CR as a surrogate marker for OS and EFS in clinical trials of novel agents cannot be applied without characterizing myeloma at the molecular level and should be used with extreme caution.

7.2 MRD Detection by Flow Cytometry

Results of multicolor flow cytometry and deep-sequencing studies suggest that among patients achieving a complete response, MRD-negative status is associated with significant improvements in PFS and OS. The UK Medical Research Council IX trial assessed the importance of achieving MRD. There was a significant improvement in OS for each log depletion in MRD level. The median OS was 1 year for ≥ 10 %, 4 years for 1 to <10 %, 5.9 years for 0.1 to <1 %, 6.8 years for 0.01 to <0.1 %, and more than 7.5 years for <0.01 % MRD level. The detection of minimal residual disease MRD in myeloma using a 0.01 % threshold ($10(-4)$) after treatment is an independent predictor of PFS [56].

8 Allogeneic Transplantation for MM

8.1 Introduction

Allogeneic hematopoietic cell transplantation (HCT) is potentially the curative treatment for multiple myeloma. However its use is limited because of high rate of treatment-related mortality and its efficacy compared with autologous HCT is not fully established. With the advent of new proteasome inhibitors and IMiDs, role of allogeneic transplant needs to be scrutinized. In subsequent sections, we will review the role of allogeneic transplant in MM.

8.2   Myeloablative HCT

Myeloablative transplants require that patients receive high-dose chemotherapy with or without total body radiation, followed by donor stem cell infusion. Myeloablative transplants are not the preferred modality and are very infrequently performed. Hence this is not discussed further in this chapter.

8.3   Syngeneic HCT

Syngeneic allogeneic transplants are from the identical twin donor and only a limited number of syngeneic transplants have been performed in multiple myeloma. The EBMT analyzed 25 syngeneic transplants and compared the results with 250 patients who underwent either autologous or allogeneic HCT (n = 125, each) HCT [57]. The TRM was substantially lower with only two patients dying due to transplant-related toxicity as compared to myeloablative allogeneic transplant. Overall survival for the patients undergoing syngenic transplants was 73 months, significantly better than that of the case-matched autologous transplants (44 months); both groups outperformed the allogeneic transplants. The Seattle Marrow Transplant Team performed syngeneic transplants on five patients with multiple myeloma [58]. Four patients responded to therapy, while one patient died one month after transplant from cytomegalovirus-associated interstitial pneumonitis. Response durations for these four patients were 6, 17, 18, and more than 72 months. These reports are useful in exploring the various treatment options but do not support the use of syngeneic HCT in place of an autologous HCT if a twin donor is available.

8.4   Non-myeloablative Allogeneic HCT

The results of non-myeloablative T-cell depleted transplants have been summarized in Table 5. Longer term follow-up of these studies is awaited. It is unclear what impact non-myeloablative HCT will have given the improved outcomes with autologous HCT after the introduction of novel agents utilized in induction, consolidation, and maintenance, in the era of novel agents. In current scenario, non-myeloablative-allogeneic transplantation remains investigational and its role needs to be validated in the era of novel agents.

8.5   Role of Auto/Allo Transplants

The role of auto–allo versus tandem autologous transplant is debatable. A meta-analysis of 1822 patients with previously untreated myeloma comparing double autologous HCT versus a single autologous HCT followed by non-myeloablative allogeneic HCT [62], allogeneic HCT was associated with

Table 5 Summary of non-myeloablative T-cell depleted transplants

Study	Previous AT	Results
EBMT [59]	$N = 413$ 44.6 % had undergone two or more prior autologous HCTs	Median PFS—9.6 months Median OS—24.7 months 5-year survival rate—30 %
Bacigalupo et al. [60]	$N = 33$ had one or more than one previous autologous transplant	CR in 62 % TRM = 13 % Median follow-up 22 months PFS = 45 % and OS = 37 %
Shimoni et al. [61]	$N = 50$	Non relapse mortality = 26 % PFS = 26 % and OS = 34 % Median follow-up time of 6.4 years

greater treatment-related mortality (relative risk [RR] 3.3; 95 % CI 2.2-4.8 (RR 1.4; 95 % CI 1.1–1.8), but similar overall survival at and beyond 36 months.

The following is a brief summary of the largest trials conducted in this setting BMT CTN Trial [63]:

- 625 patients with standard risk myeloma in this trial, 189 with an HLA-identical sibling donor were assigned to receive a myeloablative autologous HCT followed by a non-myeloablative allogeneic HCT.

Hovon 50 [64]:

- 260 patients with autologous transplant-randomly assigned to RIC sib allo ($n = 122$ patients) or maintenance with thalidomide or interferon alpha.
- Median follow-up 77 months.
- When compared with maintenance therapy, allogeneic HCT was associated with similar rates of progression-free (28 versus 22 % respectively) and overall (55 %) survival at 6 years.

French IFM [65]:

- Patients with high-risk myeloma (deletion 13 by FISH or an elevated beta-2 microglobulin level) were included in this trial.
- No benefit with autologous HCT followed by reduced-intensity allogeneic HCT compared with tandem autologous HCT [16].

Spanish PETHEMA [15]:

- Prospectively compared the use of autologous (85 patients) or reduced-intensity allogeneic (25 patients) HCT in 110 patients with myeloma who failed to achieve a complete or near complete remission after an initial autologous HCT.

- At a median follow-up after second transplantation of 5.2 years of patients who received an allogeneic HCT, there was no difference in event-free or overall survival rates.

However, the Italian study of 162 patients showed better event-free survival in patients who underwent sib matched allogeneic transplant [66].

The authors of this chapter noted that hardly any genetic data was included in these trials. Hence in the era of genomically driven personalized medicine, the role of auto/allo remains investigational and the data needs to be carefully analyzed.

8.6 Future Strategies

It is important to recognize that MM is complex disease with significant clonal heterogeneity. Transplantation helps in early reduction of clonal diversity and increases the likelihood of cure. Long-term follow-up studies show that AT can achieve profound cytoreduction and likely cure a portion of patients even before the introduction of novel drugs. Total Therapy 1 (TT1), the first tandem AT trial for myeloma, enrolled 231 patients; with a median follow-up of 17 years, 23 remain alive and progression-free with a plateau on the overall survival (OS) curve appearing around 14 years [23]. Martinez-Lopez et al. reported on 344 patients who received AT between 1989 and 1998 who had a median follow-up of 153 months. A plateau in OS appeared after 11 years and, with a further follow-up of 5 years, no relapses were observed [67]. Targeted therapy has already demonstrated some efficacy, but may merely select for resistant subclones, unless a given mutation drives the disease as recently has been described for *KRAS/NRAS* activating mutations. High-risk myeloma even with modern genetic analysis will likely remain a challenging disease to treat in years to come. AT, tandem autotransplants, auto-transplant followed by reduced-intensity allogeneic transplant and allogeneic transplant will remain an important option in the therapeutic armamentarium of myeloma. Novel immune therapeutic agent anti-CD38 antibodies, i.e., daratu-momab, checkpoint blockade inhibitors, cellular therapies, and vaccines will likely become available very soon and this can enhance the anti-myeloma response without transplant-associated risks. It is conceivable that such strategies will be complimentary and not replacement for transplant.

References

1. Stewart AK, Bergsagel PL, Greipp PR, Dispenzieri A, Gertz MA, Hayman SR et al (2007) A practical guide to defining high-risk myeloma for clinical trials, patient counseling and choice of therapy. Leukemia 21(3):529–534
2. Zhan F, Hardin J, Kordsmeier B, Bumm K, Zheng M, Tian E et al (2002) Global gene expression profiling of multiple myeloma, monoclonal gammopathy of undetermined significance, and normal bone marrow plasma cells. Blood 99(5):1745–1757

3. Fermand JP, Ravaud P, Chevret S, Divine M, Leblond V, Belanger C et al (1998) High-dose therapy and autologous peripheral blood stem cell transplantation in multiple myeloma: up-front or rescue treatment? Results of a multicenter sequential randomized clinical trial. Blood 92(9):3131–3136

4. Bergsagel DE, Ross SW, Baker DT (1962) Evaluation of new chemotherapeutic agents in the treatment of multiple myeloma. V. 1-Aminocyclopentanecarboxylic acid (NSC-1026). Cancer Chemother Rep Part 1 21:101–106

5. Alexanian R, Haut A, Khan AU, Lane M, McKelvey EM, Migliore PJ et al (1969) Treatment for multiple myeloma. Combination chemotherapy with different melphalan dose regimens. JAMA 208(9):1680–1685

6. Gay F, Hajek R, Diramondo F et al (2013) Cyclophosphamidelenalidomide-dexamethasone vs autologous transplant in newly diagnosed myeloma: a phase 3 trial. Clin Lymphoma Myeloma Leuk 13(suppl 1):S40

7. Boccadoro M, Cavallo F, Gay F, Di Raimondo F, Nagler A, Montefusco V (2013) Melphalan/prednisone/lenalidomide (MPR) versus high-dose melphalan and autologous transplantation (MEL200) plus lenalidomide maintenance or no maintenance in newly diagnosed multiple myeloma (MM) patients. J Clin Oncol 31(suppl):8509

8. Segeren CM, Sonneveld P, van der Holt B, Vellenga E, Croockewit AJ, Verhoef GE et al (2003) Overall and event-free survival are not improved by the use of myeloablative therapy following intensified chemotherapy in previously untreated patients with multiple myeloma: a prospective randomized phase 3 study. Blood 101(6):2144–2151

9. Barlogie B, Jagannath S, Desikan KR, Mattox S, Vesole D, Siegel D et al (1999) Total therapy with tandem transplants for newly diagnosed multiple myeloma. Blood 93(1):55–65

10. Barlogie B, Alexanian R, Dicke KA, Zagars G, Spitzer G, Jagannath S et al (1987) High-dose chemoradiotherapy and autologous bone marrow transplantation for resistant multiple myeloma. Blood 70(3):869–872

11. Fermand JP, Katsahian S, Divine M, Leblond V, Dreyfus F, Macro M et al (2005) High-dose therapy and autologous blood stem-cell transplantation compared with conventional treatment in myeloma patients aged 55 to 65 years: long-term results of a randomized control trial from the Group Myelome-Autogreffe. J Clin Oncol: Official J Am Soc Clin Oncol 23(36): 9227–9233

12. Blade J, Rosinol L, Sureda A, Ribera JM, Diaz-Mediavilla J, Garcia-Larana J et al (2005) High-dose therapy intensification compared with continued standard chemotherapy in multiple myeloma patients responding to the initial chemotherapy: long-term results from a prospective randomized trial from the Spanish cooperative group PETHEMA. Blood 106(12):3755–3759

13. Barlogie B, Kyle RA, Anderson KC, Greipp PR, Lazarus HM, Hurd DD et al (2006) Standard chemotherapy compared with high-dose chemoradiotherapy for multiple myeloma: final results of phase III US Intergroup Trial S9321. J Clin Oncol: Official J Am Soc Clin Oncol 24 (6):929–936

14. Attal M, Harousseau JL, Stoppa AM, Sotto JJ, Fuzibet JG, Rossi JF et al (1996) A prospective, randomized trial of autologous bone marrow transplantation and chemotherapy in multiple myeloma. Intergroupe Francais du Myelome. N Engl J Med 335(2):91–97

15. Rosinol L, Oriol A, Teruel AI, Hernandez D, Lopez-Jimenez J, de la Rubia J et al (2012) Superiority of bortezomib, thalidomide, and dexamethasone (VTD) as induction pretransplantation therapy in multiple myeloma: a randomized phase 3 PETHEMA/GEM study. Blood 120(8):1589–1596

16. Berz D, McCormack EM, Winer ES, Colvin GA, Quesenberry PJ (2007) Cryopreservation of hematopoietic stem cells. Am J Hematol 82(6):463–472

17. Moreau P, Facon T, Attal M, Hulin C, Michallet M, Maloisel F et al (2002) Comparison of 200 mg/m(2) melphalan and 8 Gy total body irradiation plus 140 mg/m(2) melphalan as conditioning regimens for peripheral blood stem cell transplantation in patients with newly diagnosed multiple myeloma: final analysis of the Intergroupe Francophone du Myelome 9502 randomized trial. Blood 99(3):731–735

18. Desikan KR, Tricot G, Dhodapkar M, Fassas A, Siegel D, Vesole DH et al (2000) Melphalan plus total body irradiation (MEL-TBI) or cyclophosphamide (MEL-CY) as a conditioning regimen with second autotransplant in responding patients with myeloma is inferior compared to historical controls receiving tandem transplants with melphalan alone. Bone Marrow Transplant 25(5):483–487

19. Blade J, Vesole DH, Gertz M (2003) High-dose therapy in multiple myeloma. Blood 102 (10):3469–3470

20. Barlogie B, Smith L, Alexanian R (1984) Effective treatment of advanced multiple myeloma refractory to alkylating agents. N Engl J Med 310(21):1353–1356

21. Harousseau JL, Milpied N, Laporte JP, Collombat P, Facon T, Tigaud JD et al (1992) Double-intensive therapy in high-risk multiple myeloma. Blood 79(11):2827–2833

22. Fermand JP, Levy Y, Gerota J, Benbunan M, Cosset JM, Castaigne S et al (1989) Treatment of aggressive multiple myeloma by high-dose chemotherapy and total body irradiation followed by blood stem cells autologous graft. Blood 73(1):20–23

23. Barlogie B, Tricot GJ, van Rhee F, Angtuaco E, Walker R, Epstein J et al (2006) Long-term outcome results of the first tandem autotransplant trial for multiple myeloma. Br J Haematol 135(2):158–164

24. Barlogie B, Tricot G, Anaissie E, Shaughnessy J, Rasmussen E, van Rhee F et al (2006) Thalidomide and hematopoietic-cell transplantation for multiple myeloma. N Engl J Med 354 (10):1021–1030

25. Barlogie B, Tricot G, Rasmussen E, Anaissie E, van Rhee F, Zangari M et al (2006) Total therapy 2 without thalidomide in comparison with total therapy 1: role of intensified induction and posttransplantation consolidation therapies. Blood 107(7):2633–2638

26. Attal M, Harousseau JL, Facon T, Guilhot F, Doyen C, Fuzibet JG et al (2003) Single versus double autologous stem-cell transplantation for multiple myeloma. N Engl J Med 349 (26):2495–2502

27. Cavo M, Tosi P, Zamagni E, Cellini C, Tacchetti P, Patriarca F et al (2007) Prospective, randomized study of single compared with double autologous stem-cell transplantation for multiple myeloma: Bologna 96 clinical study. J Clin Oncol: Official J Am Soc Clin Oncol 25 (17):2434–2441

28. Fermand JP, Alberti C, Morolleau JP (2003) Single versus tandem high dose therapy (HDT) supported with autlogous blood stem cell (ABSC) transplantation using unselected or CD34- enriched ABSC: results of a two by two designed radomized trial in 230 young aptients with multiple myeloma (MM). Hematol J 4:S59

29. Goldschmidt H (2005) Single vs double high dose therapy in multiple myeloma: second analysis of the GMMG-HD2 trial. Haematologica 90:38

30. Cavo M, Cellini C, Zamagni E (2005) Update on high dose therapy—Italian studies. Haematologica 90:39

31. Vesole DH, Tricot G, Jagannath S, Desikan KR, Siegel D, Bracy D et al (1996) Autotransplants in multiple myeloma: what have we learned? Blood 88(3):838–847

32. Awan F, Kochuparambil ST, Falconer DE, Cumpston A, Leadmon S, Watkins K et al (2013) Comparable efficacy and lower cost of PBSC mobilization with intermediate-dose cyclophosphamide and G-CSF compared with plerixafor and G-CSF in patients with multiple myeloma treated with novel therapies. Bone Marrow Transplant 48(10):1279–1284

33. Hosing C, Qazilbash MH, Kebriaei P, Giralt S, Davis MS, Popat U et al (2006) Fixed-dose single agent pegfilgrastim for peripheral blood progenitor cell mobilisation in patients with multiple myeloma. Br J Haematol 133(5):533–537

34. DiPersio JF, Stadtmauer EA, Nademanee A, Micallef IN, Stiff PJ, Kaufman JL et al (2009) Plerixafor and G-CSF versus placebo and G-CSF to mobilize hematopoietic stem cells for autologous stem cell transplantation in patients with multiple myeloma. Blood 113(23):5720–5726

35. Giralt S, Stadtmauer EA, Harousseau JL, Palumbo A, Bensinger W, Comenzo RL et al (2009) International myeloma working group (IMWG) consensus statement and guidelines regarding the current status of stem cell collection and high-dose therapy for multiple myeloma and the role of plerixafor (AMD 3100). Leukemia 23(10):1904–1912
36. Kumar S, Giralt S, Stadtmauer EA, Harousseau JL, Palumbo A, Bensinger W et al (2009) Mobilization in myeloma revisited: IMWG consensus perspectives on stem cell collection following initial therapy with thalidomide-, lenalidomide-, or bortezomib-containing regimens. Blood 114(9):1729–1735
37. Palumbo A, Bringhen S, Bruno B, Falcone AP, Liberati AM, Grasso M et al (2010) Melphalan 200 mg/m(2) versus melphalan 100 mg/m(2) in newly diagnosed myeloma patients: a prospective, multicenter phase 3 study. Blood 115(10):1873–1879
38. Anagnostopoulos A, Aleman A, Ayers G, Donato M, Champlin R, Weber D et al (2004) Comparison of high-dose melphalan with a more intensive regimen of thiotepa, busulfan, and cyclophosphamide for patients with multiple myeloma. Cancer 100(12):2607–2612
39. Fenk R, Schneider P, Kropff M, Huenerlituerkoglu AN, Steidl U, Aul C et al (2005) High-dose idarubicin, cyclophosphamide and melphalan as conditioning for autologous stem cell transplantation increases treatment-related mortality in patients with multiple myeloma: results of a randomised study. Br J Haematol 130(4):588–594
40. Badros A, Barlogie B, Siegel E, Roberts J, Langmaid C, Zangari M et al (2001) Results of autologous stem cell transplant in multiple myeloma patients with renal failure. Br J Haematol 114(4):822–829
41. Facon T, Mary JY, Hulin C, Benboubker L, Attal M, Pegourie B et al (2007) Melphalan and prednisone plus thalidomide versus melphalan and prednisone alone or reduced-intensity autologous stem cell transplantation in elderly patients with multiple myeloma (IFM 99-06): a randomised trial. Lancet 370(9594):1209–1218
42. Schmitz N, Linch DC, Dreger P, Goldstone AH, Boogaerts MA, Ferrant A et al (1996) Randomised trial of filgrastim-mobilised peripheral blood progenitor cell transplantation versus autologous bone-marrow transplantation in lymphoma patients. Lancet 347(8998):353–357
43. Ford PA, Grant SJ, Mick R, Keck G (2015) Autologous stem-cell transplantation without hematopoietic support for the treatment of hematologic malignancies in Jehovah's witnesses. J Clin Oncol: Official J Am Soc Clin Oncol 33(15):1674–1679
44. Gertz MA, Ansell SM, Dingli D, Dispenzieri A, Buadi FK, Elliott MA et al (2008) Autologous stem cell transplant in 716 patients with multiple myeloma: low treatment-related mortality, feasibility of outpatient transplant, and effect of a multidisciplinary quality initiative. Mayo Clin Proc 83(10):1131–1138
45. Jones JA, Qazilbash MH, Shih YC, Cantor SB, Cooksley CD, Elting LS (2008) In-hospital complications of autologous hematopoietic stem cell transplantation for lymphoid malignancies: clinical and economic outcomes from the Nationwide Inpatient Sample. Cancer 112(5):1096–1105
46. Bjorkstrand B, Svensson H, Goldschmidt H, Ljungman P, Apperley J, Mandelli F et al (2001) Alpha-interferon maintenance treatment is associated with improved survival after high-dose treatment and autologous stem cell transplantation in patients with multiple myeloma: a retrospective registry study from the European Group for Blood and Marrow Transplantation (EBMT). Bone Marrow Transplant 27(5):511–515
47. Davies FE, Forsyth PD, Rawstron AC, Owen RG, Pratt G, Evans PA et al (2001) The impact of attaining a minimal disease state after high-dose melphalan and autologous transplantation for multiple myeloma. Br J Haematol 112(3):814–819
48. Attal M, Lauwers-Cances V, Marit G, Caillot D, Moreau P, Facon T et al (2012) Lenalidomide maintenance after stem-cell transplantation for multiple myeloma. N Engl J Med 366 (19):1782–1791

49. Shaughnessy J, Jacobson J, Sawyer J, McCoy J, Fassas A, Zhan F et al (2003) Continuous absence of metaphase-defined cytogenetic abnormalities, especially of chromosome 13 and hypodiploidy, ensures long-term survival in multiple myeloma treated with Total Therapy I: interpretation in the context of global gene expression. Blood 101(10):3849–3856

50. McCarthy PL, Owzar K, Hofmeister CC, Hurd DD, Hassoun H, Richardson PG et al (2012) Lenalidomide after stem-cell transplantation for multiple myeloma. N Engl J Med 366 (19):1770–1781

51. Child JA, Morgan GJ, Davies FE, Owen RG, Bell SE, Hawkins K et al (2003) High-dose chemotherapy with hematopoietic stem-cell rescue for multiple myeloma. N Engl J Med 348 (19):1875–1883

52. Rajkumar SV, Fonseca R, Dispenzieri A, Lacy MQ, Witzig TE, Lust JA et al (2000) Effect of complete response on outcome following autologous stem cell transplantation for myeloma. Bone Marrow Transplant 26(9):979–983

53. Walker R, Barlogie B, Haessler J, Tricot G, Anaissie E, Shaughnessy JD Jr et al (2007) Magnetic resonance imaging in multiple myeloma: diagnostic and clinical implications. J Clin Oncol: Official J Am Soc Clin Oncol 25(9):1121–1128

54. van Rhee F, Bolejack V, Hollmig K, Pineda-Roman M, Anaissie E, Epstein J et al (2007) High serum-free light chain levels and their rapid reduction in response to therapy define an aggressive multiple myeloma subtype with poor prognosis. Blood 110(3):827–832

55. Haessler J, Shaughnessy JD Jr, Zhan F, Crowley J, Epstein J, van Rhee F et al (2007) Benefit of complete response in multiple myeloma limited to high-risk subgroup identified by gene expression profiling. Clin Cancer Res: Official J Am Assoc Cancer Res 13(23):7073–7079

56. Rawstron AC, Gregory WM, de Tute RM, Davies FE, Bell SE, Drayson MT et al (2015) Minimal residual disease in myeloma by flow cytometry: independent prediction of survival benefit per log reduction. Blood 125(12):1932–1935

57. Gahrton G, Svensson H, Bjorkstrand B, Apperley J, Carlson K, Cavo M et al (1999) Syngeneic transplantation in multiple myeloma—a case-matched comparison with autologous and allogeneic transplantation. European Group for Blood and Marrow Transplantation. Bone Marrow Transplant 24(7):741–745

58. Fefer A, Cheever MA, Greenberg PD (1986) Identical-twin (syngeneic) marrow transplantation for hematologic cancers. J Natl Cancer Inst 76(6):1269–1273

59. Auner HW, Szydlo R, van Biezen A, Iacobelli S, Gahrton G, Milpied N et al (2013) Reduced intensity-conditioned allogeneic stem cell transplantation for multiple myeloma relapsing or progressing after autologous transplantation: a study by the European Group for Blood and Marrow Transplantation. Bone Marrow Transplant 48(11):1395–1400

60. Majolino I, Davoli M, Carnevalli E, Locasciulli A, Di Bartolomeo P, Scime R et al (2007) Reduced intensity conditioning with thiotepa, fludarabine, and melphalan is effective in advanced multiple myeloma. Leuk lymphoma 48(4):759–766

61. Shimoni A, Hardan I, Ayuk F, Schilling G, Atanackovic D, Zeller W et al (2010) Allogenic hematopoietic stem-cell transplantation with reduced-intensity conditioning in patients with refractory and recurrent multiple myeloma: long-term follow-up. Cancer 116(15):3621–3630

62. Armeson KE, Hill EG, Costa LJ (2013) Tandem autologous vs autologous plus reduced intensity allogeneic transplantation in the upfront management of multiple myeloma: meta-analysis of trials with biological assignment. Bone Marrow Transplant 48(4):562–567

63. Krishnan A, Pasquini MC, Logan B, Stadtmauer EA, Vesole DH, Alyea E 3rd et al (2011) Autologous haemopoietic stem-cell transplantation followed by allogeneic or autologous haemopoietic stem-cell transplantation in patients with multiple myeloma (BMT CTN 0102): a phase 3 biological assignment trial. Lancet Oncol 12(13):1195–1203

64. Lokhorst HM, van der Holt B, Cornelissen JJ, Kersten MJ, van Oers M, Raymakers R et al (2012) Donor versus no-donor comparison of newly diagnosed myeloma patients included in the HOVON-50 multiple myeloma study. Blood 119(26):6219–6225; quiz 399

65. Garban F, Attal M, Michallet M, Hulin C, Bourhis JH, Yakoub-Agha I et al (2006) Prospective comparison of autologous stem cell transplantation followed by dose-reduced allograft (IFM99-03 trial) with tandem autologous stem cell transplantation (IFM99-04 trial) in high-risk de novo multiple myeloma. Blood 107(9):3474–3480
66. Bruno B, Rotta M, Patriarca F, Mordini N, Allione B, Carnevale-Schianca F et al (2007) A comparison of allografting with autografting for newly diagnosed myeloma. New Engl J Med 356(11):1110–1120
67. Martinez-Lopez J, Blade J, Mateos MV, Grande C, Alegre A, Garcia-Larana J et al (2011) Long-term prognostic significance of response in multiple myeloma after stem cell transplantation. Blood 118(3):529–534

Bone Disease in Multiple Myeloma

Homare Eda, Loredana Santo, G. David Roodman
and Noopur Raje

Abstract

Bone involvement represented by osteolytic bone disease (OBD) or osteopenia is one of the pathognomonic and defining characteristics of multiple myeloma (MM). Nearly 90 % of patients with MM develop osteolytic bone lesions, frequently complicated by skeletal-related events (SRE) such as severe bone pain, pathological fractures, vertebral collapse, hypercalcemia, and spinal cord compression. All of these not only result in a negative impact on quality of life but also adversely impact overall survival. OBD is a consequence of increased osteoclast (OC) activation along with osteoblast (OB) inhibition, resulting in altered bone remodeling. OC number and activity are increased in MM via cytokine deregulation within the bone marrow (BM) milieu, whereas negative regulators of OB differentiation suppress bone formation. Inhibition of osteolysis and stimulation of OB differentiation leads to reduced tumor growth in vivo. Therefore, novel agents targeting OBD are promising therapeutic strategies not only for the treatment of MM OBD but also for the treatment of MM. Several novel agents in addition to bisphosphonates are currently under investigation for their positive effect on bone remodeling via OC inhibition or OB stimulation. Future studies will look to combine or sequence all of these agents with the goal of not only alleviating morbidity from MM OBD but also capitalizing on the resultant antitumor activity.

Keywords

Multiple myeloma · Bone disease · Therapies

H. Eda · L. Santo · G. David Roodman · N. Raje (✉)
Multiple Myeloma Program, Medical Oncology, Massachusetts General Hospital,
Boston, MA, USA
e-mail: NRAJE@mgh.harvard.edu

© Springer International Publishing Switzerland 2016
A.M. Roccaro and I.M. Ghobrial (eds.), *Plasma Cell Dyscrasias*,
Cancer Treatment and Research 169, DOI 10.1007/978-3-319-40320-5_14

1   Introduction

The past two decades have seen remarkable advances in our understanding of the biology of multiple myeloma (MM) and in the introduction of novel therapies. Novel treatments including thalidomide [1], lenalidomide [2], and the proteasome inhibitor bortezomib [3] have led to significant improvements in 5-year relative overall survival, from nearly 28.8 % in the early 1990s to 34.7 % in the previous decade [4]. Although MM remains incurable, MM patients are living longer, and the focus is centered on maximizing quality of life for patients with MM.

Bone involvement represented by osteolytic bone disease (OBD) or osteopenia is one of the pathognomonic and defining characteristic of MM [5]. Although the ratio of patients presenting with bone involvement is variable, nearly 90 % of patients with MM develop osteolytic bone lesions, frequently complicated by skeletal-related events (SRE) such as severe bone pain, pathological fractures, vertebral collapse, hypercalcemia, and spinal cord compression, resulting in a need for radiation or open reduction internal fixation (ORIF) [6–10]. Importantly, 40–50 % of MM patients develop pathologic fractures, and it increases the risk of death by more than 20 % compared with patients without fractures [8, 11]. These data indicate how OBD negatively impact both patients' quality of life and survival, and highlight the importance of focusing on treatment strategies to alleviate OBD in MM.

OBD results from the disruption of the delicate balance between osteoclasts (OCs), osteocytes, osteoblasts (OBs), and bone marrow stromal cells (BMSCs) activity. MM cells stimulate OC function and inhibit OB differentiation, resulting in bone resorption and consequent OBD. The abnormal bone marrow (BM) microenvironment in OBD provides a permissive niche that enables MM cell growth [9, 12–14]. Consequently, several novel agents and combinations are aimed at restoring bone homeostasis by targeting either OC or/and OB activity. In fact, inhibition of osteolysis and stimulation of OB differentiation leads to reduced tumor growth in vivo [13, 15]. Therefore, novel agents targeting OBD are also promising therapeutic strategies for the treatment of MM. Here, we discuss the pathogenesis of OBD and focus on advances in our understanding of its biology and therapeutic implications.

2   The Biology of Bone Metabolism

Under normal physiologic states, osteocytes, OCs and OBs result in balanced bone resorption and formation maintaining normal homeostasis. In adult bone, 90–95 % of all bone cells are represented by osteocytes while OCs and OBs are less than 10 % [16]. Osteocytes act as main regulators of bone homeostasis for OCs, considered bone resorption cells, and OBs considered bone formation cells. Osteocyte viability and function is regulated by mechanical loading, several cytokines includes well as glucocorticoids [16–18]. Osteocytes secrete several cytokines which regulate the activity of both OCs and OBs such as sclerostin, dickkopf-1 (Dkk-1), the receptor activator of nuclear factor-kappa B ligand (RANKL), and osteoprotegerin (OPG) [16]. The receptor activator of nuclear factor-kappa B (RANK), its ligand RANKL, and OPG, the decoy receptor of RANKL, play a pivotal role as central regulators of OC function. RANK-RANKL signaling activates a variety of downstream signaling pathways required for OC development. It plays a significant role in stimulating OC differentiation and maturation. Interestingly, apoptotic osteocytes release apoptotic bodies expressing RANKL to stimulate OC differentiation [19]. These data suggest that osteocytes are able to recruit OCs to sites of remodeling. Osteocytes also regulate OB differentiation via sclerostin and Dkk-1 which block canonical Wnt signaling by binding to low-density lipoprotein receptor-related protein (LRP) 5 and 6 (Wnt receptors) on the surface of OBs [16]. OBs and BMSCs also express OPG and RANKL, and regulate OC differentiation. Because OPG is a Wnt canonical signaling target [20], osteocyte also regulates OC differentiation via regulation of Wnt signaling activity in OBs. On the other hand, OCs express semaphorin 4D (Sema4D) and inhibit OB differentiation [21]. These processes are well balanced in healthy bones to maintain the bones quality and mass (Fig. 1).

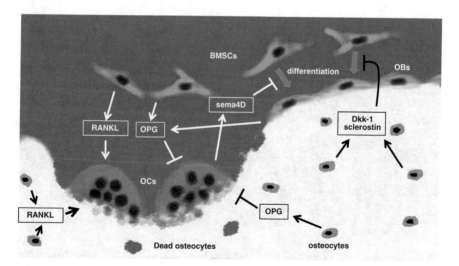

Fig. 1 Healthy Bone metabolism. Osteocytes regulate OC (osteoclast) and OB (osteoblast) differentiation. OBs also regulate OC differentiation. On the other hand, OCs can inhibit OB differentiation. These mechanisms are well balanced in healthy bones to keep the bones quality and mass

3   MM Bone Disease

In MM, the osteocyte-OC-OB axis is disrupted, stimulating bone resorption and inhibiting new bone formation with resultant development of pathognomonic osteolytic lesions (Fig. 2).

3.1   Osteoclasts in Myeloma Bone Disease

The pathogenesis of OBD in MM is primarily associated with generalized OC activation. BM biopsies from MM patients show a correlation between tumor burden, OC numbers, and resorptive surface [22, 23]. Furthermore, OC activity has positive correlation with disease activity [24, 25]. The main cytokines involved in OC differentiation and activity in MM OBD are RANKL/OPG, decoy receptor 3 (DcR3), CCL3 (also known as macrophage inflammatory protein (MIP)-1α), MIP-1β, tumour necrosis factor-alpha (TNFα), interleukin (IL)-3, IL-6, IL-11,

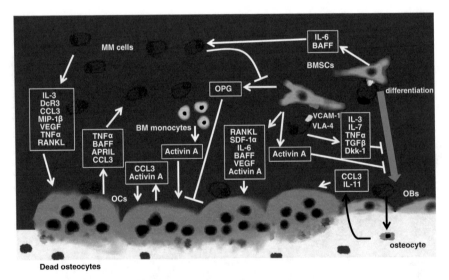

Fig. 2 Myeloma Bone Disease. MM cells produce IL-3, DcR3, CCL3, MIP-1β, VEGF, TNFα, and RANKL. MM cells also adhere to BMSCs via VLA-4 and VCAM-1 interaction, and lead to the secretion of RANKL, SDF-1a, IL-6, BAFF, VEGF, and activin A. Moreover, MM cells stimulate CCL3 and IL-11 expression in osteocytes. OCs secrete CCL3 and activin A by MM cells stimulation. These cytokines stimulate OC differentiation and activity. MM cells also inhibit OPG expression in BMSCs and OBs resulting in stimulation of OC differentiation. On the other hand, MM cells produce IL-3, IL-7, TNFα, TGFβ, and Dkk-1. MM cells also stimulate activin A expression in BMSCs. These cytokines inhibit OB differentiation. Stimulated OCs destroy bone matrix, and release several tumor growth factor from bone. Moreover, OCs and BMSCs express several cytokines. These cytokines mediate MM cell survival and proliferation

Stromal derived factor-1 alpha (SDF-1a), B-cell activating factor (BAFF), activin A, and VEGF.

MM cells stimulate OC differentiation by producing IL-3 [26], DcR3 [27, 28], CCL3, MIP-1β [29–31], VEGF [32], TNFα, [33, 34] and RANKL [35–38]. MM cells also adhere to BMSCs via very late antigen (VLA)-4 and vascular cell adhesion molecule (VCAM)-1 interaction leading to the secretion of cytokines including RANKL, SDF-1a, IL-6, BAFF, VEGF, and activin A which in turn positively affect OC differentiation and activation [9, 14, 32, 39–43]. MM cells stimulate not only RANKL expression, but also inhibit OPG expression, leading to an increase in RANKL/OPG ratio in BMSCs and OBs which in turn strongly stimulate OC differentiation [24, 44]. In addition to BMSCs and OBs, MM cells also stimulate CCL3 and pro-osteoclastogenic cytokine, IL-11 in osteocytes [45]. Moreover, OCs secrete CCL3 and activin A, and stimulate OC differentiation and activation by themselves [9, 31]. BM macrophages stimulated by IL-3 also secrete activin A [46]. All these cytokines stimulate OC differentiation and activity, and contribute to the development of MM OBD.

3.1.1 CCL3

CCL3 is a pro-inflammatory cytokine belonging to the CC chemokine subfamily. High CCL3 levels were found in MM patients' BM serum and it correlates with OBD and survival [30]. Interestingly, fibroblast growth factor receptor 3 (FGFR3) overexpression in MM with t(4,14) results in upregulation of CCL3 expression [47]. CCL3 modulates OC differentiation by binding to G-protein coupled receptors, CCR1 and CCR5, and activating ERK and AKT signaling pathways. CCL3 has the ability to stimulate OC differentiation not only from monocytes but also from immature dendritic cells by transdifferentiation [48]. In the tumor niche, MM cells and OCs are the main source for CCL3 that promotes MM cell migration and survival, along with stimulation of osteoclastogenesis [49, 50]. Vallet et al. also showed that CCL3 reduces bone formation by inhibiting OB function by ERK activation and followed by down regulation of the osteogenic transcription factor, osterix [31]. Importantly, a small molecule CCR1 antagonist inhibits CCL3-induced osteoclastogenesis and OC support of MM cells [51].

3.1.2 RANKL to OPG Ratio

Many of the cytokines which stimulate OC differentiation and activity act through RANKL and OPG. Increase of the RANKL to OPG ratio results in bone loss in several cancers and inflammatory diseases including rheumatoid arthritis [52–54]. In MM patients, BM plasma levels of RANKL are increased, whereas OPG expression is decreased compared with normal volunteers and patients with MGUS [35]. Importantly, low levels of OPG in serum correlate with advanced OBD in MM [55]. The relevance of the RANKL/OPG pathway in mediating OC differentiation and activation in MM has been further confirmed in several murine models of MM OBD. Treatment with OPG or OPG-like molecules prevented both bone destruction and MM growth in vivo [36, 56]. Interestingly, specific anti-MM strategies such as thalidomide and autologous BM transplantation improved OBD by normalizing the RANKL to OPG ratio [57, 58]. Therefore, the RANKL-OPG axis is one of the important targets in the development of novel therapeutic strategies for MM bone disease.

3.2 Bone Marrow Stromal Cells and Osteoblasts in Myeloma Bone Disease

Besides OCs, BMSCs and OBs derived from BMSCs, play an important role in the development of OBD in the presence of MM cells. MM cells stimulate OC differentiation directly by secreting OC-activating factors (OAFs) and, indirectly, by stimulating OAFs secretion such as RANKL, Activin A and VEGF in BMSCs and OBs [14, 35, 36, 59, 60]. Adhesion of MM to BMSCs leads to RANKL and VEGF secretion by BMSCs via p38 MAPK activation [59, 60]. Moreover, the sequestosome 1, p62 is an upstream regulator of p38 MAPK and NF-κB signaling pathway, activated in BMSCs by MM cell adhesion. Inhibition of p62 in BMSCs represses OC differentiation and MM cell proliferation [61]. These data suggest that p62 is a novel promising target in MM OBD. Adhesion of MM to BMSCs and immature OBs also leads to IL-6 secretion via NF-κB signaling [42, 43, 62] and X-box-binding protein 1 (XBP1) signaling [63] pathway. IL-6 stimulates MM cell proliferation and inhibition of MM plasma cell apoptosis [64] in addition to OC differentiation. Moreover, adhesion of MM cells also stimulates BAFF expression in BMSCs via NF-κB signaling [41]. BAFF is a MM cell survival factor and it rescues MM cells from apoptosis induced by IL-6 deprivation and dexamethasone via activation of NF-κB, phosphatidylinosiol-3 (PI-3) kinase/AKT, and MAPK pathways in MM cells and induction of a strong upregulation of Mcl-1 and Bcl-2 antiapoptotic proteins [65, 66]. Secreted IL-6 and BAFF also stimulates the serine/threonine kinase Pim-2 expression in MM cells via activation of NF-κB and JAK2/STAT3 pathway, resulting in MM cell survival [67]. Furthermore, MM cells stimulate activin A expression in BMSCs via Jun N-terminal kinase-dependent (JNK) activation [9]. Importantly, high activin A levels in MM patients are associated with advanced bone disease and advanced features of MM [68]. Secreted Activin A inhibits OB differentiation in addition to the growth stimulatory effects on OCs. MM cells also stimulate Pim-2 expression in BMSCs/OBs by IL-3, IL-7, TNF-a, TGF-β and activin A secretion, and inhibit OB differentiation [69].

3.2.1 Wnt Canonical Signaling in BMSCs and OBs

Wnt canonical signaling plays an important role in OB differentiation. Some Wnt proteins bind to both Frizzled and LRP 5 and 6, and activate Wnt canonical signaling. Activated Wnt signaling induces nuclear translocation of β-catenin protein resulting in stimulation of OB differentiation by activation of major OB transcription factors [70]. Wnt antagonists, such as Dkk-1, sclerostin and secreted frizzled related proteins (sFRPs) inhibit Wnt canonical signaling activity by blocking Wnt proteins binding to Wnt receptors. Thus, these Wnt antagonists act as negative regulators for OB differentiation. In MM OBD, OB differentiation is strongly inhibited. MM cells secrete several Wnt antagonists such as Dkk-1 [71], sFRP-2 [72], sFRP-3 [73] and inhibit Wnt canonical signaling. High Dkk-1 levels have been detected in MM patients' serum and have been correlated with MM bone lesions [71]. Also high circulating levels of sclerostin, encoded by the SOST gene, have been found in newly diagnosed MM patients, and correlates with MM disease stage and fractures [74]. There is a report that MM cells produce sclerostin [75], however, we and others [76] could detect very little sclerostin or SOST mRNA expression in MM cell lines. The source and role of sclerostin in MM OBD therefore remains to be defined. Importantly, Wnt antagonists inhibit OPG expression as OPG is a target of Wnt canonical signaling [20], and increase the RANKL to OPG ratio. They are responsible not only for suppression of OB differentiation and activity but also for stimulation of OC differentiation and activity in MM OBD.

3.3 Osteocytes in Myeloma Bone Disease

Osteocytes act as main regulators of bone homeostasis in healthy bone [16]. A recent study showed that MM patients have a significantly lower number of viable osteocytes than healthy controls, and that osteocyte death correlates with the presence of bone lesions [45]. Besides a lower number of viable osteocytes has been observed in the MM patients, no significant difference in the expression of sclerostin, an osteocyte marker, in biopsies of MM patients bone and healthy controls osteocyte was observed [45]. On the other hand, higher circulating levels of sclerostin have been found in newly diagnosed MM patients as mentioned before [74]. These data suggest that there might be other alternate sources of sclerostin in addition to osteocytes in MM. Moreover, MM cells stimulate osteoclastogenic cytokines, CCL3 and IL-11 expression in pre-osteocytes leading to increased OC differentiation [45]. Further investigations regarding the role of osteocytes in MM OBD are underway.

4 Treatment of Myeloma—Related Osteolytic Bone Disease

Current treatment strategies in MM have led to significant improvements in 5-year relative overall survival, but patients continue to relapse, and no definitive cure has been as yet achieved. Given the improved survival of MM patients, treatment of OBD has taken on a new relevance as the focus is now largely on quality of life. Until recently, therapeutic options for MMOBD-included bisphosphonates, radiotherapy, and surgery. These therapies are aimed at reducing the development of new osteolytic lesions and preventing SREs such as bone pain, pathological fractures, vertebral collapse, hypercalcemia, and spinal cord compression. Interestingly, several studies using novel bone-targeted agents suggest that restoring bone

Table1 Bone-Directed Therapies for Multiple Myeloma

Drug	Role	Target	Clinical Development
Bisphosphonates	FPPS inhibition (in OC)	OCs	Approved
Pamidronate	ERK activation	OBs and osteocytes	
Zoledronic acid	(in OB and osteocyte)		
etc.			
RANKL antagonist			
Denosumab	Neutralizing antibody for RANKL	OCs	Phase III clinical trials
OPG agonist			
AMGN-0007	Recombinant OPG	OCs	Phase I clinical trials
CCR1 inhibitor			
MLN3897	small-molecule CCL3 receptor antagonist	OCs	Preclinical studies
Dkk-1 antagonist			
BHQ880	Neutralizing antibody for Dkk-1	OBs	Phase II clinical trials
Sclerostin antagonist			
romosozumab	Neutralizing antibody for sclerostin	OBs	Preclinical studies
blosozumab			
Proteasome inhibitor			
bortezomib	26s proteasome inhibition	Anti-MM and OCs OB stimulation	Approved
carfilzomib	20s proteasome inhibition		
Btk inhibitor	Btk inhibition	OCs	Preclinical studies
CC-292			
PCI-32765			
LFM-A13			
Pim inhibitor	Pim inhibition	Anti-MM OB stimulation	Preclinical studies

homeostasis may lead to tumor growth inhibition. These promising preclinical results have set the stage for clinical evaluation of novel strategies targeting MM via restoring bone homeostasis. Table 1 provides a list of bone-directed agents, their roles, targets, and stage of clinical development.

4.1 Bisphosphonates

Bisphosphonates represent the standard of care for MM OBD. Nitrogen-containing bisphosphonates such as pamidronate (PAM) or zoledronic acid (ZA), more potent than PAM, reduce osteoclast activity through inhibiting farnesyl pyrophosphate synthase (FPPS) [77]. Bisphosphonates prevent OB and osteocyte apoptosis with a different mechanism from the effect on OCs [78–80]. Bisphosphonates induce ERK activation without nuclear accumulation in OBs and osteocytes. Activated ERK stimulates p90RSK and induces phosphorylation of the cytoplasmic substrates, BAD and C/EBP, which are required for OB and osteocyte survival [81].

Bisphosphonates have a well-established role in the treatment of osteoporosis [82, 83] and metastatic bone involvement from solid tumors [84–86]. In MM, treatment with bisphosphonate significantly reduces pain related to OBD and prevents SREs. Monthly infusion of PAM reduces bone pain and SREs compared with placebo [87]. PAM also significantly improved quality of life, with decreases in pain scores seen within a month. Moreover, Major et al. reported that ZA was superior to PAM for the treatment of hypercalcemia of malignancy including MM [88] although Rosen et al. reported the efficacy of ZA in preventing SREs in MM was comparable to that of PAM [84].

In addition to their role in OBD, bisphosphonates may also have an antitumor effect. The Austrian Breast and Colorectal Cancer Study Group 12 (ABCSG-12) trial showed that the administration of zoledronic acid every 6 months for 3 years reduced the risk of disease recurrence in estrogen-receptor—positive breast cancer patients [89] although no improvement was seen in the rate of disease-free survival in another study [90]. In MM, The MRC Myeloma IX trial compared ZA and oral clodronate in newly diagnosed patients and found that ZA reduced mortality by 16 % and increased median overall survival from 44.5 to 50.0 months ($P = 0.04$) [91]

4.1.1 Osteonecrosis of the Jaw

Bisphosphonate-related osteonecrosis of the jaw (BRONJ) is one of the most serious complications of bisphosphonates [92, 93]. BRONJ is traditionally defined as exposed, necrotic bone in the jaw that does not heal after 8 weeks and is generally painful. Histologically, several tissue alterations such as honeycombed-like necrotic bone with residual vital bone, inflammatory cellular elements, and hypernucleated osteoclasts are observed in BRONJ [94–96]. ZA is associated with the highest risk of BRONJ, attributed to its increased potency, and earlier studies suggested an incidence of 4–11 %, correlating with duration of exposure [97, 98]. In the MRC Myeloma IX trial, the cumulative incidence of BRONJ was 3–4 % at a median follow-up of 3.7 years [99]. It is clear that trauma, infection, and reduced vascularity including dental extractions play important roles, however, the exact etiopathogenetic mechanism of BRONJ still remains unclear. Further studies are necessary to evaluate the detailed mechanism of BRONJ development.

4.2 Denosumab

Denosumab is an OC inhibitor that plays a role in the supportive care of MM OBD. It is a monoclonal antibody, given subcutaneously, that inhibits OC activity through targeting RANKL. Denosumab is approved for increasing bone density in patients with osteoporosis and for preventing SREs in patients with metastatic bone disease [100]. It has been recently reported that denosumab causes osteosclerosis [101], and hypercalcemia has been observed following discontinuation of denosumab [102] in children. In MM, although a favorable trend was observed, denosumab was equivalent to ZA in delaying time to first on-study SRE [103]. Denosumab is not currently FDA approved for use in patients with MM; a larger, ongoing phase III study (ClinicalTrials.gov identifier: NCT01345019) is comparing it with ZA in this disease setting.

4.3 OPG Agonists

OPG is a decoy receptor for RANKL, and it blocks OC differentiation and activation. In MM patients, BM plasma levels of OPG is decreased compared with normal volunteers and patients with MGUS [35]. Importantly, low levels of OPG in serum correlate with advanced OBD in MM [55]. Treatment with OPG or OPG-like molecules prevented both bone destruction and MM growth in vivo [36, 56]. A Phase I study of a recombinant OPG construct (AMGN-0007) was conducted in MM patients with OBD, and decreased NTX/creatinine levels was observed [104].

4.4 CCR1 Inhibitors

The CCL3/CCR1 pathway stimulates OC differentiation, MM cell survival and migration, and inhibits OB differentiation suggesting that CCL3/CCR1 is a relevant target in MM OBD. Both antisense sequence and neutralizing antibody against CCL3 effectively inhibited tumor growth and restored bone remodeling in a mouse model of MM OBD [15, 105]. Similar results have been shown with a clinical grade small molecule CCR1 antagonist, MLN3897 (Millennium Pharmaceuticals) [51]. In addition to these molecules, several CCR1 antagonists were evaluated for MM OBD [106, 107]. Future clinical trials using CCR1 inhibition strategies in patients with MM OBD will help to confirm these promising preclinical results.

4.5 Anti-BAFF—Neutralizing Antibody

In MM, BAFF is expressed by monocytes, macrophages, dendritic cells, T cells, neutrophils, MM cells, and OCs [65, 108–111]. BAFF is a MM cell survival factor and rescues MM cells from apoptosis induced by IL-6 deprivation and dexamethasone via activation of NF-kB, PI-3 kinase/AKT, and MAPK kinase pathways and induction of a strong upregulation of the Mcl-1 and Bcl-2 antiapoptotic proteins [65]. In vivo—neutralizing antibodies against BAFF (LY2127399, Eli Lilly) significantly inhibit tumor burden and, importantly, reduce OBD and OC differentiation in preclinical setting [66]. On the basis of these results, a clinical trial combining BAFF-neutralizing antibody with proteasome inhibitor, bortezomib is currently ongoing, preliminary results from Raje et al. reported the treatment was well tolerated and 22 of the 48 patients enrolled achieved a partial remission or better (https://ash.confex.com/ash/2012/webprogram/Paper52052.html).

4.6   Activin A Antagonists

Activin A is secreted by BMSCs and OCs in MM OBD. Activin A stimulates OC differentiation and inhibits OB formation in MM OBD. Activin A can be targeted by a chimeric antibody RAP-011 (Acceleron Pharma), derived from the fusion of the extracellular domain of type II activin receptor (ActRIIA) and the constant domain of the murine IgG2a [112]. RAP-011 enhances OB mineralization and increases bone density in an osteoporotic mouse model. In MM, RAP-011 reversed OB inhibition, improved MM bone disease, and inhibited tumor growth in an in vivo humanized MM model [9]. In human, ACE-011 which is the humanized counterpart of RAP-011 effectively decreased bone resorption markers, C-terminal type 1 collagen telopeptide (CTX) and TRACP-5b and increased bone formation marker, serum levels of bone-specific alkaline phosphatase (BSALP) in post-menopausal women [113]. It has been shown in vitro that lenalidomide, a well known and approved treatment strategy for relapsed MM, stimulates activin A secretion on BMSCs via an Akt-mediated increase in JNK signaling [14]. Clinical trials for ACE-011 with Lenalidomide + Dexamethasone are ongoing and evaluating its role in MM (ClinicalTrials.gov identifier: NCT01562405).

4.7   Dkk-1 Antagonists

Dkk-1 plays one of the key roles in mediating OB inhibition in MM [71]. Therefore, treatment strategies to block Dkk-1 activity have been developed. In vitro assays show that inhibition of Dkk-1 via a specific neutralizing antibody promotes OB differentiation and function and reverses the negative effect of MM cells on OB differentiation [114, 115]. Moreover, in vivo studies using both murine and humanized murine models of MM-induced bone disease showed increased bone formation, OB numbers, and improvement of osteolytic lesions by Dkk-1 inhibition [115–117]. Importantly, blocking Dkk-1 also resulted in reduction of tumor growth, mainly as an indirect effect via modification of the tumor microenvironment [115]. Therefore, Dkk-1 inhibition via a neutralizing antibody restores bone homeostasis and may have an inhibitory effect on tumor growth. Currently, ongoing clinical trials combining Dkk-1 neutralizing antibody and bisphosphonates will test these promising preclinical results. In particular, ZA in combination with the proanabolic agent BHQ880, a fully human anti-Dkk-1 monoclonal antibody, has being studied in a phase I clinical trial (ClinicalTrials.gov identifier: NCT00741377). BHQ880 was also tested in a phase II clinical trial in smoldering MM (ClinicalTrials.gov identifier: NCT01302886) and preliminary results showed that BHQ880 significantly stimulated the vertebral strength by qCT from a baseline of 3 % ($P = 0.002$) (https://ash.confex.com/ash/2012/webprogram/Paper48568.html).

4.8 Sclerostin Neutralizing Antibody

Several studies have already demonstrated the importance of sclerostin in osteoporosis [118, 119], and inhibition of sclerostin represents an important strategy in the treatment of bone conditions with high catabolism. In fact, clinical trials with sclerostin neutralizing antibodies, romosozumab and blosozumab for the treatment of postmenopausal osteoporosis are ongoing and preliminary results have shown increase of bone mineral density [120–122]. In MM, higher circulating levels of sclerostin have been found in newly diagnosed MM patients, and it correlated with MM disease stage and fractures [74]. These data underscore the importance of targeting sclerostin for treatment of MM OBD. However, the source and role of sclerostin in MM OBD still remains unclear. Further studies about sclerostin's role in MM and application of sclerostin neutralizing antibody to MM OBD are expected.

4.9 Bortezomib

Bortezomib is a proteasome and NF-kB signaling pathway inhibitor with potent anti-MM activity. Bortezomib also inhibits MM-BMSC interactions, impairs osteoclastogenesis, and stimulates mesenchymal stem cell differentiation to OB and, therefore, actively modulates bone remodeling in MM [123–125]. The anabolic effects of bortezomib are associated with Runx2 upregulation via inhibition of proteasomal degradation. Runx2 is a critical transcription factor in early OB differentiation and modulates the expression of the OB-specific transcription factor osterix [125, 126]. The anti-OC effects of bortezomib are mediated by p38 inhibition at early time points and, at later time points, by impairment of NF-kB signaling and AP1 inhibition [123]. These effects have been confirmed in the clinical setting by upregulation of OB activation markers (BSALP and osteocalcin) and downregulation of bone resorption markers (CTX and TRACP-5b) as well as decrease of Dkk-1 and sRANKL in patients treated with bortezomib [127].

4.10 Carfilzomib

In contrast to bortezomib, carfilzomib is a new proteasome inhibitor that is associated with a very low incidence of peripheral neuropathy. Carfilzomib is a structural analog of the microbial natural product epoxomicin that selectively inhibits the chymotrypsin-like activity of both the constitutive proteasome and the immunoproteasome [128]. It was recently approved in July 2012 for patients with MM experiencing disease progression after prior therapy with bortezomib and an immunomodulatory drug. Carfilzomib strongly stimulates OB calcification and inhibits OC differentiation in addition to the antitumor effect [129–131]. Moreover, we showed carfilzomib reversed OB inhibition, improved MM bone disease, and inhibited tumor growth in an in vivo disseminated MM model [131]. Interestingly, we could not see upregulation of OB differentiation marker in OBs in the presence of higher concentration of carfilzomib although the concentration of carfilzomib strongly stimulates OB calcification. Further studies are necessary to evaluate the detailed mechanism of carfilzomib effect on OBs.

4.11 Bruton's Tyrosine Kinase Inhibitors

Bruton's tyrosine kinase (Btk) belongs to the Tec family of tyrosine kinases. The activation of Btk regulates B-cell development and antibodies production. Thus, Btk pathway is a potential therapeutic target in a variety of B-cell malignancies, including Waldenström's macroglobulinemia, diffuse large B-cell lymphoma, follicular lymphoma, mantle cell lymphoma and chronic lymphocytic leukemia [132]. In MM, we showed that Btk inhibitor, CC-292 strongly inhibits OC activity and improves MM OBD [131]. It decreased only INA-6 MM cell line viability in higher concentration, however, had negligible direct in vitro effects on other MM cells viability or in animal models. On the other hand, the other Btk inhibitors, PCI-32765 (ibrutinib) and LFM-A13 have shown to display some antitumor effect in MM xenograft mouse model when INA-6 MM cells were used [133, 134]. More investigations are needed to reveal the role of Btk inhibitors in the MM OBD.

4.12 Pim Inhibitor

MM cells upregulate Pim-2 expression in BMSCs/OBs and inhibit OB differentiation [69]. Meanwhile, IL-6, produced by BMSCs, BAFF, and APRIL, produced by OCs, stimulate Pim-2 expression in MM cells via activation of NF-κB and JAK2/STAT3 pathway, resulting in MM cell survival [67]. Importantly, Pim inhibitor prevents bone destruction while suppressing MM tumor burden in MM model mouse [69]. Pim-2 may become a new target for not only MM OBD but also MM treatment.

5 Conclusion

Our understanding of the biology of MM OBD was remarkably advanced in these decades. Although OCs are a critical player in the pathogenesis of bone disease, other BM microenvironmental cells such as osteocytes, OBs, and BMSCs are affected in MM and contribute to the development of MM OBD. Many novel targets for MM OBD have been discovered following these insights. Effective therapeutic strategies to overcome MM-induced OBD should target the osteocyte-OB-OC axis, combining bone-anabolic with anticatabolic agents. Such novel agents for MM OBD restoring bone balance in MM represent a novel strategy to overcome osteolytic disease and, more provocatively, to create a hostile niche for

MM tumor growth. Although there are still many unknown parts in MM OBD, further investigations will reveal these and a wide range of targeted therapies may become available to treat MM OBD more effectively in the near future.

References

1. Singhal S, Mehta J, Desikan R et al (1999) Antitumor activity of thalidomide in refractory multiple myeloma. N Engl J Med 341:1565–1571
2. Dimopoulos M, Spencer A, Attal M et al (2007) Lenalidomide plus dexamethasone for relapsed or refractory multiple myeloma. N Engl J Med 357:2123–2132
3. Richardson PG, Barlogie B, Berenson J et al (2003) A phase 2 study of bortezomib in relapsed, refractory myeloma. N Engl J Med 348:2609–2617
4. Brenner H, Gondos A, Pulte D (2008) Recent major improvement in long-term survival of younger patients with multiple myeloma. Blood 111:2521–2526
5. Raje N, Roodman GD (2011) Advances in the biology and treatment of bone disease in multiple myeloma. Clin Cancer Res 17:1278–1286
6. Coleman RE (1997) Skeletal complications of malignancy. Cancer 80:1588–1594
7. Roodman GD (2010) Pathogenesis of myeloma bone disease. J Cell Biochem 109:283–291
8. Saad F, Lipton A, Cook R, Chen YM, Smith M, Coleman R (2007) Pathologic fractures correlate with reduced survival in patients with malignant bone disease. Cancer 110:1860–1867
9. Vallet S, Mukherjee S, Vaghela N et al (2010) Activin A promotes multiple myeloma-induced osteolysis and is a promising target for myeloma bone disease. Proc Natl Acad Sci USA 107:5124–5129
10. Vallet S, Raje N (2011) Bone anabolic agents for the treatment of multiple myeloma. Cancer Microenviron 4:339–349
11. Sonmez M, Akagun T, Topbas M, et al (2008) Effect of pathologic fractures on survival in multiple myeloma patients: a case control study. J Exp Clin Cancer Res 27:11-9966-27-11
12. Podar K, Chauhan D, Anderson KC (2009) Bone marrow microenvironment and the identification of new targets for myeloma therapy. Leukemia 23:10–24
13. Edwards CM, Edwards JR, Lwin ST et al (2008) Increasing Wnt signaling in the bone marrow microenvironment inhibits the development of myeloma bone disease and reduces tumor burden in bone in vivo. Blood 111:2833–2842
14. Scullen T, Santo L, Vallet S et al (2013) Lenalidomide in combination with an activin A-neutralizing antibody: preclinical rationale for a novel anti-myeloma strategy. Leukemia 27:1715–1721
15. Choi SJ, Oba Y, Gazitt Y et al (2001) Antisense inhibition of macrophage inflammatory protein 1-alpha blocks bone destruction in a model of myeloma bone disease. J Clin Invest 108:1833–1841
16. Bonewald LF (2011) The amazing osteocyte. J Bone Miner Res 26:229–238
17. Aguirre JI, Plotkin LI, Stewart SA et al (2006) Osteocyte apoptosis is induced by weightlessness in mice and precedes osteoclast recruitment and bone loss. J Bone Miner Res 21:605–615
18. Kitase Y, Barragan L, Qing H et al (2010) Mechanical induction of PGE2 in osteocytes blocks glucocorticoid-induced apoptosis through both the beta-catenin and PKA pathways. J Bone Miner Res 25:2657–2668
19. Kogianni G, Mann V, Noble BS (2008) Apoptotic bodies convey activity capable of initiating osteoclastogenesis and localized bone destruction. J Bone Miner Res 23:915–927
20. Baron R, Kneissel M (2013) WNT signaling in bone homeostasis and disease: from human mutations to treatments. Nat Med 19:179–192

21. Negishi-Koga T, Shinohara M, Komatsu N et al (2011) Suppression of bone formation by osteoclastic expression of semaphorin 4D. Nat Med 17:1473–1480
22. Valentin-Opran A, Charhon SA, Meunier PJ, Edouard CM, Arlot ME (1982) Quantitative histology of myeloma-induced bone changes. Br J Haematol 52:601–610
23. Taube T, Beneton MN, McCloskey EV, Rogers S, Greaves M, Kanis JA (1992) Abnormal bone remodelling in patients with myelomatosis and normal biochemical indices of bone resorption. Eur J Haematol 49:192–198
24. Terpos E, Szydlo R, Apperley JF et al (2003) Soluble receptor activator of nuclear factor kappaB ligand-osteoprotegerin ratio predicts survival in multiple myeloma: proposal for a novel prognostic index. Blood 102:1064–1069
25. Politou M, Terpos E, Anagnostopoulos A et al (2004) Role of receptor activator of nuclear factor-kappa B ligand (RANKL), osteoprotegerin and macrophage protein 1-alpha (MIP-1a) in monoclonal gammopathy of undetermined significance (MGUS). Br J Haematol 126: 686–689
26. Lee JW, Chung HY, Ehrlich LA et al (2004) IL-3 expression by myeloma cells increases both osteoclast formation and growth of myeloma cells. Blood 103:2308–2315
27. Colucci S, Brunetti G, Mori G et al (2009) Soluble decoy receptor 3 modulates the survival and formation of osteoclasts from multiple myeloma bone disease patients. Leukemia 23:2139–2146
28. Brunetti G, Oranger A, Mori G et al (2010) The formation of osteoclasts in multiple myeloma bone disease patients involves the secretion of soluble decoy receptor 3. Ann N Y Acad Sci 1192:298–302
29. Abe M, Hiura K, Wilde J et al (2002) Role for macrophage inflammatory protein (MIP)-1alpha and MIP-1beta in the development of osteolytic lesions in multiple myeloma. Blood 100:2195–2202
30. Uneda S, Hata H, Matsuno F et al (2003) Macrophage inflammatory protein-1 alpha is produced by human multiple myeloma (MM) cells and its expression correlates with bone lesions in patients with MM. Br J Haematol 120:53–55
31. Vallet S, Pozzi S, Patel K et al (2011) A novel role for CCL3 (MIP-1alpha) in myeloma-induced bone disease via osteocalcin downregulation and inhibition of osteoblast function. Leukemia 25:1174–1181
32. Gupta D, Treon SP, Shima Y et al (2001) Adherence of multiple myeloma cells to bone marrow stromal cells upregulates vascular endothelial growth factor secretion: therapeutic applications. Leukemia 15:1950–1961
33. Nanes MS (2003) Tumor necrosis factor-alpha: molecular and cellular mechanisms in skeletal pathology. Gene 321:1–15
34. Kitaura H, Sands MS, Aya K et al (2004) Marrow stromal cells and osteoclast precursors differentially contribute to TNF-alpha-induced osteoclastogenesis in vivo. J Immunol 173:4838–4846
35. Giuliani N, Bataille R, Mancini C, Lazzaretti M, Barille S (2001) Myeloma cells induce imbalance in the osteoprotegerin/osteoprotegerin ligand system in the human bone marrow environment. Blood 98:3527–3533
36. Pearse RN, Sordillo EM, Yaccoby S et al (2001) Multiple myeloma disrupts the TRANCE/osteoprotegerin cytokine axis to trigger bone destruction and promote tumor progression. Proc Natl Acad Sci USA 98:11581–11586
37. Roux S, Meignin V, Quillard J et al (2002) RANK (receptor activator of nuclear factor-kappaB) and RANKL expression in multiple myeloma. Br J Haematol 117:86–92
38. Colucci S, Brunetti G, Rizzi R et al (2004) T cells support osteoclastogenesis in an in vitro model derived from human multiple myeloma bone disease: the role of the OPG/TRAIL interaction. Blood 104:3722–3730
39. Michigami T, Shimizu N, Williams PJ et al (2000) Cell-cell contact between marrow stromal cells and myeloma cells via VCAM-1 and alpha(4)beta(1)-integrin enhances production of osteoclast-stimulating activity. Blood 96:1953–1960

40. Hideshima T, Chauhan D, Hayashi T et al (2002) The biological sequelae of stromal cell-derived factor-1alpha in multiple myeloma. Mol Cancer Ther 1:539–544
41. Tai YT, Li XF, Breitkreutz I et al (2006) Role of B-cell-activating factor in adhesion and growth of human multiple myeloma cells in the bone marrow microenvironment. Cancer Res 66:6675–6682
42. Chauhan D, Uchiyama H, Akbarali Y et al (1996) Multiple myeloma cell adhesion-induced interleukin-6 expression in bone marrow stromal cells involves activation of NF-kappa B. Blood 87:1104–1112
43. Uchiyama H, Barut BA, Mohrbacher AF, Chauhan D, Anderson KC (1993) Adhesion of human myeloma-derived cell lines to bone marrow stromal cells stimulates interleukin-6 secretion. Blood 82:3712–3720
44. Sezer O, Heider U, Zavrski I, Kuhne CA, Hofbauer LC (2003) RANK ligand and osteoprotegerin in myeloma bone disease. Blood 101:2094–2098
45. Giuliani N, Ferretti M, Bolzoni M et al (2012) Increased osteocyte death in multiple myeloma patients: role in myeloma-induced osteoclast formation. Leukemia 26:1391–1401
46. Silbermann R, Bolzoni M, Storti P et al (2014) Bone marrow monocyte-/macrophage-derived activin A mediates the osteoclastogenic effect of IL-3 in multiple myeloma. Leukemia 28:951–954
47. Masih-Khan E, Trudel S, Heise C et al (2006) MIP-1alpha (CCL3) is a downstream target of FGFR3 and RAS-MAPK signaling in multiple myeloma. Blood 108:3465–3471
48. Rivollier A, Mazzorana M, Tebib J et al (2004) Immature dendritic cell transdifferentiation into osteoclasts: a novel pathway sustained by the rheumatoid arthritis microenvironment. Blood 104:4029–4037
49. Han JH, Choi SJ, Kurihara N, Koide M, Oba Y, Roodman GD (2001) Macrophage inflammatory protein-1alpha is an osteoclastogenic factor in myeloma that is independent of receptor activator of nuclear factor kappaB ligand. Blood 97:3349–3353
50. Lentzsch S, Gries M, Janz M, Bargou R, Dorken B, Mapara MY (2003) Macrophage inflammatory protein 1-alpha (MIP-1 alpha) triggers migration and signaling cascades mediating survival and proliferation in multiple myeloma (MM) cells. Blood 101:3568–3573
51. Vallet S, Raje N, Ishitsuka K et al (2007) MLN3897, a novel CCR1 inhibitor, impairs osteoclastogenesis and inhibits the interaction of multiple myeloma cells and osteoclasts. Blood 110:3744–3752
52. Mancino AT, Klimberg VS, Yamamoto M, Manolagas SC, Abe E (2001) Breast cancer increases osteoclastogenesis by secreting M-CSF and upregulating RANKL in stromal cells. J Surg Res 100:18–24
53. Moschen AR, Kaser A, Enrich B et al (2005) The RANKL/OPG system is activated in inflammatory bowel disease and relates to the state of bone loss. Gut 54:479–487
54. Romas E, Gillespie MT, Martin TJ (2002) Involvement of receptor activator of NFkappaB ligand and tumor necrosis factor-alpha in bone destruction in rheumatoid arthritis. Bone 30:340–346
55. Seidel C, Hjertner O, Abildgaard N et al (2001) Serum osteoprotegerin levels are reduced in patients with multiple myeloma with lytic bone disease. Blood 98:2269–2271
56. Croucher PI, Shipman CM, Lippitt J et al (2001) Osteoprotegerin inhibits the development of osteolytic bone disease in multiple myeloma. Blood 98:3534–3540
57. Terpos E, Politou M, Szydlo R et al (2004) Autologous stem cell transplantation normalizes abnormal bone remodeling and sRANKL/osteoprotegerin ratio in patients with multiple myeloma. Leukemia 18:1420–1426
58. Terpos E, Mihou D, Szydlo R et al (2005) The combination of intermediate doses of thalidomide with dexamethasone is an effective treatment for patients with refractory/relapsed multiple myeloma and normalizes abnormal bone remodeling, through the reduction of sRANKL/osteoprotegerin ratio. Leukemia 19:1969–1976

59. Nguyen AN, Stebbins EG, Henson M et al (2006) Normalizing the bone marrow microenvironment with p38 inhibitor reduces multiple myeloma cell proliferation and adhesion and suppresses osteoclast formation. Exp Cell Res 312:1909–1923
60. Ishitsuka K, Hideshima T, Neri P et al (2008) p38 mitogen-activated protein kinase inhibitor LY2228820 enhances bortezomib-induced cytotoxicity and inhibits osteoclastogenesis in multiple myeloma; therapeutic implications. Br J Haematol 141:598–606
61. Hiruma Y, Honjo T, Jelinek DF et al (2009) Increased signaling through p62 in the marrow microenvironment increases myeloma cell growth and osteoclast formation. Blood 113:4894–4902
62. Urashima M, Chauhan D, Uchiyama H, Freeman GJ, Anderson KC (1995) CD40 ligand triggered interleukin-6 secretion in multiple myeloma. Blood 85:1903–1912
63. Xu G, Liu K, Anderson J et al (2012) Expression of XBP1 s in bone marrow stromal cells is critical for myeloma cell growth and osteoclast formation. Blood 119:4205–4214
64. Dankbar B, Padro T, Leo R et al (2000) Vascular endothelial growth factor and interleukin-6 in paracrine tumor-stromal cell interactions in multiple myeloma. Blood 95:2630–2636
65. Moreaux J, Legouffe E, Jourdan E et al (2004) BAFF and APRIL protect myeloma cells from apoptosis induced by interleukin 6 deprivation and dexamethasone. Blood 103:3148–3157
66. Neri P, Kumar S, Fulciniti MT et al (2007) Neutralizing B-cell activating factor antibody improves survival and inhibits osteoclastogenesis in a severe combined immunodeficient human multiple myeloma model. Clin Cancer Res 13:5903–5909
67. Asano J, Nakano A, Oda A et al (2011) The serine/threonine kinase Pim-2 is a novel anti-apoptotic mediator in myeloma cells. Leukemia 25:1182–1188
68. Terpos E, Kastritis E, Christoulas D et al (2012) Circulating activin-A is elevated in patients with advanced multiple myeloma and correlates with extensive bone involvement and inferior survival; no alterations post-lenalidomide and dexamethasone therapy. Ann Oncol 23:2681–2686
69. Hiasa M, Teramachi J, Oda A et al (2015) Pim-2 kinase is an important target of treatment for tumor progression and bone loss in myeloma. Leukemia 29:207–217
70. Westendorf JJ, Kahler RA, Schroeder TM (2004) Wnt signaling in osteoblasts and bone diseases. Gene 341:19–39
71. Tian E, Zhan F, Walker R et al (2003) The role of the Wnt-signaling antagonist DKK1 in the development of osteolytic lesions in multiple myeloma. N Engl J Med 349:2483–2494
72. Oshima T, Abe M, Asano J et al (2005) Myeloma cells suppress bone formation by secreting a soluble Wnt inhibitor, sFRP-2. Blood 106:3160–3165
73. Giuliani N, Morandi F, Tagliaferri S et al (2007) Production of Wnt inhibitors by myeloma cells: potential effects on canonical Wnt pathway in the bone microenvironment. Cancer Res 67:7665–7674
74. Terpos E, Christoulas D, Katodritou E et al (2012) Elevated circulating sclerostin correlates with advanced disease features and abnormal bone remodeling in symptomatic myeloma: reduction post-bortezomib monotherapy. Int J Cancer 131:1466–1471
75. Colucci S, Brunetti G, Oranger A et al (2011) Myeloma cells suppress osteoblasts through sclerostin secretion. Blood Cancer J 1:e27
76. Delgado-Calle J, Bellido T, Roodman GD (2014) Role of osteocytes in multiple myeloma bone disease. Curr Opin Support Palliat Care 8:407–413
77. Favus MJ (2010) Bisphosphonates for osteoporosis. N Engl J Med 363:2027–2035
78. Plotkin LI, Weinstein RS, Parfitt AM, Roberson PK, Manolagas SC, Bellido T (1999) Prevention of osteocyte and osteoblast apoptosis by bisphosphonates and calcitonin. J Clin Invest 104:1363–1374
79. Kogianni G, Mann V, Ebetino F et al (2004) Fas/CD95 is associated with glucocorticoid-induced osteocyte apoptosis. Life Sci 75:2879–2895
80. Plotkin LI, Manolagas SC, Bellido T (2006) Dissociation of the pro-apoptotic effects of bisphosphonates on osteoclasts from their anti-apoptotic effects on osteoblasts/osteocytes with novel analogs. Bone 39:443–452

81. Plotkin LI, Aguirre JI, Kousteni S, Manolagas SC, Bellido T (2005) Bisphosphonates and estrogens inhibit osteocyte apoptosis via distinct molecular mechanisms downstream of extracellular signal-regulated kinase activation. J Biol Chem 280:7317–7325

82. Black DM, Cummings SR, Karpf DB et al (1996) Randomised trial of effect of alendronate on risk of fracture in women with existing vertebral fractures. Fracture Intervention Trial Research Group. Lancet 348:1535–1541

83. Black DM, Delmas PD, Eastell R et al (2007) Once-yearly zoledronic acid for treatment of postmenopausal osteoporosis. N Engl J Med 356:1809–1822

84. Rosen LS, Gordon D, Kaminski M et al (2003) Long-term efficacy and safety of zoledronic acid compared with pamidronate disodium in the treatment of skeletal complications in patients with advanced multiple myeloma or breast carcinoma: a randomized, double-blind, multicenter, comparative trial. Cancer 98:1735–1744

85. Rosen LS, Gordon D, Tchekmedyian S et al (2003) Zoledronic acid versus placebo in the treatment of skeletal metastases in patients with lung cancer and other solid tumors: a phase III, double-blind, randomized trial—the Zoledronic Acid Lung Cancer and Other Solid Tumors Study Group. J Clin Oncol 21:3150–3157

86. Saad F, Gleason DM, Murray R et al (2004) Long-term efficacy of zoledronic acid for the prevention of skeletal complications in patients with metastatic hormone-refractory prostate cancer. J Natl Cancer Inst 96:879–882

87. Berenson JR, Lichtenstein A, Porter L et al (1996) Efficacy of pamidronate in reducing skeletal events in patients with advanced multiple myeloma. Myeloma Aredia Study Group. N Engl J Med 334:488–493

88. Major P, Lortholary A, Hon J et al (2001) Zoledronic acid is superior to pamidronate in the treatment of hypercalcemia of malignancy: a pooled analysis of two randomized, controlled clinical trials. J Clin Oncol 19:558–567

89. Gnant M, Mlineritsch B, Stoeger H et al (2011) Adjuvant endocrine therapy plus zoledronic acid in premenopausal women with early-stage breast cancer: 62-month follow-up from the ABCSG-12 randomised trial. Lancet Oncol 12:631–641

90. Coleman RE, Marshall H, Cameron D et al (2011) Breast-cancer adjuvant therapy with zoledronic acid. N Engl J Med 365:1396–1405

91. Morgan GJ, Davies FE, Gregory WM et al (2010) First-line treatment with zoledronic acid as compared with clodronic acid in multiple myeloma (MRC Myeloma IX): a randomised controlled trial. Lancet 376:1989–1999

92. Raje N, Woo SB, Hande K et al (2008) Clinical, radiographic, and biochemical characterization of multiple myeloma patients with osteonecrosis of the jaw. Clin Cancer Res 14:2387–2395

93. Woo SB, Hellstein JW, Kalmar JR (2006) Narrative [corrected] review: bisphosphonates and osteonecrosis of the jaws. Ann Intern Med 144:753–761

94. Basso FG, Turrioni AP, Hebling J, de Souza Costa CA (2013) Effects of zoledronic acid on odontoblast-like cells. Arch Oral Biol 58:467–473

95. Bagan J, Scully C, Sabater V, Jimenez Y (2009) Osteonecrosis of the jaws in patients treated with intravenous bisphosphonates (BRONJ): a concise update. Oral Oncol 45:551–554

96. Wimalawansa SJ (2008) Insight into bisphosphonate-associated osteomyelitis of the jaw: pathophysiology, mechanisms and clinical management. Expert Opin Drug Saf 7:491–512

97. Dimopoulos MA, Kastritis E, Anagnostopoulos A et al (2006) Osteonecrosis of the jaw in patients with multiple myeloma treated with bisphosphonates: evidence of increased risk after treatment with zoledronic acid. Haematologica 91:968–971

98. Zervas K, Verrou E, Teleioudis Z et al (2006) Incidence, risk factors and management of osteonecrosis of the jaw in patients with multiple myeloma: a single-centre experience in 303 patients. Br J Haematol 134:620–623

99. Morgan GJ (2011) Further analyses of the Myeloma IX Study. Lancet 378:768–769

100. Yee AJ, Raje NS (2012) Denosumab, a RANK ligand inhibitor, for the management of bone loss in cancer patients. Clin Interv Aging 7:331–338

101. Kobayashi E, Setsu N (2015) Osteosclerosis induced by denosumab. Lancet 385:539-6736 (14)61338-6. Epub 2014 Oct 28
102. Gossai N, Hilgers MV, Polgreen LE, Greengard EG (2015) Critical hypercalcemia following discontinuation of denosumab therapy for metastatic giant cell tumor of bone. Pediatr Blood Cancer
103. Henry DH, Costa L, Goldwasser F et al (2011) Randomized, double-blind study of denosumab versus zoledronic acid in the treatment of bone metastases in patients with advanced cancer (excluding breast and prostate cancer) or multiple myeloma. J Clin Oncol 29:1125–1132
104. Body JJ, Greipp P, Coleman RE et al (2003) A phase I study of AMGN-0007, a recombinant osteoprotegerin construct, in patients with multiple myeloma or breast carcinoma related bone metastases. Cancer 97:887–892
105. Oyajobi BO, Franchin G, Williams PJ et al (2003) Dual effects of macrophage inflammatory protein-1alpha on osteolysis and tumor burden in the murine 5TGM1 model of myeloma bone disease. Blood 102:311–319
106. Oba Y, Lee JW, Ehrlich LA et al (2005) MIP-1alpha utilizes both CCR1 and CCR5 to induce osteoclast formation and increase adhesion of myeloma cells to marrow stromal cells. Exp Hematol 33:272–278
107. Dairaghi DJ, Oyajobi BO, Gupta A et al (2012) CCR1 blockade reduces tumor burden and osteolysis in vivo in a mouse model of myeloma bone disease. Blood 120:1449–1457
108. Novak AJ, Darce JR, Arendt BK et al (2004) Expression of BCMA, TACI, and BAFF-R in multiple myeloma: a mechanism for growth and survival. Blood 103:689–694
109. Mackay F, Browning JL (2002) BAFF: a fundamental survival factor for B cells. Nat Rev Immunol 2:465–475
110. Moore PA, Belvedere O, Orr A et al (1999) BLyS: member of the tumor necrosis factor family and B lymphocyte stimulator. Science 285:260–263
111. Moreaux J, Cremer FW, Reme T et al (2005) The level of TACI gene expression in myeloma cells is associated with a signature of microenvironment dependence versus a plasmablastic signature. Blood 106:1021–1030
112. Pearsall RS, Canalis E, Cornwall-Brady M et al (2008) A soluble activin type IIA receptor induces bone formation and improves skeletal integrity. Proc Natl Acad Sci USA 105:7082–7087
113. Ruckle J, Jacobs M, Kramer W et al (2009) Single-dose, randomized, double-blind, placebo-controlled study of ACE-011 (ActRIIA-IgG1) in postmenopausal women. J Bone Miner Res 24:744–752
114. Pozzi S, Fulciniti M, Yan H et al (2013) In vivo and in vitro effects of a novel anti-Dkk1 neutralizing antibody in multiple myeloma. Bone 53:487–496
115. Fulciniti M, Tassone P, Hideshima T et al (2009) Anti-DKK1 mAb (BHQ880) as a potential therapeutic agent for multiple myeloma. Blood 114:371–379
116. Yaccoby S, Ling W, Zhan F, Walker R, Barlogie B, Shaughnessy JD Jr (2007) Antibody-based inhibition of DKK1 suppresses tumor-induced bone resorption and multiple myeloma growth in vivo. Blood 109:2106–2111
117. Heath DJ, Chantry AD, Buckle CH et al (2009) Inhibiting Dickkopf-1 (Dkk1) removes suppression of bone formation and prevents the development of osteolytic bone disease in multiple myeloma. J Bone Miner Res 24:425–436
118. Hoeppner LH, Secreto FJ, Westendorf JJ (2009) Wnt signaling as a therapeutic target for bone diseases. Expert Opin Ther Targets 13:485–496
119. Lewiecki EM (2011) New targets for intervention in the treatment of postmenopausal osteoporosis. Nat Rev Rheumatol 7:631–638
120. McClung MR, Grauer A, Boonen S et al (2014) Romosozumab in postmenopausal women with low bone mineral density. N Engl J Med 370:412–420

121. McColm J, Hu L, Womack T, Tang CC, Chiang AY (2014) Single- and multiple-dose randomized studies of blosozumab, a monoclonal antibody against sclerostin, in healthy postmenopausal women. J Bone Miner Res 29:935–943
122. Clarke BL (2014) Anti-sclerostin antibodies: utility in treatment of osteoporosis. Maturitas 78:199–204
123. von Metzler I, Krebbel H, Hecht M et al (2007) Bortezomib inhibits human osteoclastogenesis. Leukemia 21:2025–2034
124. Zangari M, Esseltine D, Lee CK et al (2005) Response to bortezomib is associated to osteoblastic activation in patients with multiple myeloma. Br J Haematol 131:71–73
125. Mukherjee S, Raje N, Schoonmaker JA et al (2008) Pharmacologic targeting of a stem/progenitor population in vivo is associated with enhanced bone regeneration in mice. J Clin Invest 118:491–504
126. Giuliani N, Morandi F, Tagliaferri S et al (2007) The proteasome inhibitor bortezomib affects osteoblast differentiation in vitro and in vivo in multiple myeloma patients. Blood 110:334–338
127. Terpos E, Heath DJ, Rahemtulla A et al (2006) Bortezomib reduces serum dickkopf-1 and receptor activator of nuclear factor-kappaB ligand concentrations and normalises indices of bone remodelling in patients with relapsed multiple myeloma. Br J Haematol 135:688–692
128. Kuhn DJ, Chen Q, Voorhees PM et al (2007) Potent activity of carfilzomib, a novel, irreversible inhibitor of the ubiquitin-proteasome pathway, against preclinical models of multiple myeloma. Blood 110:3281–3290
129. Hurchla MA, Garcia-Gomez A, Hornick MC et al (2013) The epoxyketone-based proteasome inhibitors carfilzomib and orally bioavailable oprozomib have anti-resorptive and bone-anabolic activity in addition to anti-myeloma effects. Leukemia 27:430–440
130. Ha SW, Weitzmann MN, Beck GR Jr (2014) Bioactive silica nanoparticles promote osteoblast differentiation through stimulation of autophagy and direct association with LC3 and p62. ACS Nano 8:5898–5910
131. Eda H, Santo L, Cirstea DD et al (2014) A novel Bruton's tyrosine kinase inhibitor CC-292 in combination with the proteasome inhibitor carfilzomib impacts the bone microenvironment in a multiple myeloma model with resultant antimyeloma activity. Leukemia 28:1892–1901
132. Brown JR (2013) Ibrutinib in chronic lymphocytic leukemia and B cell malignancies. Leuk Lymphoma
133. Tai YT, Chang BY, Kong SY et al (2012) Bruton tyrosine kinase inhibition is a novel therapeutic strategy targeting tumor in the bone marrow microenvironment in multiple myeloma. Blood 120:1877–1887
134. Bam R, Ling W, Khan S et al (2013) Role of Bruton's tyrosine kinase in myeloma cell migration and induction of bone disease. Am J Hematol 88:463–471

Part III
Primary Amyloidosis, Systemic Light Chain and Heavy Chain Diseases, Plasmacytoma

Immunoglobulin Light Chain Systemic Amyloidosis

Angela Dispenzieri and Giampaolo Merlini

Abstract

Immunoglobulin light chain amyloidosis (AL) is a rare, complex disease caused by misfolded free light chains produced by a usually small, indolent plasma cell clone. Effective treatments exist that can alter the natural history, provided that they are started before irreversible organ damage has occurred. The cornerstones of the management of AL amyloidosis are early diagnosis, accurate typing, appropriate risk-adapted therapy, tight follow-up, and effective supportive treatment. The suppression of the amyloidogenic light chains using the cardiac biomarkers as guide to choose chemotherapy is still the mainstay of therapy. There are exciting possibilities ahead, including the study of oral proteasome inhibitors, antibodies directed at plasma cell clone, and finally antibodies attacking the amyloid deposits are entering the clinic, offering unprecedented opportunities for radically improving the care of this disease.

Keywords

Immunoglobulin light chain amyloidosis · Cardiac amyloidosis · Biomarkers · Chemotherapy · Immunotherapy

A. Dispenzieri
Division of Hematology, Mayo Clinic, Rochester, MN, USA

A. Dispenzieri
Division of Laboratory Medicine, Mayo Clinic, Rochester, MN, USA

G. Merlini (✉)
Amyloidosis Research and Treatment Center, Foundation IRCCS Policlinico San Matteo and Department of Molecular Medicine, University of Pavia, Pavia, Italy
e-mail: gmerlini@unipv.it

© Springer International Publishing Switzerland 2016
A.M. Roccaro and I.M. Ghobrial (eds.), *Plasma Cell Dyscrasias*,
Cancer Treatment and Research 169, DOI 10.1007/978-3-319-40320-5_15

Systemic amyloidoses are caused by conformational changes and aggregation of autologous proteins that deposit in tissues in the form of highly ordered fibrils [1]. This process causes structural and functional damage of the organs involved, and eventually leads to death, if left untreated. In recent years, our understanding of the pathogenesis of systemic amyloidoses and our ability to treat these diseases have much improved. The most common forms of systemic amyloidoses, reported in Table 1, are now treatable. Patients' survival can considerably improve, and quality of life can be restored, provided the disease is diagnosed at early stages and appropriately managed [2–4]. Thus, it is vital that physicians are aware of these diseases and are able to recognize their early clinical manifestations timely, when organ damage is still amenable to improve. To date, at least 31 different proteins have been identified as causative agents of amyloid diseases, ranging from localized cerebral amyloidosis in Alzheimer's diseases, to systemic amyloidoses such as immunoglobulin monoclonal light chain amyloidosis (AL) and transthyretin (ATTR) amyloidosis [5]. With an overall incidence of 8.9 new cases per million person/year, immunoglobulin light chain (AL) amyloidosis is the most common form of systemic amyloidosis in Western countries [6, 7]. This disease is usually acquired, although a familial form, linked to the Ser131Cys mutation in the kappa light chain constant region has been recently reported [8]. In this disease entity, a plasma cell clone is responsible for the production of monoclonal immunoglobulin light chains, which undergo aggregation and form amyloid deposits either systemically or, rarely, locally [9]. The latter condition is defined as localized AL amyloidosis and accounts for 5–8 % of all AL cases [10]. The common examples of localized amyloidosis are tracheobronchial, urinary tract, cutaneous, lymph node, and nodular cutaneous involvement [11]. Approximately 5–8 % of cases of amyloidosis are localized AL amyloidosis.

Table 1 Most common types of systemic amyloidosis (for the updated, complete list of amyloid proteins, see Ref. [5])

Type	Abbreviation	Precursor protein	Organs involved
Immunoglobulin light chain amyloidosis	AL	Monoclonal light chain	Heart, kidneys, liver, GI tract, peripheral nerves, autonomic nerves, soft tissues
Transthyretin amyloidosis, hereditary Wild-type transthyretin (senile) amyloidosis, acquired	ATTRm ATTRwt	Variant transthyretin, >100 mutations Wild-type transthyretin	Peripheral nerves, autonomic nerves, heart, eye, leptomeninges, infrequently kidneys Age-related, usually males (age > 65 years) primarily cardiac involvement
Reactive amyloidosis, acquired	AA	Serum amyloid A	Kidneys, GI tract, spleen, liver, autonomic nerves
Apolipoprotein A-1 amyloidosis, hereditary	AApoAI	Variant apolipoprotein AI	Heart, liver, kidneys, skin, larynx, testes

1 The Biology of the Disease

The plasma cell clone in systemic AL amyloidosis is generally indolent and of modest size (median of bone marrow plasma cells: 9 %) [12] and less than 1 % of AL patients without multiple myeloma at diagnosis eventually progress to multiple myeloma over time [13]. The degree of bone marrow infiltration and plasma cell clonality, with or without hypercalcemia, renal failure, anemia, and lytic bone lesions attributable to clonal expansion of plasma cells (CRAB criteria) [14–16], the percentage of circulating peripheral blood plasma cells [17], serum levels of amyloidogenic free light chains [18–20] and other markers of plasma cell burden [20] are of prognostic value [21].

Amyloidogenic plasma cells frequently display aneuploidy due to numerical chromosomal alterations [22]. Translocations affecting the 14q32 locus of immunoglobulin heavy chains are present in the majority of cases (>75 %) [23]. Particularly frequent are t(11;14)(q13;q32) [23] and t(4;14)(p16.3;q32) [24], present in 55 and 14 % of cases, respectively. In contrast, hyperdiploidy is relatively uncommon with respect to other plasma cell disorders and is observed in only 11 % of AL cases [25]. Recently, gain of 1q21, which is present in approximately 20 % of AL cases, has been identified as an independent adverse prognostic factor in AL amyloidosis patients treated with standard chemotherapy [26]. In patients treated with bortezomib-based regimens, t(4;14), t(14;16), del(17p), and gain of 1q21 conferred no adverse prognosis, while translocation t(11;14) was associated with adverse outcome. Cyclin D1 levels were found to be associated with preferential secretion of free light chains only [27]. A genome-wide association study has shown similarities in inherited susceptibility between AL amyloidosis and MM [28]. Whole exome sequencing showed that the mutational landscape of amyloidosis resembles myeloma with no disease defining mutations but a variety of mutations occurring in different pathways such as RAS and NF-kB [29].

The amyloidogenic potential of LCs and their organ targeting are determined by mutations and specific structural features [30–32]. Disease-associated VL gene segments also were found, IGVL6-57 (previously named 6a) and IGVL3-1 (formerly 3r) [33–35], and the frequency of their involvement in LC rearrangements was such to give reason for the λ predominance (75 %) phenomenon [34]. LCs with the V region derived from rearrangement of *IGVL6-57* gene segment were significantly more likely to be observed in patients with predominant or exclusive kidney involvement at diagnosis [33–35], while *IGVL1-44*, was found associated with a fivefold increase in the odds of dominant heart involvement [36]. Amyloid kappa LC had more GI tract and liver involvement [27], with the κI family targeting soft tissue and bone [37].

Recently, cases of heavy chain and of light + heavy chain amyloidosis or AHL amyloidosis—in which both the light and heavy chain of a monoclonal protein contribute to the formation of amyloid deposits have been reported [38–40]. To date, there is no evidence for clear difference in prognosis or presentation between AL and AH amyloidosis.

The mechanisms of tissue damage and organ dysfunction caused by the process of amyloid formation and deposition are under intense investigation. The available evidence indicates that organ dysfunction and damage may result from the combined effects of the alteration of the macroscopic and microscopic tissue architecture caused by the amyloid deposits and the intrinsic toxicity of soluble amyloidogenic precursors [41–54]. Key players in this process appear to be the immunoglobulin light chain fibril precursors. Exposure to physiologic levels of light chains purified from patients with severe amyloid cardiomyopathy, in the absence of amyloid fibrils, can cause rapid, within minutes, diastolic dysfunction in isolated mouse hearts [43]. Furthermore, the injection of amyloidogenic light chains, obtained from patients with severe amyloid heart involvement, resulted in cardiac dysfunction, cell death, and early mortality in zebrafish [42]. More recently, it has been reported that the exposure of *C. elegans* to cardiotoxic LC produced immediate inhibition of the pumping of the pharynx, which is evolutionary related to the vertebrate heart [55]. The cardiotoxic LC leads to oxidative stress and impairs cell function [45], eventually resulting in apoptosis through the noncanonical activation of the p38α MAPK pathway [41, 42]. Interestingly, the MAPK pathway is involved in the regulation of B-type natriuretic peptide transcription. Complementary evidence that prefibrillar species are involved in the toxicity in AL amyloidosis comes from substantiated clinical findings. Hematologic response to chemotherapy was shown to translate into significant improvement of organ function well before the resolution of amyloid deposits [56, 57]. These earlier observations have been subsequently supported by the discovery that chemotherapy-induced reduction of immunoglobulin free light chains, parallel the decrease of biochemical markers of cardiac dysfunction, despite unchanged myocardial amyloid deposits at echocardiography [52].

2   Clinical Manifestations

Fatigue, which may be severe, is present in two-thirds of AL patients at presentation and is usually associated with anorexia and dysgeusia resulting in unintentional weight loss in more than 50 % of cases. Malnutrition, assessed by BMI and serum transthyretin concentration, at diagnosis is a frequent comorbidity in AL amyloidosis (20 %) that affects the prognosis [58, 59].

Systemic AL amyloidosis is a truly protean condition [60], amyloid LC can target virtually every organ, with the exception of the brain, producing heterogeneous clinical manifestations. A few manifestations, including indented macroglossia, periorbital purpura and the shoulder pad sign, can be regarded as almost pathognomonic (with few exceptions [61]) for systemic AL amyloidosis (Fig. 1). They should raise the clinical suspicion of systemic amyloidosis and quickly direct the physician toward a correct diagnosis. However, these manifestations are rather uncommon, being present in no more than 15–20 % of cases, and usually are associated with very advanced disease. Involvement of soft tissues can also manifest as carpal tunnel syndrome due to amyloid deposition within the carpal

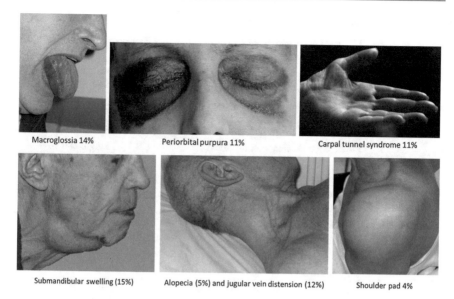

Macroglossia 14%   Periorbital purpura 11%   Carpal tunnel syndrome 11%

Submandibular swelling (15%)   Alopecia (5%) and jugular vein distension (12%)   Shoulder pad 4%

Fig. 1 Prototypic clinical manifestations in AL amyloidosis. They are not frequent, and usually they express an advanced disease

canal [62]. This condition is often bilateral and can precede the clinical onset of other organ involvement by many years. In the clinical series of patients with systemic AL amyloidosis followed at our Center (Table 2), the most frequently affected organs are kidneys and heart [4]. Renal involvement [63–66] results almost invariably in proteinuria, which can be prominent and can lead to severe hypoalbuminemia and important peripheral edema and ascites. More than 40 % of AL patients present with nephrotic syndrome at diagnosis and approximately 20 % eventually develop terminal kidney failure and require dialysis. Progression of renal damage depends on residual organ function as well as on the severity of proteinuria [67, 68]. This can, however, be prevented by effective therapy [68], which underlines the paramount importance of an early diagnosis and timely treatment initiation.

Heart involvement is the leading cause of death in AL: most of the patients die due to congestive heart failure and 25 % die from sudden cardiac death due to fatal arrhythmias or electromechanical dissociation. Complex ventricular arrhythmias on 24-h ECG Holter monitoring correlate with sudden death and are an independent prognostic factor [69]. Conduction disturbances are also frequently observed and negatively influence prognosis [70, 71]. The echocardiographic appearances seen in the advanced stages of cardiac amyloidosis are fairly pathognomonic as there are few, if any, similar-appearing adult cardiac diseases. The classic findings are increased wall thickness, low ventricular volume, and occasional dynamic left ventricular outflow obstruction that might be confused with hypertrophic cardiomyopathy [72]. Global mean values of peak systolic tissue velocity, systolic

Table 2 Clinical presentation of AL amyloidosis

Organ or syndrome	Overt clinical presentation	Biomarkers
General symptoms 80 %	Unexplained, severe, fatigue	BMI, serum transthyretin concentration
	Weight loss	
Heart 74 %	Heart failure	NT-proBNP > 332 ng/L (100 % sensitivity)
	Arrhythmias	
	Restrictive cardiac wall thickening	BNP > 73 ng/L (89 % sensitivity)
	Low electrocardiographic voltage	hsTnT
	Late gadolinium enhancement and characteristic T1 mapping at MRI	
Kidney 65 %	Nephrotic syndrome	Proteinuria > 0.5 g/d (predominantly albumin)
	Peripheral edema	
	Ascites	
	Renal failure	
Liver 20 %	Hepatomegaly without scan defects	Elevation of ALP in the absence of other causes
PNS/ANS 15/14 %	Symmetric ascending axonal peripheral neuropathy	
	Postural hypotension	
	Bladder and bowel dysfunction	
	Erectile dysfunction	
Soft tissues 17 %	Carpal tunnel syndrome	
	Purpura (periorbital)	
	Macroglossia	
	Claudication of the jaw	
	Muscular pseudohypertrophy	
	Articular deposits	

ALP alkaline phosphatase; *ANS* autonomous nervous system; and *PNS* peripheral nervous system
*Data from 1339 patients diagnosed at the Pavia Amyloidosis Research and Treatment Center
Adapted from Merlini and Palladini: Differential diagnosis of monoclonal gammopathy of undetermined significance. Hematology Am Soc Hematol Educ Program 2012 with permission from the American Society of Hematology (License Number: 3466630213342)

strain rate, and systolic strain are substantially lower in patients with cardiac amyloidosis than in those with amyloidosis and normal wall thickness or in healthy individuals. Longitudinal systolic strain echocardiography is the most accurate technique for detection of systolic dysfunction in amyloidosis. Doppler myocardial imaging can be used to detect impaired left ventricular systolic function even when no evidence of cardiac involvement exists on standard 2D and Doppler echocardiography [73]. Strain rate imaging allows for precise characterization of the mechanics of myocardial contraction and relaxation, which increases the sensitivity of this technique [74]. ECG findings in cardiac amyloidosis may include a low QRS voltage pattern (QRS amplitude, <1 mV in all the precordial leads or <0.05 mV in all the standard limb leads; 56 %), pseudoinfarction patterns (60 %), supraventricular arrhythmias (mainly atrial fibrillation) [75], atrioventricular or intra- and interventricular conduction defects, and unusual axis deviations. The presence of a low-voltage ECG, despite increased left ventricular (LV) wall thickening on echocardiography, is highly suggestive of cardiac AL amyloidosis, and a typical voltage:mass ratio has been described [76]. Although the precise reasons for the low-voltage ECG are not known, myocyte death and cardiac toxicity exerted by circulating light chains are possible contributing factors [76].

Cardiac MRI (CMR) shows increased myocardial mass, atrial structure, as well as atrial and ventricular function and other typical morphological features of restrictive cardiomyopathy. Additional findings of amyloidosis on CMR rely on tissue characterization: late gadolinium enhancement (LGE) [77], abnormally prolonged T1 times (before or after contrast), and an expansion of the extracellular volume [78, 79].

Direct imaging of amyloid fibrils, using positron emission tomographic tracers of C-11 Pittsburgh B compound [80] and F-18 florbetapir [81] seem promising and is currently under investigation. These direct amyloid imaging agents offer the potential quantitation of amyloid burden and identification of early cardiac involvement before overt cardiac structural changes [82].

Approximately 20 % of AL patients present with liver involvement, resulting in hepatomegaly and/or elevated serum alkaline phosphatase levels [4, 83]. Hyperbilirubinemia is infrequent and, when present, often indicates a poor prognosis [69–71]. Rarely, hepatic amyloidosis can lead to spontaneous liver rupture, which is usually fatal although successful combined liver–kidney transplant has been reported [84]. The spleen is generally affected by amyloid deposition, in some cases to a large extent, but splenic involvement is rarely of clinical relevance with hyposplenism [85] rarely resulting into splenic rupture [86].

Peripheral/autonomous nervous system is involved in about 14 % of patients [4] in the form of a predominantly fiber length sensitive, axonal, symmetrical, and progressive neuropathy [87]. When peripheral neuropathy is the dominant syndrome, a differential diagnosis between AL and hereditary (particularly TTR) amyloidosis is mandatory. The presence of amyloid autonomic neuropathy manifests as postural hypotension, erectile dysfunction, and gastrointestinal symptoms (constipation, diarrhea, or an alternation thereof). The latter symptoms can also be the consequence of amyloid deposition within the gastrointestinal tract, which is clinically evident in 8 % of cases in the Pavia series. Amyloid deposition, can occur also in cutis, muscle, respiratory tract, genitourinary system, and lymph nodes.

Consensus criteria for the definition of organ involvement have been recently updated [68, 88–90].

3   Diagnosis

The protean clinical features of AL amyloidosis can mimic common diseases of the elderly making the clinical suspicion difficult and translating into missed or very late diagnosis. Clinical alertness is critical. Combinations such as nephrotic syndrome and heart failure, simultaneous peripheral and autonomic neuropathy in nondiabetic patients, "left ventricular hypertrophy" on echocardiography without consistent electrocardiographic evidence or low limb lead voltages, hepatomegaly with normal imaging or albuminuria in patients with monoclonal gammopathy of undetermined significance (MGUS) or myeloma, should raise suspicion of amyloidosis [3]. However, clinical manifestations of AL amyloidosis reflect advanced organ damage, and it is vital to anticipate irreversible organ dysfunction. Early diagnosis requires switching from traditional symptoms- and signs-bound diagnostics to sensitive biomarkers signaling presymptomatic organ damage. The progressive, clinically silent, involvement of heart and kidneys can be detected early by simple, widely available, biomarkers. The amino-terminal pro-natriuretic peptide type B (NT-proBNP) is the most sensitive, although not specific, marker for amyloid cardiomyopathy. Concentration >332 ng/L can signal amyloid heart involvement months, if not years, before it becomes clinically overt. Similarly, urinary albumin >0.5/day is also a very early and sensitive markers of kidney involvement. At the Pavia Amyloidosis Center, virtually all (97 %) of patients with AL amyloidosis have either NT-proBNP >332 ng/L and/or albuminuria >0.5 g/day at presentation.

AL amyloidosis should be included in the differential diagnosis of: nondiabetic nephrotic syndrome, nonischemic cardiomyopathy with hypertrophic pattern on echocardiography; increased NT-proBNP in the absence of primary heart disease; hepatomegaly and/or increased alkaline phosphatase levels with no imaging abnormalities of the liver; peripheral and/or autonomic neuropathy; unexplained facial or neck purpura or macroglossia; association of monoclonal component with unexplained fatigue, weight loss, edema, or paresthesia.

Diagnosis is based on the histological demonstration of amyloid deposits and determination of the amyloid type. Subcutaneous abdominal fat aspiration is the simplest and least invasive diagnostic procedure. Its sensitivity is approximately 70–80 % in AL [91, 92]. Biopsy of the bone marrow combined with abdominal subcutaneous fat aspiration identifies amyloid deposits in 85 % of patients with amyloidosis. Labial salivary gland biopsy is also simple and yields a high diagnostic sensitivity. Amyloid deposits are found in the labial salivary glands of almost 60 % of patients with systemic amyloidosis and negative abdominal fat aspirate, and the sequential biopsy of these two sites has a negative predictive value of 91 %, thus limiting the need for an organ biopsy to less than 10 % of patients [93]. Gastroduodenal biopsy can be informative [94]. The biopsy of the involved organs can be performed if amyloidosis is still suspected but biopsies of alternative sites are negative. In the absence of a hematostatic disorder and/or uncontrolled hypertension, bleeding risk during kidney biopsy is not increased in patients with systemic amyloidosis and kidney biopsy can be performed safely [95]. Endomyocardial biopsy, although invasive and expensive, is usually safe and highly informative [96, 97]. Liver biopsy was reported to be associated with 4 % bleeding [98] that may be fatal. Transjugular liver biopsy is recommended in the rare event that liver biopsy is the only way to document amyloid deposits.

Confirmation of amyloid type is critical, since a dozen of proteins can cause systemic amyloidosis [5], each requiring distinct therapy. Incorrect amyloid typing results in catastrophic therapeutic consequences, such as exposing to useless and toxic chemotherapy subjects with hereditary or ATTRwt amyloidosis. Given the substantial overlap in disease manifestations of the most common types of systemic amyloidosis, clinical evaluation is of little help in differential diagnosis. Even in patients with MGUS, cardiomyopathy caused by V122I mutant transthyretin (carrier rate 4 % in Afro-Caribbeans) or by wild-type transthyretin in elderly men should be carefully considered in differential diagnosis. It must be kept in mind that identifying amyloid deposits in a patient with a monoclonal component is not conclusive evidence of AL amyloidosis, due to the high prevalence of monoclonal gammopathies particularly in the elderly. Also, the absence of a family history does not exclude the hereditary amyloidoses, due to the variable penetrance of these diseases. Tissue deposits should be typed preferentially using mass spectrometry (a current standard) [99–101], if not available, immunoelectron microscopy [92, 102], or immunohistochemistry performed in specialized laboratories [103] can be used. Gene sequencing is needed when familial amyloidosis is possible: such as those with isolated neuropathic or cardiac disease (transthyretin amyloidosis), isolated renal involvement (fibrinogen amyloidosis), corneal lattice dystrophy, progressive bilateral facial paralysis and cutis laxa (gelsolin amyloidosis), dry mouth/gastrointestinal/kidney/liver involvement (lysozyme amyloidosis), and renal/liver/cardiac involvement in relatively asymptomatic patients (apolipoprotein-A1 amyloidosis) [3].

The identification of the amyloidogenic clone requires serum and urine immunofixation combined with FLC quantification and bone marrow analysis [104, 105]. Half of all amyloidogenic PC clones produce LC only, with typically modest bone marrow infiltrate (median 5–10 %). Lambda clones dominate kappa ones by 4:1, unlike the 2:3 ratio in myeloma. Fluorescence in situ hybridization of bone marrow PC and investigations to rule out symptomatic myeloma, including skeletal survey, should be done at baseline. Immunophenotyping by multiparameter flow cytometry may be useful to detect the clone and in assessing the prognosis [15].

4 Assessing the Risk and Response to Therapy

Patients with AL amyloidosis are fragile due to amyloid multi-organ involvement. Assessing the severity of organ damage is essential for prognostication and for designing the treatment with the best risk/benefit ratio (Table 3). Simple parameters like poor performance status, New York Heart Association class ≥ 3 and low

Table 3 Response criteria in AL amyloidosis

Response	Definition
Hematologic response	
Complete response	Negative serum and urine immunofixation and normal FLC ratio
Very good partial response	FLC < 40 mg/L
Partial response	FLC decrease >50 % compared to baseline
No response	All other patients
Cardiac response	Decrease of NT-proBNP by >30 % and 300 ng/L (if baseline NT-proBNP > 650 ng/L), or at least a 2 point decrease of NYHA class (if baseline NYHA class is III or IV)
Renal response	At least 30 % decrease in proteinuria or drop below 0.5 g/24 h, in the absence of renal progression defined as a >25 % decrease in eGFR
Hepatic response	50 % decrease in abnormal alkaline phosphatase value or decrease in liver size radiographically at least 2 cm

eGFR estimated glomerular filtration rate; *dFLC* difference between involved (amyloidogenic) and uninvolved circulating free light chain; *FLC* circulating free light chain; *NT-proBNP* N-terminal pro-natriuretic peptide type B; *NYHA* New York Heart Association

Very good partial and partial hematologic response are valuable in patients with baseline dFLC > 50 mg/L. All patients are evaluable for complete remission if they have abnormal FLC ratio and /or positive immunofixation of serum and/or urine at baseline. Subjects with an intact monoclonal (M) protein > 10 g/L but with dFLC < 50 mg/L at baseline achieve a partial response if the M protein decreases by at least 50 %

systolic blood pressure (<100 mmHg) are useful bedside indicators of poor outcome [106].

The presence and severity of cardiac involvement determine the survival [2]. The severity of amyloid heart involvement can be quantified through the biomarkers of cardiac dysfunction, N-terminal natriuretic peptide type B (NT-proBNP), and cardiac damage, troponins (cTn) [53, 78–80]. The Mayo staging system using NT-proBNP (>332 ng/L) and cardiac troponin T/troponin I (cTnT, >0.035 ng/mL; cTnI, >0.1 ng/mL) [107], is the most robust method for risk stratification. Renal function (especially when eGFR <30 ml/min) affects cardiac biomarkers concentration and the Mayo staging is not directly applicable for patients in renal failure. BNP is more useful than NT-proBNP in these patients [108]. High sensitivity troponin may be sued as a single marker, in lieu of troponin and NT-proBNP in the future, but validation studies are needed [109]. Serum FLC are prognostic [18, 27] and have been incorporated in the Mayo cardiac staging system [20]. A European study has shown that patients with stage III and very high concentration of NT-proBNP (>8500 ng/L) and systolic blood pressure <100 mmHg have a very short survival, with a median of few weeks, and they tolerate poorly chemotherapy with no time to benefit from it [110]. There is no treatment that at present can help these patients, except cardiac transplantation in selected cases. Troponin is also at the base of risk assessment for eligibility to stem cell transplantation [111, 112]. Recently, it has been reported that bone marrow plasma cells > 10 % confers a poor prognosis independently from cardiac biomarkers and FLC [16]. This marker can be used to select patients who need induction therapy prior to stem cell transplantation. Other characteristic of the clone determined by FISH analysis [113] can be useful for selecting therapy. Recently, gain of 1q21, which is present in approximately 20 % of AL cases, has been identified as an independent adverse prognostic factor in AL amyloidosis patients treated with standard chemotherapy [26]. In patients treated with bortezomib-based regimens, t(4;14), t(14;16), del(17p), and gain of 1q21 conferred no adverse prognosis, while translocation t(11;14) was associated with adverse outcome [114]. These findings highlight that the prognostic impact of cytogenetic markers largely depends on the administered therapy and should therefore be judged only in the context of a specific therapy [28].

Criteria for hematologic, cardiac, and renal responses have been established and validated throughout international collaboration [66, 115] (Table 3). The criteria for liver response have not been validated and they have been defined through consensus [116]. There is general agreement among the experts that therapy should aim at obtaining at least a hematology very good partial response [117].

5   Treatment

Therapeutic strategies for AL have mostly been based on customization of treatments used for patients with multiple myeloma. The paucity of prospective trials, especially phase III trials, is a major limitation. Aside from providing the best supportive care possible, the treatment goals are to achieve: (1) at least a hematologic very good partial response, which is defined as a dFLC <40 mg/L; and (2) a cardiac response, which is defined as a 30 % reduction in NT-proBNP from a starting level of 650 pg/mL or higher [52, 115]. In general, the deeper the hematologic response, the higher is the likelihood of achieving an organ response and better overall survival though there may be exceptions for those patients with less amyloidogenic/ toxic light chains [37, 118–123]. The pursuit of VGPR/CR must be balanced by the morbidity and mortality of any given regimen given the frail state of many of these patients [115, 124]. Organ responses can occur with a hematologic partial response in as many as 30–56 % of patients. When interpreting therapeutic trials for patients with AL, a challenge with organ response as a measure in many studies is that organ response is time dependent, i.e., it can be much delayed [124]. Reports with less than 24 months follow-up often have lower organ response rates due to inadequate follow-up.

At present, the mainstay of treatment is the destruction of the underlying plasma cell clone, which in turn reduces or eliminates the amyloidogenic clonal immunoglobulin light chain. It had been assumed that the amyloid fibrils detected in tissue biopsies were the source of tissue injury and dysfunction and that chemotherapy produced improvement in organ function by shifting the equilibrium from fibril formation to fibril dissolution. That hypothesis has been challenged with the hypothesis that the clonal amyloidogenic light chains form toxic soluble intermediates responsible for the tissue damage [125, 126]. In every day clinical practice, this pathophysiologic debate is less relevant since there are currently no approved drugs that directly attack and/or dissolve the amyloid. The approach of using molecules and/or antibodies directed against serum amyloid protein or antibodies directed at the tertiary structure of the amyloid may be treatments of the future [127–129].

Whether long-term outcomes will differ depending on the means of arriving at a complete hematologic response is unknown [130]. This is most notable in the context of high-dose chemotherapy with autologous stem cell transplant versus standard dose melphalan and dexamethasone. For patients achieving hematologic CR, the 5-year OS is about 70 % regardless of the treatment modality used to achieve this depth of response [131–133]. For patients undergoing ASCT and achieving CR, 10-year survival rates approach 60 % [132]. In a retrospective analysis studying patients who achieved CR, there was a trend toward better OS among patients treated with ASCT as their primary treatment [124], but this finding is confounded by the fact that patients undergoing ASCT are highly selected and fit at baseline.

5.1   Indications for Therapy

Treatment should be initiated immediately in virtually all patients with systemic AL. The rare exception is that of a patient who has blood and bone marrow consistent with monoclonal gammopathy of undetermined significance or asymptomatic myeloma and an incidental finding of a positive Congo Red of the bone marrow. As long as there is no evidence of amyloid affecting major organs, this rare type of patient may not require immediate chemotherapy, but they should be fully staged and followed no less frequently than every 3 months with amyloid directed review of systems, serum immunoglobulin free light chains, alkaline phosphatase, troponin, NT-proBNP, and creatinine as well as spot urine for albumin.

5.2   Initial Therapy for Patients with Systemic AL

Clinical trials should always be considered in the frontline setting if available. In routine practice, the first question asked is whether a patient is a candidate for high-dose chemotherapy with autologous peripheral blood stem cell support (ASCT), not specifically because it is the best therapy, but because it is the therapy that is most restrictive and that requires the most planning (Fig. 2). Our opinion is that among those young patients with low risk disease, ASCT is an excellent option with potential for long event-free survivals. There are, however, no randomized trial data to support that it is superior therapy; on the contrary, if the one small phase 3 French study addressing this question was accepted without critical analysis, one would conclude that ASCT is inferior to Mel-Dex [130].

Initial Therapy for Patients Not Undergoing Stem Cell Transplantation

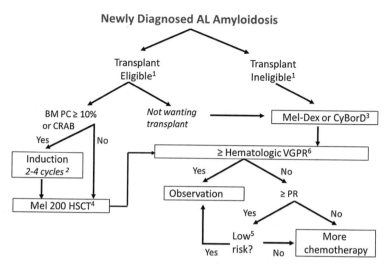

Fig. 2 Nonstudy treatment algorithm for patients with newly diagnosed AL amyloidosis. Note: many of the recommendations in this algorithm have not yet been supported by clinical trials; level of evidence is clearly indicated in text. Taken with permission from Dispenzieri et al., Mayo Clinic Proceedings [134]. *dFLC* difference between involved and uninvolved serum free light chain levels. [1]To be transplant eligible, the following criteria should be met: "physiologic" age ≤ 70 years; performance Score ≤ 2; troponin T < 0.06 ng/ml, systolic BP > −90 mm Hg; creatinine clearance ≥ 30 ml/min (unless on chronic dialysis), NYHA Class I/II, no more than two major organs significantly involved (liver, heart, kidney, or autonomic nerve). [2]Induction also used if delay in proceeding to ASCT or as clinically indicated. [3]If hematologic parameter not decreased by >50 % at 2 months, consider changing therapy. [4]For Age > 70 or CrCl < 30, use melphalan 140 mg/m². [5]Mayo 2012 stage I or II. [6]Day 100 ASCT or after 4–6 cycles of chemotherapy

5.2.1   Alkylator-Based Therapy

Table 4 demonstrates expected outcomes with standard chemotherapy. Melphalan and prednisone doubled the OS as compared to colchicine in two subsequent randomized trials, making it the standard therapy for most patients with AL until the mid-2000s [135, 136]. Although only 18 % of patients responded to melphalan and prednisone, organ responders enjoyed a median survival of 89 months, whereas nonresponders had a median survival of 15 months [137]. Multiagent alkylator-based therapy (VBMCP) did not improve OS [138], but replacing prednisone with dexamethasone improved response rates and better OS [139] (Table 5).

In 2004, Palladini et al. reported their experience with melphalan and dexamethasone among patients who were not transplant candidates. Hematologic response rates of 67 %—including 33 % complete responses–and organ response rates of 48 % were reported [139]. These patients had a median OS of 5.1 years and progression-free survival of 3.8 years [133]. As will be described in section on ASCT, the value of melphalan and dexamethasone was further validated in a prospective study of 100 patients randomized ASCT with high-dose melphalan compared to oral melphalan and dexamethasone [130]. In this highly

Table 4 Standard Chemotherapy for AL

	N	No Prior Rx (%)	≥2 organs (%)	OHR/CR (%)	Organ response (%)	Median f/u (mo)	Median Survival (m)
MP [135, 136, 138, 140, 141]	∼200[a]	Majority	NA	28	20–30	NA	18–29
VBMCP [138]	49	100	NR	29 /NR	30	35	29
Melphalan IV [142]	20[b]			50	...		∼50
Dex [143]	19	26	NR	53 /31	16	27	11
Dex [144]	25	100	NR	40/12	12	18	13.8
Dex [145]	23	43	52	NR	35	33	24
Dex-IFN [146]	93	84	71	31/14	35	41	31
VAD [142, 147–151]	32[b]	NR	NR	42–50	...	NR	...
Mel-Dex [133, 139]	46	100	76	67/33	48	60	61
Mel-Dex [130]	50	100	68	72/24	39	36	60
Mel-Dex 20 [152]	140[b]	100	NR	51/12	>20	60	20
Mel-Dex [153]	40[b]	100	80	58/13	NR	NR	10.5
Mel-IV-Dex [154]	61[b]	100	92	44/11	25	27	17.5
Mel-Dex [155]	70[b]	0	>50	26/8	NR	17	66 % at 2 year

Taken with permission from Dispenzieri et al., Mayo Clinic Proceedings [134]
[a]Conglomeration of multiple trials
[b]Case series/reports

selected population, on an intention-to-treat basis, the median survival for melphalan and dexamethasone treated patients was 57 months.

In contrast, two other phase 2 studies examining melphalan and dexamethasone had markedly inferior results with 3-month mortality rates of 23 and 28 % and median overall survivals of 10.5 and 17.5 months [153, 154]. These two series included patients with severely impaired cardiac function as assessed by soluble cardiac biomarkers demonstrating the relationship between patient selection and outcome [172].

The historical concern for myelodysplastic syndrome among AL patients receiving oral alkylator has been attenuated by more recent data demonstrating rates of myelodysplasia of 2.4 % [133, 139] rather than the historical rates of 7 % of the total patient population and a 42-month actuarial risk of myelodysplasia or acute leukemia of 21 % [173]. This lower rate is attributed to the modest total dose of melphalan administered (median, 288 mg; range, 48–912 mg), even considering the additional cycles delivered in relapsing patients [133, 139].

Table 5 Immune modulatory derivatives in patients with AL

Regimen	N	No prior Rx (%)	≥2 organs (%)	OHR/CR (%)	Organ response (%)	Median f/u (mo)	OS
Thal 200–800 mg [156]	16	6	31	25/0	0	NR	NR
Thal/Dex [157]	31	0	61	48/0	26	32	NR
Thal 200–800 [158]	12	58	67	0	11	2[a]	NR
Thal 50–200 [159]	18	28	50	0	11	6[a]	NR
CTX/Thal/Dex [160]	65[c]	41	≥50	74/21	33	18	2-year 77 %
Mel-Dex-thal [161]	22	86	NR	36/5	18	28	1-year 20 %
Len ± Dex [162]	22	43	57	43/5	26	17	2-year 50 %
Len ± Dex [163]	69	6	52	47[c]/16	21	NR	NR[b]
Len ± Dex [164]	24	0	NR	38/0	4	23	1-year 50 %
Len-Mel-Dex [165]	26	100	62	58/23	50	19	2-year 81 %
Len-Mel-Dex [166]	25	92	≥50	58/8	8	17	1-year 58 %
Len-Mel-Dex [167]	16	69	≥50	43/7	1	34	3-year 70 % PFS 24 mo
Len-Cycl-Dex [168]	21	0	86	62/5	15	38	3-year 50 % PFS 13 mo
Len-Cycl-Dex [169]	35	69	54	60/11	29	32	38 mo PFS 28 mo
Len-Cycl-Dex [170]	37	65	54	55/8	22	29	3-year ∼33 % 17 mo
Pom-Dex [171]	33	0	<2	48/3	15	28	28 mo PFS 14 mo

Taken with permission from Dispenzieri et al., Mayo Clinic Proceedings [134]

Rx treatment; *AE* adverse events; *Cardiac* cardiac involvement; *Dex* dexamethasone; *f/u* follow-up; *mo* months; *IFN* interferon; *Thal* thalidomide; *Len* lenalidomide

[a]Median time on treatment

[b]Case series, not a clinical trial

[c]Partial response rate based on first 34 patients treated. No information on the additional 35

5.2.2 Immune Modulator Drug Therapy

Thalidomide, as a single agent, has a heightened toxicity in patients with amyloidosis and no hematologic or organ responses has been reported [156, 159]. In contrast, in combination with dexamethasone, 48 % of 31 patients achieved hematologic response, with eight (26 %) organ responses. Median time to response was 3.6 months (range, 2.5–8.0 months). Treatment-related toxicity was frequent (65 %), and symptomatic bradycardia was common (26 %) [157]. All of these patients were previously treated.

In contrast, the UK group reported on prospective, observational studies of the combination of thalidomide with cyclophosphamide and dexamethasone [160]. A hematological response occurred in 74 % of 65 evaluable patients including complete hematological responses in 21 %. With a median follow-up of 22 months, median-estimated OS from commencement of treatment was 41 months. Toxicity was not adequately assessed because this was not a clinical trial, and further study of this combination has shown it to be less well tolerated than previously thought [174]. Palladini et al. treated 22 newly diagnosed patients with cardiac involvement with the combination of melphalan, thalidomide, and dexamethasone [161]. Despite a hematologic response rate of 36 %, only 20 % of patients were alive for 1 year and toxicity was significant.

Most of the lenalidomide data comes from trials that combine both previously untreated and previously treated patients with AL [115, 131, 132]. This makes interpretation of data in the newly diagnosed population difficult, especially because newly diagnosed patients with AL paradoxically have inferior survival than do previously treated AL patients due to the initial 30–40 % death rate that occurs within the first 3–6 months of diagnosis [115, 175]. With lenalidomide and dexamethasone, overall hematologic response occurred in 38–47 % of patients, with CR in 5–16 % and a median OS ranging from 1 to 2 years. These and other trials have demonstrated that the starting dose of lenalidomide should be no higher than 15 mg per day given on a 1–21 every 28-day schedule. As lenalidomide has been used to treat AL, serious cardiac and renal toxicity have been reported, making it imperative to consider drug toxicity rather than "disease progression" if patients on lenalidomide deteriorate [115, 174, 176–178]. With the use of IMiDs in patients with AL, NT-proBNP and troponin not infrequently rise. Whether this rise is true cardiac toxicity or an epiphenomenon is unclear, but reversible clinical deterioration has been shown in patients treated with lenalidomide [176].

The most promising of the lenalidomide, alkylator, dexamethasone combinations was that of melphalan, lenalidomide, and dexamethasone which was employed in 26 newly diagnosed patients with AL [165]. The population was highly selected since enrollment required an ECOG performance status of 0 or 1. Fifty-eight percent of patients achieved a PR including 23 % who achieved a CR. In contrast, when Dinner et al. used this regimen in a less highly selected patient population, both CR and OS were substantially lower [166]. The Boston group tested this same regimen in patients with newly diagnosed and previously treated AL, and also found lower CR rates, but fairly comparable OS [167].

Results with cyclophosphamide, lenalidomide, and dexamethasone do not appear as favorable, but selection criteria for these studies were less restrictive [115, 168]. Applying these study results to the newly diagnosed population is also challenging since two of the studies included both newly diagnosed and previously treated patients, and the third included only previously treated patients. In these studies, hematologic response rates were around 60 % with CR rates of only 5–11 %. Median OS for both newly diagnosed and previously treated was 17–38 months [115, 168].

The newest immune modulator drug (IMiD), pomalidomide has been combined with dexamethasone, and produced a hematologic response rate of 41 %, including a 43 % hematologic response rate in IMiD refractory patients [115]. All patients had received prior therapy, so the regimen has not been tested in the first line setting. The 1-year overall and progression-free survival were 77 and 59 %, respectively.

5.2.3   Proteasome Inhibitor Therapy

Bortezomib appears to be a highly active treatment in patients with AL, but to date there are very limited safety (or efficacy) data generated from prospective clinical trials. There is a paucity of high-quality data, but the enthusiasm for its use resulted in the publication of a number of case series included in Table 6.

The largest prospective clinical trial (CAN2007) evaluated single-agent bortezomib, but included only a highly selected patient population [181–183]. Patients were excluded if they had no prior therapy, advanced cardiac disease (NYHA III or IV) or baseline hypotension [181–183]. The CAN2007 trial evaluated two schedules of therapy, that is the standard twice weekly (days 1, 4, 8, 11, every 21 days) and a once weekly (days 1, 8, 15, and 22 every 35 days) schedule. The once weekly schedule was preferred in terms of toxicity and dose delivered. Hematologic response rates were comparable at 67 and 68 %, respectively. The CR rates favored the once weekly schedule over the twice weekly schedule 37 % versus 24 %. Median overall survival for the group was 63 months.

The only prospective randomized trial for newly diagnosed AL patients that incorporates bortezomib ± dexamethasone required that patients be transplant eligible, such that they could be randomized to either two cycles of bortezomib before proceeding to ASCT or to immediate ASCT (see discussion in ASCT section) [179]. In this highly selected population, the therapy was well tolerated.

The third prospective trial was a pilot for 10 patients with AL and an underlying lymphoproliferative disorder [181]. Most patients had prior therapy. The hematologic response rate was 78 %, but there were no CRs, and 90 % of patients were alive at 13 months.

The remainder of the data comes from small retrospective studies and includes patients treated either with single-agent bortezomib or in combination with dexamethasone as part of clinical practice. Once again, there is a mix of patients without clearly specified cardiac risk. The earliest case series included 94 patients, mostly relapsed or refractory; the overall hematologic response rate was 72 % including a CR rate of 25 % and organ response rate of 30 % [186]. A subsequent

Table 6 Proteasome inhibitors in patients with AL

Regimen	N	No prior Rx (%)	≥2 organs (%)	OHR/CR (%)	Organ response (%)	Median f/u (mo)	OS
Bor-Dex x 2 + ASCT [179] versus ASCT [179]	56	100	59	86/68 versus 48/36	>65 versus >25	28	2-year 95 % versus 2-year 69 %
Bor-Mel-Dex versus Mel-Dex [180]	35 35	100	NR	76/NR 58/NR	NR	14	1-year 86 %
Bor [181–183]	70	0	>44	63(33)[b]	24[c]	52	4-year 67 %
Bor-Ritux Dex [184]	10	60	40	78/0	0	13	1-year 90 %
Bor-Mel-Dex [185]	17	100	NR	94/56	NR	11	NR
Bor ± dex [186]	94[a]	19	NR	72/25	30	12	1-year 76 %
Bor + dex [187]	26[a]	69	65	54/31	12	15	Med 19 mo
Bor-Mel-Dex [188] versus Mel-Dex	87[a, d] 87[a, d]	100	≥ 50	69/42 51/19	NR	26	3-year 58 % 3-year 45 %
Bor-Ctx-Dex [189] versus Thal-Ctx-Dex	69[a, d] 69[a, d]	100	NR	71/40 80/25	NR	13 25	1-year 65 % 1-year 67 %
Bor-Ctx-Dex [190]	17[a]	58	82	94/71	NR	21	21-mo 71 %
Bor-Ctx-Dex [191]	20[a]	100	NR	90/65	46	14	2-year 98 %
Bor-Ctx-Dex [191]	23[a]	0		74/22			
Bor-Ctx-Dex [192]	60[a, e]	100	NR	68/17	32	12	1-year 57 %
Bor-Mel-Pred [193]	19[a]	100	90	84/37	47	8	2-year 39 %

Taken with permission from Dispenzieri et al., Mayo Clinic Proceedings [134]

Rx treatment; *AE* adverse events; *Cardiac* cardiac involvement; *Dex* dexamethasone; *f/u* follow-up; *mo* months

[a]Case series, not a clinical trial

[b]Excluding the Phase I patients

[c]The denominator ($n = 62$) for this calculation includes some of the 18 dose escalation pts since that group contained 5 of the 15 organ responses

[d]Matched case-control studies

[e]Retrospective look at patients with Stage III (Mayo 2004) disease

retrospective study, had a lower overall response rate, but a comparable CR rate; [187] the median survival, however was more modest at 19 months [187] rather than a 1-year OS of 76 % [186].

5.2.4 Bortezomib, Alkylator, and Corticosteroid Combinations

The fourth prospective clinical trial incorporating bortezomib included both newly diagnosed and relapsed patients. It has only been reported in abstract form and is therefore difficult to interpret [185]. The combination of melphalan, dexamethasone, and bortezomib has produced response rates of 94 %, but the follow-up is short, and toxicity data are lacking [185]. The remaining reports of combinations of alkylator and bortezomib are all case series [169, 191, 193] and two case-control series [183, 192]. Case series of cyclophosphamide, dexamethasone, and bortezomib have also been published with response rates of 93 % [169, 191], but safety data are again sparse.

A case-controlled study comparing the outcome of 87 patients treated with bortezomib plus MDex (BMDex) with that of 87 controls treated with MDex was performed, matching on presence of cardiac involvement and renal involvement, Mayo Clinic cardiac stage (2004), NT-proBNP above or below 8500 ng/L, systolic blood pressure above or below 100 mm Hg, treatment with full dose dexamethasone (40 mg days 1–4), eGFR above or below 30 ml/min per 1.72 m^2, and dFLC above or below 180 mg/L [183]. This study revealed a higher rate of complete responses with the BMDex (42 % vs. 19 %), but no significant survival advantage for the group as a whole (58 % vs. 45 %, $p = 0.4$) or for the highest risk patients [183]. With a median follow-up of 26 months, separation of the survival curves did not occur in patient groups with NT-proBNP >8500 pg/L and/or NYHA class >II. The only subgroup receiving bortezomib that fared significantly better than its case-matched cohort was the lowest risk patients, but this observation may be confounded by the fact that the BMDex patients were from a later period–after 2009 (78 % vs. 32 %)—a time when more treatment options were available and possibly lead time bias related to earlier recognition in a later cohort. Moreover, in toto, only 18 of the MDex patients received bortezomib as second line therapy. The authors concluded that intermediate-risk patients who are not fit enough to receive high-dose dexamethasone are likely to obtain the greatest advantage from the addition of bortezomib to MDex.

The other matched case-control study was performed by Venner et al. These authors compared 69 patients treated with cyclophosphamide, bortezomib, and dexamethasone (CVD) to 69 patients treated with cyclophosphamide, thalidomide, and dexamethasone (CTD) in the frontline setting [192]. Patients were matched based on Mayo cardiac stage (2004), and they aimed to have similar proportions of patients with high dFLC and ultrahigh NT-proBNP, i.e., 8500 ng/L. Their practice was to change regimens if a 90 % reduction in dFLC was not achieved after three cycles of therapy. A higher percentage of the CTD patients were switched to an alternate therapy (20 % vs. 1 %). All but one of the CTD patients received bortezomib containing regimen as second line. On an intention-to-treat basis, the overall response rates were 71 % versus 80 % in the CVD and CTD arms, respectively, (*P* = 0.32). A higher complete response (CR) rate was observed in the CVD arm (40.5 %) versus CTD (24.6 %), *P* = 0.046. Approximately 25 % of patients died within 3 months of starting therapy. One-year OS was 65 and 67 % for CVD and CTD, respectively, (*P* = 0.87) with median respective follow-up times of 13 and 25 months. There was no difference in overall survival by treatment even when patients were considered by whether or not they had very high NT-proBNP; however, the median PFS was 28.0 and 14.0 m for CVD and CTD, respectively, (*P* = 0.04).

In a recent analysis of patients with newly diagnosed Mayo 2004 Stage III patients, the 1- and 2-year overall survivals were estimated for patients treated with different regimens [194]. The anticipated 1- and 2-year OS rates with various regimens were as follows: CRd, approximately 40 and 20–24 %; CTD/ Mel-Dex, 46 and 29 %; MRD, 22 and 22 %; and VCD, 57 and 51 %. Caveats to this analysis are that the majority of these data were gleaned from small numbers of patients on observational studies treated over a long period of time rather than prospective clinical trials, making selection and reporting bias important confounders.

5.2.5   Non-ASCT Therapy for AL Patients with Underlying Lymphoproliferative Disease or IgM Monoclonal Gammopathy

IgM-associated AL amyloidosis is a rare clinical entity with distinctive clinical characteristics. Many cases may be "localized forms" in which there is only nodal involvement or soft tissue involvement without any visceral involvement. Many of these cases can merely be observed, but observed more aggressively if there is a circulating monoclonal protein and especially if there are circulating monotypic serum immunoglobulin free light chains. Chemotherapy is more often reserved for those cases in which there is typical amyloid deposition in viscera and/or nervous system. Historically, regimens have been borrowed from both the myeloma and the Waldenström macroglobulinemia armamentarium, but not tested systematically given the rarity of IgM-associated AL. These treatments have included single agent or combinations of cladrabine, fludarabine, rituximab, chorambucil, cyclophosphamide, vincristine, doxorubicin, oral melphalan, corticosteroids, and ASCT [181, 195–197].

In a retrospective series of 77 patients, there was a 32 % response rate with no CRs, and it appeared that the oral alkylators had the lowest response rates [197]. Overall survival was 49 months. In another series of 15 patients, the 3-year OS was 58 % [196]. Until the incorporation of bortezomib, complete hematologic responses had been rare, but patients have achieved organ responses and overall survivals comparable to patients with pure plasma cell disorders.

There are two reports of incorporating bortezomib into the treatment of these patients. The first is a pilot from Palladini et al. They treated 10 patients with IgM AL with rituximab, bortezomib, and dexamethasone [181]. Hematologic response was achieved in 78 % of patients, including three refractory to previous rituximab. Two patients had normalization of their kappa to lambda ratio, but none achieved a negative immunofixation. With a median follow-up of 13 months, one patient died.

The second report including bortezomib was that of eight Japanese patients who were treated with CyBorD [198]. Four patients had complete remissions (CR), two had very good partial responses, and two had partial responses. Five of six patients (83 %) had organ responses in the heart and/or kidney.

Bendamustine and ibrutinib may also be candidates for study in this patient population.

5.2.6   ASCT for AL Amyloidosis

The initial positive reports of ASCT came from Comenzo et al. [199]. The concept of selection bias was initially raised [172], but then settled with a case-control study [159] and favorable long-term outcomes [200, 201]. The most commonly used conditioning regimen is melphalan 200 mg/m^2 although doses of 100–140 mg/m^2 have been used in sicker patients. With upfront ASCT without any induction therapy, hematologic responses have been reported anywhere from 32 to 68 % and complete hematologic responses from 16 to 50 % [130, 131, 199, 201–204]. Organ response is time dependent, and a median time to response can take up to 1 year even among patients achieving hematologic CR [124]. Organ response rates range anywhere from 31 to 64 %. Patients with the deepest hematologic responses are more likely to have long-term survival [131, 201].

The French MDex versus ASCT phase 3 trial was a prospective randomized study of 100 patients randomized to ASCT with high-dose melphalan conditioning compared to oral MDex [130]. Dose modified melphalan was used based on the risk factors of the period [205], rather than the more reliable soluble biomarker methods of the present. In this selected population, there was no difference between the two arms for hematologic response, and the landmark analysis performed to correct for the unexpectedly high early mortality associated with ASCT also showed no difference in OS. On an intention-to-treat basis, the median survival for MDex was 57 months versus 22 months for the ASCT arm. This important study is limited by its small size for a disease that is as heterogeneous as AL. Among the 50 patients randomized to receive ASCT, only 37 actually received the planned transplant and 9 of those died within 100 days, indicating an unacceptably high (24 %) treatment-related mortality (TRM), leaving only 28 patients for the landmark analysis. In contrast, of the 50 patients randomized to melphalan and dexamethasone, 43 patients received three or more cycles of therapy. Based on the small sample size and unexpectedly high TRM in this phase III trial, consideration must be given to the evidence obtained from patients reported from prospective single arm studies, case-control series, observational studies, and registry studies numbering in the thousands (Table 7) [130, 131, 201, 204, 206].

The CIBMTR registry has recently reported on 1532 patients with AL treated with ASCT from multiple institutions—albeit within 24 months of their diagnosis. They found a 100-day mortality which has reduced from 20 to 11 to 5 % from the respective time periods of 1995–2000, 2001–2006, and 2007–2012 [216]. The middle interval was a comparable time period as the randomized French study, and

Table 7 Trials and case series of ASCT for Immunoglobulin Light Chain Amyloidosis

Regimen	N	Mel dose (mg/m^2)	TRM (%)	OHR/CR (%)	Median FU (mo)	Overall survival
Moreau [207]	21	140–200[b]	43	NR/14	14	4-year 57 %
Goodman [208]	92	80–200[b]	23	37/20	NR	Med 5.3 year
Vesole [204]	107	>130[b]	27	32/16	NR	2-year 56 %
Gertz[c] [209]	28	200	14	NR/NR	30	3-year 62 %
Jaccard[c] [130]	50	140–200	24	52/24	36	2-year 48
Mollee [210]	20	140–200[b]	35	50/25	18	3-year 56 %
Perz[c] [211]	24	100–200	13	54/46	31	3-year 83 %
Perfetti [212]	22	100–200	14	55/36	73	5-year 56 %
Cohen[c] [213]	42	100–200	4	60/20[d]	31	2-year 81 %
Landau[c] [214]	40	100–200	10	55/27[d]	45	3-year 82 %
Kim [215]	24	100–200	0	92/42[e]	NR	2-year 90 %
Cibeira [201]	421	100–200	11	NR/34	48	Med 6.3 year
Dispenzieri [200]	454	100–200[b]	9	80/40	60	5-year 66 %
D'Souza [206]	1536[f]	140–200	5–20	61/33	61	5-year 55-77 %

Taken with permission from Dispenzieri et al., Mayo Clinic Proceedings [134]

Mel melphalan; *TRM* transplant related mortality; *OHR* overall hematologic response; *CR* complete hematologic response; *FU* follow-up; *med* median

[a]All responses in table are ITT

[b]Alternate regimens including Mel/TBI and/or BEAM some patients

[c]Clinical trial

[d]Response rates before consolidation. For Cohen study [213] post-dexamethasone ± thalidomide OHR and CR increased to 60 and 21; for Landau study [214] after bortezomib and dexamethasone consolidation, OR and CR increased to 79 and 58 %

[e]All but one received induction treatment

[f]Registry data that may include patients from other series; the range of TRM and OS are period based, with the more recent period (2007–2012) having the lower TRM and higher OS whereas the oldest time period (1995–2000) having the higher TRM and lower OS

those 595 CIBMTR patients treated with ASCT had a 5-year OS rate of 61 % (95 %CI 57–65 %), and not 22 % as in the French study. Importantly, the survival rate continued to improve into the next interval of 2007–2012, with a 5-year OS rate of 77 % (95 %CI 72, 82 %).

5.2.7 Selection of Candidates for ASCT

As mentioned, the risk of TRM for patients receiving unattenuated high-dose melphalan approaches 50 %. At the Mayo Clinic a troponin T of greater than 0.06 ng/mL is used as an exclusion factor given a 28 % 100 day all-cause mortality among such patients in contrast to a 7 % all-cause mortality among those with a value below that threshold [111]. Another important contraindication for ASCT is low systolic blood pressure [210]. In our experience, systolic blood pressure of less than 90 mmHg is associated with a 3-month TRM of 14 % (manuscript in progress); patients with systolic blood pressure of 100 mmHg do not fare much better and should therefore be scrutinized carefully before recommending for ASCT. Patients with significantly impaired creatinine clearance are at risk for ASCT-associated renal failure [217]. Based on the existing ASCT data, the French randomized trial data, and data emerging from other therapies, we recommend not offering ASCT to those patients with high-risk features (Fig. 2), which include advanced age, troponin T $\geq$ 0.06 mcg/L, blood pressure <90 mmHg, significant involvement of more than two organs, and creatinine clearance <30 ml/min [218]. Collecting stem cells for storage can be considered in selected younger high-risk patients.

Another approach considered by some is a less-restrictive patient selection for ASCT but attenuated dosing of melphalan conditioning. Consistently, this approach resulted in lower hematologic response rates including lower CR rates [159, 201] despite reasonable TRM rates as compared to the full-dose melphalan conditioning (See below how induction and/or consolidation may prove to be exceptions to this rule). The lower OS rates in the attenuated melphalan patients are not surprising since these patients are more frail prior to starting therapy, but dose intensity of melphalan has also been shown to be important . In the Boston University cohort of 421 patients, patients receiving attenuated dose melphalan had an event-free survival of 21 months, which was less than half that of their full-dose melphalan counterparts [201].

Our interpretation of the literature is that the long-term EFS appears to be unsurpassed if ASCT is performed in select patents at high-volume transplant centers that are experienced enough with managing AL to have a low TRM [131, 159, 201] especially if patients achieve a CR [200, 201]. In contrast, for those patients who have significant comorbidity related to their AL meriting consideration of reduction of conditioning melphalan dose intensity, based on data from the randomized control trial and single arm outcomes from both Mayo Clinic and Boston University, transplant is likely not a preferred initial option [111, 130, 131, 201].

5.2.8 Induction Therapy Pre-ASCT

To date, the use of induction chemotherapy prior to HDM/SCT has been evaluated in only four prospective studies dealing specifically with this issue (Table 8). The trial that included bortezomib was considered positive, and the other three were negative [219]. We and others have shown that patients undergoing ASCT who achieve CR without induction have exceedingly good outcomes, i.e., 10-year OS of more than 70 % [200]. In an analysis of the rates of CR and VGPR among AL patients going directly to ASCT, patients with BM PC $\leq$ 10, the respective rates were 44 and 13 %; whereas, for those patients with BMPC $\geq$ 10 %, the respective rates were only 25 and 11 %. In both groups the 6-year OS for these CR patients was 88–89 % (manuscript in progress). These data would suggest that at least half of the patients with low tumor burden may not require additional therapy prior to ASCT.

Table 8 Induction and consolidation pre- and post-ASCT[b]

	N	No Prior Rx (%)	≥2 organs (%)	OHR/CR (%)	Median f/u (mo)	Overall survival
Induction						
B-Dex x 2 +ASCT [179] versus ASCT [179]	28 28	100	59	86/68 versus 48/36	NR	2-year 95 % versus 2-year 69 %
Oral MEL +ASCT [220] versus ASCT	48 52	100	74	NR/17 NR/21	45	5-year 39 % 5-year 51 %
B-Dex x 2 +ASCT [221]	35	97	86	77[a]/57	36	5-year 84 %
VAD [211]	28	89	54	43/39	31	3-year 71 %
Consolidation						
Tandem ASCT [222]	53	85	>44	NR/60	43	4-year 80 %[b]
Tandem ASCT [223]	68	87	62	6/NR	47–51	Med 68 m/47 m[c]
ASCT → thal-dex [213]	42	100–200	4	60/20[d]	31	2-year 81 %
ASCT → bortez [214]	40	100–200	10	55/27[d]	45	3-year 82 %

Taken with permission from Dispenzieri et al., Mayo Clinic Proceedings [134]
[a]VGPR or better
[b]This figure also includes the 9 patients who never received any ASCT due to inadequate stem cell collection; all other figures are based on the 53 who received at least 1 ASCT
[c]For those patients with coexistent MM
[d]For patients with coexistent multiple myeloma

Huang et al. have reported on the use of two cycles of bortezomib (1.3 mg/m^2/dose) and dexamethasone (40 mg/dose) on days 1, 4, 8, 11 every 21 days as induction versus no pretreatment prior to risk-adjusted melphalan and ASCT [219]. The primary endpoint was achieved with 65 % of BD + ASCT patients and 36 % of the no BD + ASCT achieving a CR by 1 year. More importantly, however, the respective 2-year OS rates were 95 and 69 %, and the respective 2-year PFS rates were 81 and 51 %. Two-year renal survival rates among the "no BD + ASCT" group were surprisingly low at 62 %. However, on multivariate analysis, only troponin I—and not induction—was predictive of overall survival. There was only a trend toward benefit with BD induction, potentially due to small sample size.

Another test of bortezomib induction prior to ASCT had comparable CR rates. In this study, 35 patients have been treated with biweekly bortezomib and dexamethasone for two cycles as part of a phase II study [221]. Five patients who were transplant eligible at enrolment had clinical deterioration during induction necessitating withdrawal prior to ASCT. Those who underwent ASCT had bortezomib also included as part of their conditioning regimen. By intention-to-treat CR and VGPR rates were 55 and 16 %, respectively.

In another prospective trial, which included 100 newly diagnosed patients considered candidates for ASCT, patients were randomized either to two cycles of oral melphalan and prednisone prior to ASCT or to immediate ASCT [203]. With a median follow-up of 45 months, the OS was no different between the two groups. Fewer patients received ASCT in the induction group because of disease progression during the oral chemotherapy phase of the study; this was particularly notable for patients with cardiac involvement. There was a trend toward an OS disadvantage with oral melphalan and prednisone among patients with cardiac involvement.

Similarly, a phase II trial from Perz et al. [211] indicated that administering vincristine, doxorubicin, and dexamethasone (VAD) for 2–6 cycles before HDM/SCT did not increase the hematologic response rate. Twenty-eight patients were included in the trial, but only 24 made it to stem cell chemomobilization and ASCT. Three-year OS from ASCT was 71 % on an ITT basis. The authors concluded that this therapy seemed to be equivalent to that seen without prior induction therapy.

5.2.9   Consolidation Therapy Post-ASCT

There are two chemotherapy trials and two tandem transplant trials addressing consolidative chemotherapy in AL post-ASCT (Table 8). The two phase II trials testing consolidative chemotherapy were from Memorial Sloan Kettering. In these trials patients not achieving CR received consolidative thalidomide ± dexamethasone [213] or bortezomib ± dexamethasone [214]. In the former study, 31 patients began consolidative therapy, with 52 % completing 9 months of treatment, and 42 % achieving a deeper hematological response. By intention-to-treat, overall hematological response rate was 71 % (36 % complete response) with 44 % having organ responses [213]. In the latter study, 17 of 23 patients undergoing ASCT received consolidative bortezomib and dexamethasone; overall 74 % achieved a CR, and 58 % had organ responses [214].

Sanchorawala et al. performed a prospective trial testing whether a second consolidative (tandem) ASCT could induce CR in patients in who had not achieved CR at 6 months after first ASCT with 200 mg/m^2 melphalan [132]. Sixty-two patients were enrolled, 9 did not receive first ASCT due to complications of collection or inadequate collection, 4 died within 100 days of first ASCT, and 27 achieved a CR 6 months after the first ASCT. Seventeen had a second ASCT with one dying within 100 days and five achieving a CR after second ASCT. The other nine who had not achieved CR with first ASCT did not proceed to second ASCT due to patient choice or excessive nonhematologic toxicities during first ASCT. The overall CR rate was 56 % by ITT and 60 % if one only includes the 53 patients who received at least one ASCT.

The second tandem trial included older and/or slightly sicker patients with attenuated melphalan conditioning (100 mg/m^2 per transplant) followed by consolidative ASCT [167]. Fifty-nine were labeled as "AL only" because they had fewer than 30 % bone marrow plasma cells and no CRAB, and nine were called "AL with MM." The "AL with MM" group received induction with thalidomide and dexamethasone and was scheduled to receive maintenance with thalidomide and dexamethasone post second ASCT, but it is unclear if patient any made it to the maintenance phase. Just under half of the "AL only" group received a second ASCT, and two of nine with "AL with MM" received second ASCT. The OS was 68 months and 47 months for the "AL only" and "AL with MM," respectively, and median PFS was 38 months and 16 months [167].

The body of literature that demonstrates inferior survival among those not achieving the deepest responses would support the concept of consolidative therapy post-ASCT among poor responders [115]. Whether the attainment of deeper response is purely "prognostic"—a demonstration of poor chemosensitivity resulting in shortened survival—or whether deeper response can serve as a goal that will alter a patient's subsequent outcome has not yet been proven. The logic of the second supposition, however, is appealing from a pathogenic standpoint, i.e., that the circulating free light chain is the source of organ damage either through direct toxicity or through fibril formation; reducing the "toxin" should improve outcomes. Under the same premise, we recommend post-ASCT consolidation therapy in patients not achieving at least a VGPR at day 100 post-ASCT.

5.2.10   ASCT in Patients on Hemodialysis

Once a patient with AL has started dialysis, it is highly unlikely that renal function will ever return without a renal allograft. ASCT can be performed safely in these patients, as long there is attention to dose adjustment of melphalan and supportive care medications. If there is even mild cardiac disease, the level of soluble cardiac biomarkers will be higher due to the impaired glomerular filtration rate, and the patient's cardiac status should be evaluated by other functional means to determine ASCT eligibility. All data supporting these recommendations are from case series [217] and personal experience, but TRM in selected patients ranges from 6 to 13 % [217]. Comparable CR rates have been observed—53 % in one series—but the median OS in this same series was only 25 months. The eight patients with CR, however, had a median OS of 4.5 years.

5.2.11   Allogeneic Hematopoietic Stem Cell Transplantation

Allogeneic hematopoietic stem cell transplantation is not a standard therapy for patients with AL. There are no prospective clinical trials, only small case series [224, 225]. The European Group for Blood and Marrow Transplantation registry reported 19 patients with AL who underwent allogeneic ($n = 15$) or syngeneic ($n = 4$) hematopoietic stem cell transplantation between 1991 and 2003 [226]. With a median follow-up time of 19 months, overall and progression-free survival rates were 60 and 53 % at 1 year, respectively. Forty percent of patients died of TRM.

5.2.12   Treating Relapsed or Refractory AL

Overall, patients receiving second line therapy do better than patients receiving first line therapy due to the very high death rate that occurs within the first 6 months of diagnosis. Clearly getting a rapid and deep hematologic response is better than not, but patients who are physically more resilient survive to receive second or higher line therapy. The tables contain a mix of newly diagnosed and previously treated

Treatment of AL – off study

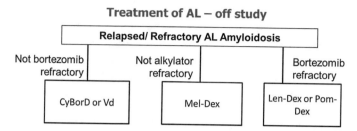

Fig. 3 Nonstudy treatment algorithm for transplant-eligible patients with relapsed or refractory AL amyloidosis. Taken with permission from Dispenzieri et al., Mayo Clinic Proceedings [134]. Note: many of the recommendations in this algorithm have not yet been supported by clinical trials; level of evidence is clearly indicated in text

patients. Patients not refractory to bortezomib should receive a bortezomib containing regimen. Those not alkylator refractory are candidates for melphalan and dexamethasone. For those patients who are bortezomib refractory, lenalidomide and dexamethasone or pomalidomide and dexamethasone are recommended (Fig. 3).

5.3   Supportive Therapy for AL

5.3.1   Supportive care for cardiac AL

There are special considerations among patients with cardiac amyloidosis. These patients typically have severe diastolic dysfunction with a nondilated ventricle leading to increased filling pressures, often with low cardiac output. The use of standard medical therapy for heart failure with reduced ejection fraction, specifically beta blockers and ACE inhibitors or ARBs often worsen patients' clinical status. Diuretics are the mainstay of care with the best results achieved with a combination of loop diuretics and spironolactone. Metolazone or periodic thoracentesis may be considered in select cases [156]. Beta blockade may cause profound hypotension and low cardiac output and should be avoided.

Patients with cardiac amyloid are at risk for intracardiac thrombi [227, 228]; in one study 35 % of patients with AL who had transesophageal echocardiograms had atrial thrombus, the majority of which were located in the right or left atrial appendages [228]. Anticoagulation should be considered recognizing that life-threatening bleeding is a potential risk.

For those patients with atrial fibrillation, rate control can be a challenge since beta blockade and calcium channel blockers are often poorly tolerated. Digoxin has been considered contraindicated in cardiac amyloidosis due to concerns regarding digoxin binding and an increased risk of toxicity [229], but digoxin is often preferable over calcium channel blockers and beta blockers for rate control in atrial fibrillation. Nondihydropyridine calcium channel blockers should be avoided due to its associated bradycardia and negative inotropic effects [230]. In our experience amiodarone is often helpful for rhythm control, and selected patients may benefit from atrioventricular node ablation with permanent pacing. Patients with cardiac amyloidosis are susceptible to malignant arrhythmias including ventricular tachycardia, ventricular fibrillation, and pulseless electrical activity [231, 232]. The role of implantable cardioverter-defibrillators is controversial in these patients, since both successes and failures have been documented [128, 232–234]. Although appropriate ICD device therapy has been observed in patients with AL cardiac amyloid, studies to date have not demonstrated a survival advantage [235]. A study of implanted cardiac rhythm recorders found that sudden death in AL is commonly due to pulseless electrical activity, often preceded by bradycardia [236]. Given the absence of randomized studies, the role of ICD therapy for primary prevention in cardiac AL remains unclear.

5.3.2   Supportive Care for Renal AL

Among patients with renal involvement, which is nephrotic syndrome in the majority, the major problem is third space fluid distribution due to hypoalbuminemia. This may be further exacerbated by coexisting cardiomyopathy. Diuretics are the mainstay of therapy. It is not unusual for nephrologists to institute an angiotensin converting enzyme inhibitor based on their management of diabetic nephropathy. There are no data to support this intervention in AL. Adequate suppression of the underlying clone is the most important maneuver to improve renal function [237]. Patients on dialysis may struggle with hypotension which can be successfully managed with predialysis midodrine.

5.3.3   Supportive Care for AL Involving the Nerves

Amyloidosis patients with neuropathy typically have small fiber involvement which can be treated symptomatically with amitriptyline, nortriptyline, gabapentin, pregabalin, or duloxetine. Topical preparations that include various combinations of lidocaine, ketamine, and/or amitriptyline may also provide relief. For patients with neuropathy due to carpal tunnel syndrome, carpal tunnel release or carpal tunnel braces are of benefit. The autonomic insufficiency can be very difficult to manage, especially among patients with severe nephrotic syndrome or severe cardiomyopathy. Fludrocortisone and salt tablets are only useful in a minority of these patients since they may aggravate congestive heart failure or peripheral edema. The alpha-1 receptor agonist midodrine or the anticholinergic pyridostigmine can improve neurogenic orthostatic hypotension [238] and metoclopramide, used in diabetic gastroparesis, can help with gastric emptying.

5.4   Organ Transplantation

Solid organ transplantation is a controversial intervention among patients with AL. Because the disease is systemic and presumably incurable, there is concern that the amyloid will either reoccur in the transplanted organ or progress in another organ resulting in a poor outcome. The best outcomes have occurred in the setting of careful patient selection, excluding patients with clinically evident multi-organ involvement, and among those who received chemotherapy to eradicate the clone either before or after the solid organ transplantation.

The results of cardiac orthotopic cardiac transplantation are mixed [115]. Recommendations are derived from fewer than 100 transplants described in eight series. Five-year OS rates range from 18 to 65 %. Key determinants for the best outcomes include limiting candidates to those who have lower tumor burden and clinical organ involvement limited to the heart and administering chemotherapy that is effective against the clone. The majority of patients do not satisfy these criteria and even those who do satisfy these criteria who are placed on a transplant list do not survive long enough to receive an orthotopic heart.

Many of the reports of renal transplantation for amyloidosis combine AL with AA amyloidosis making outcomes for the former condition difficult to discern [115]. Options include cadaveric and living donor transplantations. Given the limited cadaveric donor pool and the risk of recurrence or death related to their underlying AL, the vast majority of renal transplants have been done with living donors. Five-year overall survival rates have ranged between 67–78 % in carefully selected patients, once again favoring those patients with limited disease and tumor burden and those who receive highly effective chemotherapy, including ASCT. It is our current practice to offer renal allografting to AL patients with ESRD who have already achieved CR most typically after ASCT.

Unlike hereditary amyloidosis, liver transplantation is rarely performed for patients with AL amyloidosis [115, 239, 240]. Outcomes are poor as illustrated by 1-year and 5-year OS rates of 32 and 22 % in a series of 9 patients transplanted in the UK.

6 Future Directions

There is unprecedented interest in AL, which has resulted in improved outcomes for these patients. Clearly, more work needs to be done, especially in the realms of earlier diagnosis, of salvaging the 35 % of patients who appear destined to die within the first 6 months of their diagnosis, and in more innovative therapies. Physicians caring for patients with AL have been borrowing and customizing therapies used for patients with multiple myeloma with varying degrees of success. There are exciting possibilities ahead, including the study of oral proteasome inhibitors, antibodies directed at CD38 or CS-1, and other novel therapies that are showing promise in patients with multiple myeloma. There are three antibodies in clinical trials that attack the amyloid itself and may be paradigm shifting (NCT01707264, NCT01777243, NCT02245867, and NCT02312206). The role of organ transplant or ventricular assist devices may hold promise as well.

References

1. Merlini G, Bellotti V (2003) Molecular mechanisms of amyloidosis. N Engl J Med 349 (6):583–596. doi:10.1056/NEJMra023144349/6/583
2. Merlini G, Palladini G (2008) Amyloidosis: is a cure possible? Ann Oncol 19 Suppl 4: iv63–66
3. Merlini G, Wechalekar AD, Palladini G (2013) Systemic light chain amyloidosis: an update for treating physicians. Blood 121(26):5124–5130. doi:10.1182/blood-2013-01-453001
4. Merlini G, Palladini G (2012) Differential diagnosis of monoclonal gammopathy of undetermined significance. Hematol Am Soc Hematol Educ Program 2012:595–603. doi:10. 1182/asheducation-2012.1.595
5. Sipe JD, Benson MD, Buxbaum JN, Ikeda S, Merlini G, Saraiva MJ, Westermark P (2014) Nomenclature 2014: amyloid fibril proteins and clinical classification of the amyloidosis. Amyloid 21(4):221–224. doi:10.3109/13506129.2014.964858
6. Kyle RA, Linos A, Beard CM, Linke RP, Gertz MA, O'Fallon WM, Kurland LT (1992) Incidence and natural history of primary systemic amyloidosis in Olmsted County, Minnesota, 1950 through 1989. Blood 79(7):1817–1822
7. Pinney JH, Smith CJ, Taube JB, Lachmann HJ, Venner CP, Gibbs SD, Dungu J, Banypersad SM, Wechalekar AD, Whelan CJ, Hawkins PN, Gillmore JD (2013) Systemic amyloidosis in England: an epidemiological study. Br J Haematol 161(4):525–532. doi:10. 1111/bjh.12286
8. Benson MD, Liepnieks JJ, Kluve-Beckerman B (2015) Hereditary systemic immunoglobulin light-chain amyloidosis. Blood 125(21):3281–3286. doi:10.1182/blood-2014-12-618108
9. Merlini G, Stone MJ (2006) Dangerous small B-cell clones. Blood 108(8):2520–2530
10. Dispenzieri A, Gertz MA, Buadi F (2012) What do I need to know about immunoglobulin light chain (AL) amyloidosis? Blood Rev 26(4):137–154. doi:10.1016/j.blre.2012.03.001
11. Biewend ML, Menke DM, Calamia KT (2006) The spectrum of localized amyloidosis: a case series of 20 patients and review of the literature. Amyloid 13(3):135–142. doi:10.1080/ 13506120600876773
12. Gertz MA, Kyle RA, Greipp PR (1989) The plasma cell labeling index: a valuable tool in primary systemic amyloidosis. Blood 74(3):1108–1111
13. Rajkumar SV, Gertz MA, Kyle RA (1998) Primary systemic amyloidosis with delayed progression to multiple myeloma. Cancer 82(8):1501–1505. doi:10.1002/(SICI)1097-0142 (19980415)82:8<1501:AID-CNCR11>3.0.CO;2-8
14. Perfetti V, Colli Vignarelli M, Anesi E, Garini P, Quaglini S, Ascari E, Merlini G (1999) The degrees of plasma cell clonality and marrow infiltration adversely influence the prognosis of AL amyloidosis patients. Haematologica 84(3):218–221
15. Paiva B, Vidriales MB, Perez JJ, Lopez-Berges MC, Garcia-Sanz R, Ocio EM, de Las Heras N, Cuello R, de Coca AG, Pardal E, Alonso J, Sierra M, Barez A, Hernandez J, Suarez L, Galende J, Mateos MV, San Miguel JF (2011) The clinical utility and prognostic value of multiparameter flow cytometry immunophenotyping in light-chain amyloidosis. Blood 117(13):3613–3616. doi:10.1182/blood-2010-12-324665
16. Kourelis TV, Kumar SK, Gertz MA, Lacy MQ, Buadi FK, Hayman SR, Zeldenrust S, Leung N, Kyle RA, Russell S, Dingli D, Lust JA, Lin Y, Kapoor P, Rajkumar SV, McCurdy A, Dispenzieri A (2013) Coexistent multiple myeloma or increased bone marrow plasma cells define equally high-risk populations in patients with immunoglobulin light chain amyloidosis. J Clin Oncol 31(34):4319–4324. doi:10.1200/JCO.2013.50.8499
17. Pardanani A, Witzig TE, Schroeder G, McElroy EA, Fonseca R, Dispenzieri A, Lacy MQ, Lust JA, Kyle RA, Greipp PR, Gertz MA, Rajkumar SV (2003) Circulating peripheral blood plasma cells as a prognostic indicator in patients with primary systemic amyloidosis. Blood 101(3):827–830. doi:10.1182/blood-2002-06-16982002-06-1698
18. Dispenzieri A, Lacy MQ, Katzmann JA, Rajkumar SV, Abraham RS, Hayman SR, Kumar SK, Clark R, Kyle RA, Litzow MR, Inwards DJ, Ansell SM, Micallef IM, Porrata LF,

Elliott MA, Johnston PB, Greipp PR, Witzig TE, Zeldenrust SR, Russell SJ, Gastineau D, Gertz MA (2006) Absolute values of immunoglobulin free light chains are prognostic in patients with primary systemic amyloidosis undergoing peripheral blood stem cell transplantation. Blood 107(8):3378–3383

19. Wechalekar A (2009) A new staging system for AL amyloidosis incorporating serum free light chains, cardiac troponin-T and NT-proBNP. Blood 114:abstr. 2796

20. Kumar S (2009) A novel prognostic staging system for light chain amyloidosis (AL) incorporating markers of plasma cell burden and organ involvement. Blood 114: abstr. 2797

21. Merlini G, Seldin DC, Gertz MA (2011) Amyloidosis: pathogenesis and new therapeutic options. J Clin Oncol 29(14):1924–1933

22. Fonseca R, Ahmann GJ, Jalal SM, Dewald GW, Larson DR, Therneau TM, Gertz MA, Kyle RA, Greipp PR (1998) Chromosomal abnormalities in systemic amyloidosis. Br J Haematol 103(3):704–710

23. Hayman SR, Bailey RJ, Jalal SM, Ahmann GJ, Dispenzieri A, Gertz MA, Greipp PR, Kyle RA, Lacy MQ, Rajkumar SV, Witzig TE, Lust JA, Fonseca R (2001) Translocations involving the immunoglobulin heavy-chain locus are possible early genetic events in patients with primary systemic amyloidosis. Blood 98(7):2266–2268

24. Perfetti V, Coluccia AM, Intini D, Malgeri U, Vignarelli MC, Casarini S, Merlini G, Neri A (2001) Translocation T(4;14)(p16.3;q32) is a recurrent genetic lesion in primary amyloidosis. Am J Pathol 158(5):1599–1603

25. Bochtler T, Hegenbart U, Heiss C, Benner A, Moos M, Seckinger A, Pschowski-Zuck S, Kirn D, Neben K, Bartram CR, Ho AD, Goldschmidt H, Hose D, Jauch A, Schonland SO (2011) Hyperdiploidy is less frequent in AL amyloidosis compared with monoclonal gammopathy of undetermined significance and inversely associated with translocation t (11;14). Blood 117(14):3809–3815. doi:10.1182/blood-2010-02-268987

26. Bochtler T, Hegenbart U, Kunz C, Benner A, Seckinger A, Dietrich S, Granzow M, Neben K, Goldschmidt H, Ho AD, Hose D, Jauch A, Schonland SO (2014) Gain of chromosome 1q21 is an independent adverse prognostic factor in light chain amyloidosis patients treated with melphalan/dexamethasone. Amyloid 21(1):9–17. doi:10.3109/13506129.2013.854766

27. Kumar S, Dispenzieri A, Katzmann JA, Larson DR, Colby CL, Lacy MQ, Hayman SR, Buadi FK, Leung N, Zeldenrust SR, Ramirez-Alvarado M, Clark RJ, Kyle RA, Rajkumar SV, Gertz MA (2010) Serum immunoglobulin free light-chain measurement in primary amyloidosis: prognostic value and correlations with clinical features. Blood 116 (24):5126–5129. doi:10.1182/blood-2010-06-290668

28. Weinhold N, Forsti A, da Silva Filho MI, Nickel J, Campo C, Hoffmann P, Nothen MM, Hose D, Goldschmidt H, Jauch A, Langer C, Hegenbart U, Schonland SO, Hemminki K (2014) Immunoglobulin light-chain amyloidosis shares genetic susceptibility with multiple myeloma. Leukemia. doi:10.1038/leu.2014.208

29. Boyle EM, Walker BA, Rowczienio D, Wardell CP, Murison A, Mikulasova A, Sachchithanantham S, Baginska A, Mahmood S, Gillmore JD, Lachmann HJ, Hawkins PN, Leleu X, Davies FE, Morgan GJ, Wechalekar A (2014) Exome sequencing to define a genetic signature of plasma cells in systemic AL amyloidosis. Blood 124(21)

30. Blancas-Mejia LM, Tischer A, Thompson JR, Tai J, Wang L, Auton M, Ramirez-Alvarado M (2014) Kinetic control in protein folding for light chain amyloidosis and the differential effects of somatic mutations. J Mol Biol 426(2):347–361. doi:10.1016/j.jmb.2013.10.016

31. Bellotti V, Mangione P, Merlini G (2000) Review: Immunoglobulin light chain amyloidosis - The archetype of structural and pathogenic variability. J Struct Biol 130(2–3):280–289

32. Prokaeva T, Spencer B, et al (2010) Contribution of light chain variable region genes to organ tropism and survival in AL amyloidosis. Amyloid 17(S1):62, Abstract OP-046

33. Comenzo RL, Zhang Y, Martinez C, Osman K, Herrera GA (2001) The tropism of organ involvement in primary systemic amyloidosis: contributions of Ig V-L germ line gene use and clonal plasma cell burden. Blood 98(3):714–720

34. Perfetti V, Casarini S, Palladini G, Vignarelli MC, Klersy C, Diegoli M, Ascari E, Merlini G (2002) Analysis of V lambda-J lambda expression in plasma cells from primary (AL) amyloidosis and normal bone marrow identifies 3r (lambda III) as a new amyloid-associated germline gene segment. Blood 100(3):948–953

35. Abraham RS, Geyer SM, Price-Troska TL, Allmer C, Kyle RA, Gertz MA, Fonseca R (2003) Immunoglobulin light chain variable (V) region genes influence clinical presentation and outcome in light chain-associated amyloidosis (AL). Blood 101(10):3801–3808

36. Perfetti V, Palladini G, Casarini S, Navazza V, Rognoni P, Obici L, Invernizzi R, Perlini S, Klersy C, Merlini G (2012) The repertoire of lambda light chains causing predominant amyloid heart involvement and identification of a preferentially involved germline gene, IGLV1-44. Blood 119(1):144–150. doi:10.1182/blood-2011-05-355784

37. Poshusta TL, Sikkink LA, Leung N, Clark RJ, Dispenzieri A, Ramirez-Alvarado M (2009) Mutations in specific structural regions of immunoglobulin light chains are associated with free light chain levels in patients with Al amyloidosis. PLoS ONE 4(4):e5169

38. Grogg KL, Aubry MC, Vrana JA, Theis JD, Dogan A (2013) Nodular pulmonary amyloidosis is characterized by localized immunoglobulin deposition and is frequently associated with an indolent B-cell lymphoproliferative disorder. Am J Surg Pathol 37 (3):406–412. doi:10.1097/PAS.0b013e318272fe19

39. Nasr SH, Said SM, Valeri AM, Sethi S, Fidler ME, Cornell LD, Gertz MA, Dispenzieri A, Buadi FK, Vrana JA, Theis JD, Dogan A, Leung N (2013) The diagnosis and characteristics of renal heavy-chain and heavy/light-chain amyloidosis and their comparison with renal light-chain amyloidosis. Kidney Int 83(3):463–470. doi:10.1038/ki.2012.414

40. Picken MM (2013) Non-light-chain immunoglobulin amyloidosis: time to expand or refine the spectrum to include light + heavy chain amyloidosis? Kidney Int 83(3):353–356. doi:10. 1038/ki.2012.433

41. Shi J, Guan J, Jiang B, Brenner DA, Del Monte F, Ward JE, Connors LH, Sawyer DB, Semigran MJ, Macgillivray TE, Seldin DC, Falk R, Liao R (2010) Amyloidogenic light chains induce cardiomyocyte contractile dysfunction and apoptosis via a non-canonical p38alpha MAPK pathway. Proc Natl Acad Sci USA 107(9):4188–4193. doi:10.1073/pnas. 0912263107

42. Mishra S, Guan J, Plovie E, Seldin DC, Connors LH, Merlini G, Falk RH, MacRae CA, Liao R (2013) Human amyloidogenic light chain proteins result in cardiac dysfunction, cell death, and early mortality in zebrafish. Am J Physiol Heart Circ Physiol 305(1):H95–103. doi:10.1152/ajpheart.00186.2013

43. Liao R, Jain M, Teller P, Connors LH, Ngoy S, Skinner M, Falk RH, Apstein CS (2001) Infusion of light chains from patients with cardiac amyloidosis causes diastolic dysfunction in isolated mouse hearts. Circulation 104(14):1594–1597

44. Guan J, Mishra S, Shi J, Plovie E, Qiu Y, Cao X, Gianni D, Jiang B, Del Monte F, Connors LH, Seldin DC, Lavatelli F, Rognoni P, Palladini G, Merlini G, Falk RH, Semigran MJ, Dec GW, Macrae CA, Liao R (2013) Stanniocalcin1 is a key mediator of amyloidogenic light chain induced cardiotoxicity. Basic Res Cardiol 108(5):378. doi:10. 1007/s00395-013-0378-5

45. Brenner DA, Jain M, Pimentel DR, Wang B, Connors LH, Skinner M, Apstein CS, Liao R (2004) Human amyloidogenic light chains directly impair cardiomyocyte function through an increase in cellular oxidant stress. Circ Res 94(8):1008–1010

46. Walsh DM, Klyubin I, Fadeeva JV, Cullen WK, Anwyl R, Wolfe MS, Rowan MJ, Selkoe DJ (2002) Naturally secreted oligomers of amyloid beta protein potently inhibit hippocampal long-term potentiation in vivo. Nature 416(6880):535–539. doi:10.1038/416535a

47. Reixach N, Deechongkit S, Jiang X, Kelly JW, Buxbaum JN (2004) Tissue damage in the amyloidoses: Transthyretin monomers and nonnative oligomers are the major cytotoxic

species in tissue culture. Proc Natl Acad Sci USA 101(9):2817–2822. doi:10.1073/pnas. 0400062101040006210l

48. Laurén J, Gimbel DA, Nygaard HB, Gilbert JW, Strittmatter SM (2009) Cellular prion protein mediates impairment of synaptic plasticity by amyloid-beta oligomers. Nature 457 (7233):1128–1132. doi:10.1038/nature07761

49. Ren R, Hong Z, Gong H, Laporte K, Skinner M, Seldin DC, Costello CE, Connors LH, Trinkaus-Randall V (2010) Role of glycosaminoglycan sulfation in the formation of immunoglobulin light chain amyloid oligomers and fibrils. J Biol Chem 285(48):37672– 37682. doi:10.1074/jbc.M110.149575

50. Laganowsky A, Liu C, Sawaya MR, Whitelegge JP, Park J, Zhao M, Pensalfini A, Soriaga AB, Landau M, Teng PK, Cascio D, Glabe C, Eisenberg D (2012) Atomic view of a toxic amyloid small oligomer. Science 335(6073):1228–1231. doi:10.1126/science.1213151

51. Walsh DM, Selkoe DJ (2007) A beta oligomers—a decade of discovery. J Neurochem 101 (5):1172–1184. doi:10.1111/j.1471-4159.2006.04426.x

52. Palladini G, Lavatelli F, Russo P, Perlini S, Perfetti V, Bosoni T, Obici L, Bradwell AR, D'Eril GM, Fogari R, Moratti R, Merlini G (2006) Circulating amyloidogenic free light chains and serum N-terminal natriuretic peptide type B decrease simultaneously in association with improvement of survival in AL. Blood 107(10):3854–3858

53. Palladini G, Campana C, Klersy C, Balduini A, Vadacca G, Perfetti V, Perlini S, Obici L, Ascari E, d'Eril GM, Moratti R, Merlini G (2003) Serum N-terminal pro-brain natriuretic peptide is a sensitive marker of myocardial dysfunction in AL amyloidosis. Circulation 107 (19):2440–2445

54. Sousa MM, Cardoso I, Fernandes R, Guimaraes A, Saraiva MJ (2001) Deposition of transthyretin in early stages of familial amyloidotic polyneuropathy: evidence for toxicity of nonfibrillar aggregates. Am J Pathol 159(6):1993–2000

55. Diomede L, Rognoni P, Lavatelli F, Romeo M, del Favero E, Cantu L, Ghibaudi E, di Fonzo A, Corbelli A, Fiordaliso F, Palladini G, Valentini V, Perfetti V, Salmona M, Merlini G (2014) A Caenorhabditis elegans-based assay recognizes immunoglobulin light chains causing heart amyloidosis. Blood 123(23):3543–3552. doi:10.1182/blood-2013-10-525634

56. Comenzo RL, Vosburgh E, Simms RW, Bergethon P, Sarnacki D, Finn K, Dubrey S, Faller DV, Wright DG, Falk RH, Skinner M (1996) Dose-intensive melphalan with blood stem cell support for the treatment of AL amyloidosis: one-year follow-up in five patients. Blood 88(7):2801–2806

57. Dember LM, Sanchorawala V, Seldin DC, Wright DG, LaValley M, Berk JL, Falk RH, Skinner M (2001) Effect of dose-intensive intravenous melphalan and autologous blood stem-cell transplantation on al amyloidosis-associated renal disease. Ann Intern Med 134(9 Pt 1):746–753. doi:200105010 00011

58. Caccialanza R, Palladini G, Klersy C, Cena H, Vagia C, Cameletti B, Russo P, Lavatelli F, Merlini G (2006) Nutritional status of outpatients with systemic immunoglobulin light-chain amyloidosis 1. Am J Clin Nutr 83(2):350–354

59. Caccialanza R, Palladini G, Klersy C, Cereda E, Bonardi C, Cameletti B, Montagna E, Russo P, Foli A, Milani P, Lavatelli F, Merlini G (2011) Nutritional status independently affects quality of life of patients with systemic immunoglobulin light-chain (AL) amyloidosis. Ann Hematol. doi:10.1007/s00277-011-1309-x

60. Obici L, Perfetti V, Palladini G, Moratti R, Merlini G (2005) Clinical aspects of systemic amyloid diseases. Biochim Biophys Acta 1753(1):11–22

61. Cowan AJ, Skinner M, Berk JL, Sloan JM, O'Hara C, Seldin DC, Sanchorawala V (2011) Macroglossia - not always AL amyloidosis. Amyloid 18(2):83–86. doi:10.3109/13506129. 2011.560217

62. Prokaeva T, Spencer B, Kaut M, Ozonoff A, Doros G, Connors LH, Skinner M, Seldin DC (2007) Soft tissue, joint, and bone manifestations of AL amyloidosis: clinical presentation, molecular features, and survival. Arthritis Rheum 56(11):3858–3868. doi:10.1002/art.22959

63. Gertz MA, Lacy MQ, Dispenzieri A (2002) Immunoglobulin light chain amyloidosis and the kidney. Kidney Int 61(1):1–9. doi:10.1046/j.1523-1755.2002.00085.x
64. Gertz MA, Leung N, Lacy MQ, Dispenzieri A, Zeldenrust SR, Hayman SR, Buadi FK, Dingli D, Greipp PR, Kumar SK, Lust JA, Rajkumar SV, Russell SJ, Witzig TE (2009) Clinical outcome of immunoglobulin light chain amyloidosis affecting the kidney. Nephrol Dial Transplant 24(10):3132–3137. doi:10.1093/ndt/gfp201
65. Bergesio F, Ciciani AM, Manganaro M, Palladini G, Santostefano M, Brugnano R, Di Palma AM, Gallo M, Rosati A, Tosi PL, Salvadori M (2008) Renal involvement in systemic amyloidosis: an Italian collaborative study on survival and renal outcome. Nephrol Dial Transplant 23(3):941–951. doi:10.1093/ndt/gfm684
66. Palladini G, Hegenbart U, Milani P, Kimmich C, Foli A, Ho AD, Vidus Rosin M, Albertini R, Moratti R, Merlini G, Schonland S (2014) A staging system for renal outcome and early markers of renal response to chemotherapy in AL amyloidosis. Blood. doi:10.1182/blood-2014-04-570010
67. Leung N, Dispenzieri A, Lacy MQ, Kumar SK, Hayman SR, Fervenza FC, Cha SS, Gertz MA (2007) Severity of baseline proteinuria predicts renal response in immunoglobulin light chain-associated amyloidosis after autologous stem cell transplantation. Clin J Am Soc Nephrol 2(3):440–444. doi:10.2215/CJN.02450706
68. Palladini G, Hegenbart U, Milani P, Kimmich C, Foli A, Ho AD, Rosin MV, Albertini R, Moratti R, Merlini G, Schoenland S (2014) A staging system for renal outcome and early markers of renal response to chemotherapy in AL amyloidosis. Blood 124(15):2325–2332. doi:10.1182/blood-2014-04-570010
69. Park MA, Mueller PS, Kyle RA, Larson DR, Plevak MF, Gertz MA (2003) Primary (AL) hepatic amyloidosis: clinical features and natural history in 98 patients. Medicine (Baltimore) 82(5):291–298. doi:10.1097/01.md.0000091183.93122.c7
70. Peters RA, Koukoulis G, Gimson A, Portmann B, Westaby D, Williams R (1994) Primary amyloidosis and severe intrahepatic cholestatic jaundice. Gut 35(9):1322–1325
71. Rubinow A, Koff RS, Cohen AS (1978) Severe intrahepatic cholestasis in primary amyloidosis: a report of four cases and a review of the literature. Am J Med 64(6):937–946
72. Falk RH, Quarta CC (2015) Echocardiography in cardiac amyloidosis. Heart Fail Rev 20(2):125–131. doi:10.1007/s10741-014-9466-3
73. Buss SJ, Emami M, Mereles D, Korosoglou G, Kristen AV, Voss A, Schellberg D, Zugck C, Galuschky C, Giannitsis E, Hegenbart U, Ho AD, Katus HA, Schonland SO, Hardt SE (2012) Longitudinal left ventricular function for prediction of survival in systemic light-chain amyloidosis: incremental value compared with clinical and biochemical markers. J Am Coll Cardiol 60(12):1067–1076. doi:10.1016/j.jacc.2012.04.043
74. Nesbitt GC, Mankad S (2009) Strain and strain rate imaging in cardiomyopathy. Echocardiography 26(3):337–344. doi:10.1111/j.1540-8175.2008.00867.x
75. Rahman JE, Helou EF, Gelzer-Bell R, Thompson RE, Kuo C, Rodriguez ER, Hare JM, Baughman KL, Kasper EK (2004) Noninvasive diagnosis of biopsy-proven cardiac amyloidosis. J Am Coll Cardiol 43(3):410–415
76. Rapezzi C, Merlini G, Quarta CC, Riva L, Longhi S, Leone O, Salvi F, Ciliberti P, Pastorelli F, Biagini E, Coccolo F, Cooke RM, Bacchi-Reggiani L, Sangiorgi D, Ferlini A, Cavo M, Zamagni E, Fonte ML, Palladini G, Salinaro F, Musca F, Obici L, Branzi A, Perlini S (2009) Systemic cardiac amyloidoses: disease profiles and clinical courses of the 3 main types. Circulation 120(13):1203–1212. doi:10.1161/CIRCULATIONAHA.108.843334
77. Maceira AM, Joshi J, Prasad SK, Moon JC, Perugini E, Harding I, Sheppard MN, Poole-Wilson PA, Hawkins PN, Pennell DJ (2005) Cardiovascular magnetic resonance in cardiac amyloidosis. Circulation 111(2):186–193. doi:10.1161/01.CIR.0000152819.97857.9D
78. Banypersad SM, Sado DM, Flett AS, Gibbs SD, Pinney JH, Maestrini V, Cox AT, Fontana M, Whelan CJ, Wechalekar AD, Hawkins PN, Moon JC (2013) Quantification of myocardial extracellular volume fraction in systemic Al amyloidosis: an equilibrium contrast

cardiovascular magnetic resonance study. Circ Cardiovasc Imaging 6(1):34–39. doi:10.1161/CIRCIMAGING.112.978627

79. Fontana M, Chung R, Hawkins PN, Moon JC (2015) Cardiovascular magnetic resonance for amyloidosis. Heart Fail Rev 20(2):133–144. doi:10.1007/s10741-014-9470-7

80. Antoni G, Lubberink M, Estrada S, Axelsson J, Carlson K, Lindsjo L, Kero T, Langstrom B, Granstam SO, Rosengren S, Vedin O, Wassberg C, Wikstrom G, Westermark P, Sorensen J (2013) In vivo visualization of amyloid deposits in the heart with 11C-PIB and PET. J Nucl Med 54(2):213–220. doi:10.2967/jnumed.111.102053

81. Dorbala S, Vangala D, Semer J, Strader C, Bruyere JR Jr, Di Carli MF, Moore SC, Falk RH (2014) Imaging cardiac amyloidosis: a pilot study using F-florbetapir positron emission tomography. Eur J Nucl Med Mol Imaging. doi:10.1007/s00259-014-2787-6

82. Merlini G, Narula J, Arbustini E (2014) Molecular imaging of misfolded protein pathology for early clues to involvement of the heart. Eur J Nucl Med Mol Imaging. doi:10.1007/s00259-014-2832-5

83. Russo P, Palladini G, Foli A, Zenone Bragotti L, Milani P, Nuvolone M, Obici L, Perfetti V, Brugnatelli S, Invernizzi R, Merlini G (2011) Liver involvement as the hallmark of aggressive disease in light chain amyloidosis: distinctive clinical features and role of light chain type in 225 patients. Amyloid 18(Suppl 1):92–93. doi:10.3109/13506129.2011.574354033

84. Mosconi G, Scolari MP, Feliciangeli G, Zanetti A, Zanelli P, Buscaroli A, Piccari M, Faenza S, Ercolani G, Faenza A, Pinna AD, Stefoni S (2006) Combined liver-kidney transplantation with preformed anti-HLA antibodies: a case report. Transplant Proc 38(4):1125–1126. doi:10.1016/j.transproceed.2006.03.045

85. Di Sabatino A, Carsetti R, Corazza GR (2011) Post-splenectomy and hyposplenic states. Lancet. doi:10.1016/S0140-6736(10)61493-6

86. Renzulli P, Schoepfer A, Mueller E, Candinas D (2009) Atraumatic splenic rupture in amyloidosis. Amyloid 16(1):47–53. doi:10.1080/13506120802676922

87. Matsuda M, Gono T, Morita H, Katoh N, Kodaira M, Ikeda S (2011) Peripheral nerve involvement in primary systemic AL amyloidosis: a clinical and electrophysiological study. Eur J Neurol 18(4):604–610. doi:10.1111/j.1468-1331.2010.03215.x

88. Gertz M, Comenzo R, Falk R, Fermand J, Hazenberg B, Hawkins P, Merlini G, Moreau P, Ronco P, Sanchorawala V, Sezer O, Solomon A, Grateau G (2005) Definition of organ involvement and treatment response in immunoglobulin light chain amyloidosis (AL): a consensus opinion from the 10th international symposium on amyloid and amyloidosis, Tours, France, 18-22 April 2004. Am J Hematol 79(4):319–328

89. Palladini G, Dispenzieri A, Gertz MA, Kumar S, Wechalekar A, Hawkins PN, Schonland S, Hegenbart U, Comenzo R, Kastritis E, Dimopoulos MA, Jaccard A, Klersy C, Merlini G (2012) New criteria for response to treatment in immunoglobulin light chain amyloidosis based on free light chain measurement and cardiac biomarkers: impact on survival outcomes. J Clin Oncol 30(36):4541–4549. doi:10.1200/JCO.2011.37.7614

90. Gertz MA, Merlini G (2010) Definition of organ involvement and response to treatment in AL amyloidosis: an updated consensus opinion. Amyloid 17(S1):48–49

91. Palladini G, Verga L, Corona S, Obici L, Morbini P, Lavatelli F, Donadei S, Sarais G, Roggeri L, Foli A, Russo P, Bragotti LZ, Paulli M, Minoli L, Magrini U, Merlini G (2010) Diagnostic performance of immuno-electron microscopy of abdominal fat in systemic amyloidoses. Amyloid 17:59–60

92. Fernandez de Larrea C, Verga L, Morbini P, Klersy C, Lavatelli F, Foli A, Obici L, Milani P, Capello GL, Paulli M, Palladini G, Merlini G (2015) A practical approach to the diagnosis of systemic amyloidoses. Blood. doi:10.1182/blood-2014-11-609883

93. Foli A, Palladini G, Caporali R, Verga L, Morbini P, Obici L, Russo P, Sarais G, Donadei S, Montecucco C, Merlini G (2011) The role of minor salivary gland biopsy in the diagnosis of systemic amyloidosis: results of a prospective study in 62 patients. Amyloid 18:80–82

94. Yilmaz M, Unsal A, Sokmen M, Harmankaya O, Alkim C, Kabukcuoglu F, Ozagari A (2012) Duodenal biopsy for diagnosis of renal involvement in amyloidosis. Clin Nephrol 77 (2):114–118. doi:10.5414/CN107139

95. Soares SM, Fervenza FC, Lager DJ, Gertz MA, Cosio FG, Leung N (2008) Bleeding complications after transcutaneous kidney biopsy in patients with systemic amyloidosis: single-center experience in 101 patients. Am J Kidney Dis 52(6):1079–1083. doi:10.1053/j.ajkd.2008.05.022

96. Arbustini E, Merlini G, Gavazzi A, Grasso M, Diegoli M, Fasani R, Bellotti V, Marinone G, Morbini P, Dal Bello B (1995) Cardiac immunocyte-derived (AL) amyloidosis: an endomyocardial biopsy study in 11 patients. 130(3 Pt 1):528–536

97. Pellikka PA, Holmes DR Jr, Edwards WD, Nishimura RA, Tajik AJ, Kyle RA (1988) Endomyocardial biopsy in 30 patients with primary amyloidosis and suspected cardiac involvement. Arch Intern Med 148(3):662–666

98. Park MA, Mueller PS, Kyle RA, Larson DR, Plevak MF, Gertz MA (2003) Primary (AL) hepatic amyloidosis—clinical features and natural history in 98 patients. Medicine 82 (5):291–298

99. Lavatelli F, Perlman DH, McComb ME, Theberge R, Seldin DC, Connors LH, Merlini G, Skinner M, Costello CE (2006) A proteomic approach to the study of systemic amyloidoses. Amyloid 13(Suppl. 1):13

100. Vrana JA, Gamez JD, Madden BJ, Theis JD, Bergen HR 3rd, Dogan A (2009) Classification of amyloidosis by laser microdissection and mass spectrometry-based proteomic analysis in clinical biopsy specimens. Blood 114(24):4957–4959

101. Theis JD, Dasari S, Vrana JA, Kurtin PJ, Dogan A (2013) Shotgun-proteomics-based clinical testing for diagnosis and classification of amyloidosis. J Mass Spectrom 48(10):1067–1077. doi:10.1002/jms.3264

102. Arbustini E, Morbini P, Verga L, Concardi M, Porcu E, Pilotto A, Zorzoli I, Garini P, Anesi E, Merlini G (1997) Light and electron microscopy immunohistochemical characterization of amyloid deposits. Amyloid 4(3):157–170

103. Schonland SO, Hegenbart U, Bochtler T, Mangatter A, Hansberg M, Ho AD, Lohse P, Rocken C (2012) Immunohistochemistry in the classification of systemic forms of amyloidosis: a systematic investigation of 117 patients. Blood 119(2):488–493. doi:10.1182/blood-2011-06-358507

104. Palladini G, Russo P, Bosoni T, Verga L, Sarais G, Lavatelli F, Nuvolone M, Obici L, Casarini S, Donadei S, Albertini R, Righetti G, Marini M, Graziani MS, Melzi D'Eril GV, Moratti R, Merlini G (2009) Identification of amyloidogenic light chains requires the combination of serum-free light chain assay with immunofixation of serum and urine. Clin Chem 55(3):499–504

105. Katzmann JA, Kyle RA, Benson J, Larson DR, Snyder MR, Lust JA, Rajkumar SV, Dispenzieri A (2009) Screening panels for detection of monoclonal gammopathies. Clin Chem 55(8):1517–1522

106. Wechalekar AD, Schonland SO, Kastritis E, Gillmore JD, Dimopoulos MA, Lane T, Foli A, Foard D, Milani P, Rannigan L, Hegenbart U, Hawkins PN, Merlini G, Palladini G (2013) A European collaborative study of treatment outcomes in 346 patients with cardiac stage III AL amyloidosis. Blood 121(17):3420–3427. doi:10.1182/blood-2012-12-473066

107. Dispenzieri A, Gertz MA, Kyle RA, Lacy MQ, Burritt MF, Therneau TM, McConnell JP, Litzow MR, Gastineau DA, Tefferi A, Inwards DJ, Micallef IN, Ansell SM, Porrata LF, Elliott MA, Hogan WJ, Rajkumar SV, Fonseca R, Greipp PR, Witzig TE, Lust JA, Zeldenrust SR, Snow DS, Hayman SR, McGregor CG, Jaffe AS (2004) Prognostication of survival using cardiac troponins and N-terminal pro-brain natriuretic peptide in patients with primary systemic amyloidosis undergoing peripheral blood stem cell transplantation. Blood 104(6):1881–1887

108. Palladini G, Foli A, Milani P, Russo P, Albertini R, Lavatelli F, Obici L, Perlini S, Moratti R, Merlini G (2012) Best use of cardiac biomarkers in patients with AL amyloidosis and renal failure. Am J Hematol 87(5):465–471. doi:10.1002/ajh.23141

109. Dispenzieri A, Gertz MA, Kumar SK, Lacy MQ, Kyle RA, Saenger AK, Grogan M, Zeldenrust SR, Hayman SR, Buadi F, Greipp PR, Leung N, Russell SR, Dingli D, Lust JA, Rajkumar SV, Jaffe AS (2014) High sensitivity cardiac troponin T in patients with immunoglobulin light chain amyloidosis. Heart 100(5):383–388. doi:10.1136/heartjnl-2013-304957

110. Wechalekar A, Schonland SO, Kastritis E, Hawkins PN, Dimopoulos MA, Russo P, Lane T, Foli A, Foard D, Milani P, Rannigan L, Hegenbart U, Gillmore JD, Merlini G, Palladini G (2011) European collaborative study of treatment outcomes in 347 patients with systemic AL amyloidosis with Mayo stage III disease. Blood 118(21):454–455

111. Gertz M, Lacy M, Dispenzieri A, Hayman S, Kumar S, Buadi F, Leung N, Litzow M (2008) Troponin T level as an exclusion criterion for stem cell transplantation in light-chain amyloidosis. Leukemia & lymphoma 49(1):36–41

112. Gertz MA, Lacy MQ, Dispenzieri A, Kumar SK, Dingli D, Leung N, Hogan WJ, Buadi FK, Hayman SR (2013) Refinement in patient selection to reduce treatment-related mortality from autologous stem cell transplantation in amyloidosis. Bone Marrow Transplant 48 (4):557–561. doi:10.1038/bmt.2012.170

113. Warsame R, Kumar SK, Gertz MA, Lacy MQ, Buadi FK, Hayman SR, Leung N, Dingli D, Lust JA, Ketterling RP, Lin Y, Russell S, Hwa L, Kapoor P, Go RS, Zeldenrust SR, Kyle RA, Rajkumar SV, Dispenzieri A (2015) Abnormal FISH in patients with immunoglobulin light chain amyloidosis is a risk factor for cardiac involvement and for death. Blood Cancer J 5:e310. doi:10.1038/bcj.2015.34

114. Bochtler T, Hegenbart U, Kunz C, Granzow M, Benner A, Seckinger A, Kimmich C, Goldschmidt H, Ho AD, Hose D, Jauch A, Schonland SO (2015) Translocation t(11;14) with is associated adverse outcome in patients with newly diagnosed AL amyloidosis when treated with bortezomib-based regimens. J Clin Oncol 33(12):1371–1378. doi:10.1200/JCO.2014.57.4947

115. Palladini G, Dispenzieri A, Gertz MA, Kumar S, Wechalekar A, Hawkins PN, Schonland S, Hegenbart U, Comenzo R, Kastritis E, Dimopoulos MA, Jaccard A, Klersy C, Merlini G (2012) New criteria for response to treatment in immunoglobulin light chain amyloidosis based on free light chain measurement and cardiac biomarkers: impact on survival outcomes. J Clinical Oncol: Off J Amer Soc Clinical Oncol 30(36):4541–4549. doi:10.1200/JCO.2011.37.7614

116. Gertz MA, Comenzo R, Falk RH, Fermand JP, Hazenberg BP, Hawkins PN, Merlini G, Moreau P, Ronco P, Sanchorawala V, Sezer O, Solomon A, Grateau G (2005) Definition of organ involvement and treatment response in immunoglobulin light chain amyloidosis (AL): a consensus opinion from the 10(th) international symposium on amyloid and amyloidosis. Am J Hematol 79(4):319–328

117. Merlini G, Comenzo RL, Seldin DC, Wechalekar A, Gertz MA (2014) Immunoglobulin light chain amyloidosis. Expert Rev Hematol 7(1):143–156. doi:10.1586/17474086.2014.858594

118. Perfetti V, Casarini S, Palladini G, Vignarelli MC, Klersy C, Diegoli M, Ascari E, Merlini G (2002) Analysis of V(lambda)-J(lambda) expression in plasma cells from primary (AL) amyloidosis and normal bone marrow identifies 3r (lambdaIII) as a new amyloid-associated germline gene segment. Blood 100(3):948–953. doi:10.1182/blood-2002-01-0114

119. Stevens FJ, Weiss DT, Solomon A (1999) Structural bases of light chain related pathology. In: Zanetti M, Capra JD (eds) The Antibodies, vol 5. Harwood Academic Publishers, Amsterdam, pp 175–208

120. Hurle MR, Helms LR, Li L, Chan W, Wetzel R (1994) A role for destabilizing amino acid replacements in light-chain amyloidosis. Proc Natl Acad Sci USA 91(12):5446–5450

121. Stevens PW, Raffen R, Hanson DK, Deng YL, Berrios-Hammond M, Westholm FA, Murphy C, Eulitz M, Wetzel R, Solomon A et al (1995) Recombinant immunoglobulin variable domains generated from synthetic genes provide a system for in vitro characterization of light-chain amyloid proteins. Protein Sci 4(3):421–432. doi:10.1002/pro.5560040309

122. Connors LH, Jiang Y, Budnik M, Theberge R, Prokaeva T, Bodi KL, Seldin DC, Costello CE, Skinner M (2007) Heterogeneity in primary structure, post-translational modifications, and germline gene usage of nine full-length amyloidogenic kappa1 immunoglobulin light chains. Biochemistry 46(49):14259–14271

123. Randles EG, Thompson JR, Martin DJ, Ramirez-Alvarado M (2009) Structural alterations within native amyloidogenic immunoglobulin light chains. J Mol Biol 389(1):199–210

124. Kaufman GP, Dispenzieri A, Gertz MA, Lacy MQ, Buadi FK, Hayman SR, Leung N, Dingli D, Lust JA, Lin Y, Kapoor P, Go RS, Zeldenrust SR, Kyle RA, Rajkumar SV, Kumar SK (2015) Kinetics of organ response and survival following normalization of the serum free light chain ratio in AL amyloidosis. Am J Hematol 90(3):181–186. doi:10.1002/ajh.23898

125. Trinkaus-Randall V, Walsh MT, Steeves S, Monis G, Connors LH, Skinner M (2005) Cellular response of cardiac fibroblasts to amyloidogenic light chains. Am J Pathol 166 (1):197–208

126. Mishra S, Guan J, Plovie E, Seldin DC, Connors LH, Merlini G, Falk RH, MacRae CA, Liao R (2013) Human amyloidogenic light chain proteins result in cardiac dysfunction, cell death, and early mortality in zebrafish. Am J Physiol Heart Circ Physiol 305(1):H95–103. doi:10.1152/ajpheart.00186.2013

127. Pepys MB, Herbert J, Hutchinson WL, Tennent GA, Lachmann HJ, Gallimore JR, Lovat LB, Bartfai T, Alanine A, Hertel C, Hoffmann T, Jakob-Roetne R, Norcross RD, Kemp JA, Yamamura K, Suzuki M, Taylor GW, Murray S, Thompson D, Purvis A, Kolstoe S, Wood SP, Hawkins PN (2002) Targeted pharmacological depletion of serum amyloid P component for treatment of human amyloidosis. Nature 417(6886):254–259

128. Bodin K, Ellmerich S, Kahan MC, Tennent GA, Loesch A, Gilbertson JA, Hutchinson WL, Mangione PP, Gallimore JR, Millar DJ, Minogue S, Dhillon AP, Taylor GW, Bradwell AR, Petrie A, Gillmore JD, Bellotti V, Botto M, Hawkins PN, Pepys MB (2010) Antibodies to human serum amyloid P component eliminate visceral amyloid deposits. Nature 468 (7320):93–97

129. Wall JS, Kennel SJ, Stuckey AC, Long MJ, Townsend DW, Smith GT, Wells KJ, Fu Y, Stabin MG, Weiss DT, Solomon A (2010) Radioimmunodetection of amyloid deposits in patients with AL amyloidosis. Blood 116(13):2241–2244. doi:10.1182/blood-2010-03-273797

130. Jaccard A, Moreau P, Leblond V, Leleu X, Benboubker L, Hermine O, Recher C, Asli B, Lioure B, Royer B, Jardin F, Bridoux F, Grosbois B, Jaubert J, Piette JC, Ronco P, Quet F, Cogne M, Fermand JP (2007) High-dose melphalan versus melphalan plus dexamethasone for AL amyloidosis. New Engl J Med 357(11):1083–1093

131. Gertz MA, Lacy MQ, Dispenzieri A, Hayman SR, Kumar SK, Leung N, Gastineau DA (2007) Effect of hematologic response on outcome of patients undergoing transplantation for primary amyloidosis: importance of achieving a complete response. Haematologica 92 (10):1415–1418

132. Sanchorawala V, Skinner M, Quillen K, Finn KT, Doros G, Seldin DC (2007) Long-term outcome of patients with AL amyloidosis treated with high-dose melphalan and stem-cell transplantation. Blood 110(10):3561–3563

133. Palladini G, Russo P, Nuvolone M, Lavatelli F, Perfetti V, Obici L, Merlini G (2007) Treatment with oral melphalan plus dexamethasone produces long-term remissions in AL amyloidosis. Blood 110(2):787–788

134. Dispenzieri A, Buadi F, Kumar SK, Reeder C, etc. (2015) The treatment of AL amyloidosis: Mayo stratification of myeloma and risk-adapted Therapy (mSMART) Consensus Statement. Mayo Clin Proc 90(8):1054–1081

135. Kyle RA, Gertz MA, Greipp PR, Witzig TE, Lust JA, Lacy MQ, Therneau TM (1997) A trial of three regimens for primary amyloidosis: colchicine alone, melphalan and prednisone, and melphalan, prednisone, and colchicine. N Engl J Med 336(17):1202–1207

136. Skinner M, Anderson J, Simms R, Falk R, Wang M, Libbey C, Jones LA, Cohen AS (1996) Treatment of 100 patients with primary amyloidosis: a randomized trial of melphalan, prednisone, and colchicine versus colchicine only. Am J Med 100(3):290–298

137. Gertz MA, Kyle RA, Greipp PR (1991) Response rates and survival in primary systemic amyloidosis. Blood 77(2):257–262

138. Gertz MA, Lacy MQ, Lust JA, Greipp PR, Witzig TE, Kyle RA (1999) Prospective randomized trial of melphalan and prednisone versus vincristine, carmustine, melphalan, cyclophosphamide, and prednisone in the treatment of primary systemic amyloidosis. J Clin Oncol 17(1):262–267

139. Palladini G, Perfetti V, Obici L, Caccialanza R, Semino A, Adami F, Cavallero G, Rustichelli R, Virga G, Merlini G (2004) Association of melphalan and high-dose dexamethasone is effective and well tolerated in patients with AL (primary) amyloidosis who are ineligible for stem cell transplantation. Blood 103(8):2936–2938

140. Kyle RA, Greipp PR, Garton JP, Gertz MA (1985) Primary systemic amyloidosis. Comparison of melphalan/prednisone versus colchicine. Am J Med 79(6):708–716

141. Kyle RA, Greipp PR (1978) Primary systemic amyloidosis: comparison of melphalan and prednisone versus placebo. Blood 52(4):818–827

142. Lachmann HJ, Gallimore R, Gillmore JD, Carr-Smith HD, Bradwell AR, Pepys MB, Hawkins PN (2003) Outcome in systemic AL amyloidosis in relation to changes in concentration of circulating free immunoglobulin light chains following chemotherapy. Br J Haematol 122(1):78–84

143. Gertz MA, Lacy MQ, Lust JA, Greipp PR, Witzig TE, Kyle RA (1999) Phase II trial of high-dose dexamethasone for previously treated immunoglobulin light-chain amyloidosis. Am J Hematol 61(2):115–119

144. Gertz MA, Lacy MQ, Lust JA, Greipp PR, Witzig TE, Kyle RA (1999) Phase II trial of high-dose dexamethasone for untreated patients with primary systemic amyloidosis. Med Oncol 16(2):104–109

145. Palladini G, Anesi E, Perfetti V, Obici L, Invernizzi R, Balduini C, Ascari E, Merlini G (2001) A modified high-dose dexamethasone regimen for primary systemic (AL) amyloidosis. Br J Haematol 113(4):1044–1046

146. Dhodapkar MV, Hussein MA, Rasmussen E, Solomon A, Larson RA, Crowley JJ, Barlogie B (2004) Clinical efficacy of high-dose dexamethasone with maintenance dexamethasone/alpha interferon in patients with primary systemic amyloidosis: results of United States Intergroup Trial Southwest Oncology Group (SWOG) S9628. Blood 104 (12):3520–3526

147. Levy Y, Belghiti-Deprez D, Sobel A (1988) Treatment of AL amyloidosis without myeloma. Ann Med Interne 139(3):190–193

148. Wardley AM, Jayson GC, Goldsmith DJ, Venning MC, Ackrill P, Scarffe JH (1998) The treatment of nephrotic syndrome caused by primary (light chain) amyloid with vincristine, doxorubicin and dexamethasone. Br J Cancer 78(6):774–776

149. van Gameren I, Hazenberg BP, Jager PL, Smit JW, Vellenga E (2002) AL amyloidosis treated with induction chemotherapy with VAD followed by high dose melphalan and autologous stem cell transplantation. Amyloid 9(3):165–174

150. Ichida M, Imagawa S, Ohmine K, Komatsu N, Hatake K, Ozawa K, Miura Y (2000) Successful treatment of multiple myeloma–associated amyloidosis by interferon-alpha, dimethyl sulfoxide, and VAD (vincristine, adriamycin, and dexamethasone). Int J Hematol 72(4):491–493

151. Gono T, Matsuda M, Shimojima Y, Ishii W, Koyama J, Sakashita K, Koike K, Hoshii Y, Ikeda S (2004) VAD with or without subsequent high-dose melphalan followed by autologous stem cell support in AL amyloidosis: Japanese experience and criteria for patient selection. Amyloid 11(4):245–256

152. Palladini G, Milani P, Foli A, Obici L, Lavatelli F, Nuvolone M, Caccialanza R, Perlini S, Merlini G (2014) Oral melphalan and dexamethasone grants extended survival with minimal toxicity in AL amyloidosis: long-term results of a risk-adapted approach. Haematologica 99 (4):743–750. doi:10.3324/haematol.2013.095463

153. Lebovic D, Hoffman J, Levine BM, Hassoun H, Landau H, Goldsmith Y, Maurer MS, Steingart RM, Cohen AD, Comenzo RL (2008) Predictors of survival in patients with systemic light-chain amyloidosis and cardiac involvement initially ineligible for stem cell transplantation and treated with oral melphalan and dexamethasone. Br J Haematol 143 (3):369–373

154. Dietrich S, Schonland SO, Benner A, Bochtler T, Kristen AV, Beimler J, Hund E, Zorn M, Goldschmidt H, Ho AD, Hegenbart U (2010) Treatment with intravenous melphalan and dexamethasone is not able to overcome the poor prognosis of patients with newly diagnosed systemic light chain amyloidosis and severe cardiac involvement. Blood 116(4):522–528. doi:10.1182/blood-2009-11-253237

155. Sanchorawala V, Seldin DC, Berk JL, Sloan JM, Doros G, Skinner M (2010) Oral cyclic melphalan and dexamethasone for patients with AL amyloidosis. Clin Lymphoma Myeloma Leuk 10(6):469–472. doi:10.3816/CLML.2010.n.081

156. Seldin DC, Choufani EB, Dember LM, Wiesman JF, Berk JL, Falk RH, O'Hara C, Fennessey S, Finn KT, Wright DG, Skinner M, Sanchorawala V (2003) Tolerability and efficacy of thalidomide for the treatment of patients with light cahin-associated (AL) amyloidosis. Clinical Lymphoma 3(4):241–246

157. Palladini G, Perfetti V, Perlini S, Obici L, Lavatelli F, Caccialanza R, Invernizzi R, Comotti B, Merlini G (2005) The combination of thalidomide and intermediate-dose dexamethasone is an effective but toxic treatment for patients with primary amyloidosis (AL). Blood 105(7):2949–2951

158. Dispenzieri A, Lacy MQ, Rajkumar SV, Geyer S, Witzig TE, Fonseca R, Lust JA, Greipp PR, Kyle RA, Gertz MA (2003) Poor tolerance to high doses of thalidomide in patients with primary systemic amyloidosis. Amyloid 10(4):257–261

159. Dispenzieri A, Lacy MQ, Geyer SM, Greipp PR, Witzig TE, Lust JA, Zeldenrust SR, Rajkumar SV, Kyle RA, Fonseca R, Gertz MA (2004) Low dose single agent thalidomide is tolerated in patients with primary systemic amyloidosis, but responses are limited. ASH Annual Meeting Abstracts 104(11):4920

160. Wechalekar AD, Goodman HJ, Lachmann HJ, Offer M, Hawkins PN, Gillmore JD (2007) Safety and efficacy of risk-adapted cyclophosphamide, thalidomide, and dexamethasone in systemic AL amyloidosis. Blood 109(2):457–464

161. Palladini G, Russo P, Lavatelli F, Nuvolone M, Albertini R, Bosoni T, Perfetti V, Obici L, Perlini S, Moratti R, Merlini G (2009) Treatment of patients with advanced cardiac AL amyloidosis with oral melphalan, dexamethasone, and thalidomide. Ann Hematol 88(4):347–350

162. Dispenzieri A, Lacy MQ, Zeldenrust SR, Hayman SR, Kumar SK, Geyer SM, Lust JA, Allred JB, Witzig TE, Rajkumar SV, Greipp PR, Russell SJ, Kabat B, Gertz MA (2007) The activity of lenalidomide with or without dexamethasone in patients with primary systemic amyloidosis. Blood 109(2):465–470

163. Sanchorawala V, Wright DG, Rosenzweig M, Finn KT, Fennessey S, Zeldis JB, Skinner M, Seldin DC (2007) Lenalidomide and dexamethasone in the treatment of AL amyloidosis: results of a phase 2 trial. Blood 109(2):492–496

164. Palladini G, Russo P, Foli A, Milani P, Lavatelli F, Obici L, Nuvolone M, Brugnatelli S, Invernizzi R, Merlini G (2012) Salvage therapy with lenalidomide and dexamethasone in

patients with advanced AL amyloidosis refractory to melphalan, bortezomib, and thalidomide. Ann Hematol 91(1):89–92. doi:10.1007/s00277-011-1244-x

165. Moreau P, Jaccard A, Benboubker L, Royer B, Leleu X, Bridoux F, Salles G, Leblond V, Roussel M, Alakl M, Hermine O, Planche L, Harousseau JL, Fermand JP (2010) Lenalidomide in combination with melphalan and dexamethasone in patients with newly diagnosed AL amyloidosis: a multicenter phase 1/2 dose-escalation study. Blood 116 (23):4777–4782

166. Dinner S, Witteles W, Afghahi A, Witteles R, Arai S, Lafayette R, Schrier S, Liedtke M (2013) Lenalidomide, melphalan and dexamethasone in an immunoglobulin light chain amyloidosis patient population with high rates of advanced cardiac involvement. Haematologica 98(10):1593–1599. doi:10.3324/haematol.2013.084574

167. Sanchorawala V, Patel JM, Sloan JM, Shelton AC, Zeldis JB, Seldin DC (2013) Melphalan, lenalidomide and dexamethasone for the treatment of immunoglobulin light chain amyloidosis: results of a phase II trial. Haematologica 98(5):789–792. doi:10.3324/haematol.2012.075192

168. Palladini G, Russo P, Milani P, Foli A, Lavatelli F, Nuvolone M, Perlini S, Merlini G (2013) A phase II trial of cyclophosphamide, lenalidomide and dexamethasone in previously treated patients with AL amyloidosis. Haematologica 98(3):433–436. doi:10.3324/haematol.2012.073593

169. Kumar SK, Hayman SR, Buadi FK, Roy V, Lacy MQ, Gertz MA, Allred J, Laumann KM, Bergsagel LP, Dingli D, Mikhael JR, Reeder CB, Stewart AK, Zeldenrust SR, Greipp PR, Lust JA, Fonseca R, Russell SJ, Rajkumar SV, Dispenzieri A (2012) Lenalidomide, cyclophosphamide, and dexamethasone (CRd) for light-chain amyloidosis: long-term results from a phase 2 trial. Blood 119(21):4860–4867. doi:10.1182/blood-2012-01-407791

170. Kastritis E, Terpos E, Roussou M, Gavriatopoulou M, Pamboukas C, Boletis I, Marinaki S, Apostolou T, Nikitas N, Gkortzolidis G, Michalis E, Delimpasi S, Dimopoulos MA (2012) A phase 1/2 study of lenalidomide with low-dose oral cyclophosphamide and low-dose dexamethasone (RdC) in AL amyloidosis. Blood 119(23):5384–5390. doi:10.1182/blood-2011-12-396903

171. Dispenzieri A, Buadi F, Laumann K, LaPlant B, Hayman SR, Kumar SK, Dingli D, Zeldenrust SR, Mikhael JR, Hall R, Rajkumar SV, Reeder C, Fonseca R, Bergsagel PL, Stewart AK, Roy V, Witzig TE, Lust JA, Russell SJ, Gertz MA, Lacy MQ (2012) Activity of pomalidomide in patients with immunoglobulin light-chain amyloidosis. Blood 119 (23):5397–5404. doi:10.1182/blood-2012-02-413161

172. Dispenzieri A, Lacy MQ, Kyle RA, Therneau TM, Larson DR, Rajkumar SV, Fonseca R, Greipp PR, Witzig TE, Lust JA, Gertz MA (2001) Eligibility for hematopoietic stem-cell transplantation for primary systemic amyloidosis is a favorable prognostic factor for survival. J Clinical Oncol: Off J Amer Soc Clinical Oncol 19(14):3350–3356

173. Gertz MA, Kyle RA (1990) Acute leukemia and cytogenetic abnormalities complicating melphalan treatment of primary systemic amyloidosis. Arch Intern Med 150(3):629–633

174. Gillmore J, Cocks K, Gibbs SDJ, Sattianayagam PT, Lane T, Lachmann H, Schey S, Cavenagh JD, Oakervee H, Morgan GJ, Mehta AB, Bourne S, Skinner E, Booth G, Hawkins PN, Wechalekar AD (2009) Cyclophosphamide, thalidomide and dexamethasone (CTD) versus melphalan plus dexamethasone (MD) for newly-diagnosed systemic AL amyloidosis—results from the UK amyloidosis treatment trial. ASH Annual Meeting Abstracts 114(22):2869

175. Kumar SK, Gertz MA, Lacy MQ, Dingli D, Hayman SR, Buadi FK, Short-Detweiler K, Zeldenrust SR, Leung N, Greipp PR, Lust JA, Russell SJ, Kyle RA, Rajkumar SV, Dispenzieri A (2011) Recent improvements in survival in primary systemic amyloidosis and the importance of an early mortality risk score. Mayo Clin Proc 86(1):12–18. doi:10.4065/mcp.2010.0480

176. Dispenzieri A, Dingli D, Kumar SK, Rajkumar SV, Lacy MQ, Hayman S, Buadi F, Zeldenrust S, Leung N, Detweiler-Short K, Lust JA, Russell SJ, Kyle RA, Gertz MA (2010)

Discordance between serum cardiac biomarker and immunoglobulin-free light-chain response in patients with immunoglobulin light-chain amyloidosis treated with immune modulatory drugs. Am J Hematol 85(10):757–759

177. Tapan U, Seldin DC, Finn KT, Fennessey S, Shelton A, Zeldis JB, Sanchorawala V (2010) Increases in B-type natriuretic peptide (BNP) during treatment with lenalidomide in AL amyloidosis. Blood 116(23):5071–5072. doi:10.1182/blood-2010-09-305136

178. Specter R, Sanchorawala V, Seldin DC, Shelton A, Fennessey S, Finn KT, Zeldis JB, Dember LM (2011) Kidney dysfunction during lenalidomide treatment for AL amyloidosis. Nephrol Dial Transplant 26(3):881–886. doi:10.1093/ndt/gfq482

179. Huang X, Wang Q, Chen W, Zeng C, Chen Z, Gong D, Zhang H, Liu Z (2014) Induction therapy with bortezomib and dexamethasone followed by autologous stem cell transplantation versus autologous stem cell transplantation alone in the treatment of renal AL amyloidosis: a randomized controlled trial. BMC Med 12:2. doi:10.1186/1741-7015-12-2

180. Kastritis E, Leleu X, Arrnulf B, Zamagni E, Mollee P, Cibeira MT, Schonland S, Moreau P, Hajek R, Jaccard A, Nicolas-Virelizier E, Filshie R, Augustson B, Mateos MV, Milani P, Dimopoulos M, Hachulla E, Fermand JP, Foli A, Palumbo A, Sonneveld P, Johnsen E, Merlini G, Palladini G (2014) A randomized phase III trial of melphalan and dexamethasone (MDex) versus bortezomib, melphalan and dexamethasone (BMDex) for untreated patients with AL amyloidosis. Blood 124(21):35

181. Reece DE, Hegenbart U, Sanchorawala V, Merlini G, Palladini G, Blade J, Fermand JP, Hassoun H, Heffner L, Vescio RA, Liu K, Enny C, Esseltine DL, van de Velde H, Cakana A, Comenzo RL (2011) Efficacy and safety of once-weekly and twice-weekly bortezomib in patients with relapsed systemic AL amyloidosis: results of a phase 1/2 study. Blood 118 (4):865–873. doi:10.1182/blood-2011-02-334227

182. Reece DE, Sanchorawala V, Hegenbart U, Merlini G, Palladini G, Fermand JP, Vescio RA, Liu X, Elsayed YA, Cakana A, Comenzo RL (2009) Weekly and twice-weekly bortezomib in patients with systemic AL amyloidosis: results of a phase 1 dose-escalation study. Blood 114(8):1489–1497

183. Reece DE, Hegenbart U, Sanchorawala V, Merlini G, Palladini G, Blade J, Fermand JP, Hassoun H, Heffner L, Kukreti V, Vescio RA, Pei L, Enny C, Esselltine DL, van de Velde H, Cakana A, Comenzo RL (2014) Long-term follow-up from a phase 1/2 study of single-agent bortezomib in relapsed systemic AL amyloidosis. Blood 124(16):2498–2506. doi:10.1182/blood-2014-04-568329

184. Palladini G, Foli A, Russo P, Milani P, Obici L, Lavatelli F, Merlini G (2011) Treatment of IgM-associated AL amyloidosis with the combination of rituximab, bortezomib, and dexamethasone. Clin Lymphoma Myeloma Leuk 11(1):143–145. doi:10.3816/CLML.2011. n.033

185. Gasparetto C, Sanchorawala V, Snyder RM, Matous J, Terebelo HR, Janakiraman N, Mapara MY, Webb C, Abrams J, Zonder JA (2010) Use of melphalan (M)/dexamethasone (D)/bortezomib in AL amyloidosis. J Clin Oncol (Meeting Abstracts) 28 (15_suppl):8024-

186. Kastritis E, Wechalekar AD, Dimopoulos MA, Merlini G, Hawkins PN, Perfetti V, Gillmore JD, Palladini G (2010) Bortezomib with or without dexamethasone in primary systemic (light chain) amyloidosis. J Clin Oncol 28(6):1031–1037

187. Lamm W, Willenbacher W, Lang A, Zojer N, Muldur E, Ludwig H, Schauer-Stalzer B, Zielinski CC, Drach J (2011) Efficacy of the combination of bortezomib and dexamethasone in systemic AL amyloidosis. Ann Hematol 90(2):201–206. doi:10.1007/s00277-010-1062-6

188. Palladini G, Milani P, Foli A, Vidus Rosin M, Basset M, Lavatelli F, Nuvolone M, Obici L, Perlini S, Merlini G (2014) Melphalan and dexamethasone with or without bortezomib in newly diagnosed AL amyloidosis: a matched case-control study on 174 patients. Leukemia 28(12):2311–2316. doi:10.1038/leu.2014.227

189. Venner CP, Gillmore JD, Sachchithanantham S, Mahmood S, Lane T, Foard D, Rannigan L, Gibbs SD, Pinney JH, Whelan CJ, Lachmann HJ, Hawkins PN, Wechalekar AD (2014) A

matched comparison of cyclophosphamide, bortezomib and dexamethasone (CVD) versus risk-adapted cyclophosphamide, thalidomide and dexamethasone (CTD) in AL amyloidosis. Leukemia 28(12):2304–2310. doi:10.1038/leu.2014.218

190. Mikhael JR, Schuster SR, Jimenez-Zepeda VH, Bello N, Spong J, Reeder CB, Stewart AK, Bergsagel PL, Fonseca R (2012) Cyclophosphamide-bortezomib-dexamethasone (CyBorD) produces rapid and complete hematologic response in patients with AL amyloidosis. Blood 119(19):4391–4394. doi:10.1182/blood-2011-11-390930

191. Venner CP, Lane T, Foard D, Rannigan L, Gibbs SD, Pinney JH, Whelan CJ, Lachmann HJ, Gillmore JD, Hawkins PN, Wechalekar AD (2012) Cyclophosphamide, bortezomib, and dexamethasone therapy in AL amyloidosis is associated with high clonal response rates and prolonged progression-free survival. Blood 119(19):4387–4390. doi:10.1182/blood-2011-10-388462

192. Jaccard A, Comenzo RL, Hari P, Hawkins PN, Roussel M, Morel P, Macro M, Pellegrin JL, Lazaro E, Mohty D, Mercie P, Decaux O, Gillmore J, Lavergne D, Bridoux F, Wechalekar AD, Venner CP (2014) Efficacy of bortezomib, cyclophosphamide and dexamethasone in treatment-naive patients with high-risk cardiac AL amyloidosis (Mayo Clinic stage III). Haematologica 99(9):1479–1485. doi:10.3324/haematol.2014.104109

193. Lee JY, Lim SH, Kim SJ, Lee GY, Lee JE, Choi JO, Kim JS, Kim HJ, Lee SY, Min JH, Jeon ES, Kim K (2014) Bortezomib, melphalan, and prednisolone combination chemotherapy for newly diagnosed light chain (AL) amyloidosis. Amyloid: Int J Exp Clinical Investigation: Off J Int Soc Amyloidosis 21(4):261–266. doi:10.3109/13506129.2014.960560

194. Wechalekar AD, Schonland SO, Kastritis E, Gillmore JD, Dimopoulos MA, Lane T, Foli A, Foard D, Milani P, Rannigan L, Hegenbart U, Hawkins PN, Merlini G, Palladini G (2013) A European collaborative study of treatment outcomes in 346 patients with cardiac stage III AL amyloidosis. Blood 121(17):3420–3427. doi:10.1182/blood-2012-12-473066

195. Gertz MA, Kyle RA (2003) Amyloidosis with IgM monoclonal gammopathies. Semin Oncol 30(2):325–328

196. Sanchorawala V, Blanchard E, Seldin DC, O'Hara C, Skinner M, Wright DG (2006) AL amyloidosis associated with B-cell lymphoproliferative disorders: frequency and treatment outcomes. Am J Hematol 81(9):692–695

197. Wechalekar AD, Lachmann HJ, Goodman HJ, Bradwell A, Hawkins PN, Gillmore JD (2008) AL amyloidosis associated with IgM paraproteinemia: clinical profile and treatment outcome. Blood 112(10):4009–4016. doi:10.1182/blood-2008-02-138156

198. Kikukawa Y, Yuki H, Hirata S, Ide K, Nakata H, Miyakawa T, Matsuno N, Nosaka K, Yonemura Y, Kawaguchi T, Hata H, Mitsuya H, Okuno Y (2015) Combined use of bortezomib, cyclophosphamide, and dexamethasone induces favorable hematological and organ responses in Japanese patients with amyloid light-chain amyloidosis: a single-institution retrospective study. Int J Hematol 101(2):133–139. doi:10.1007/s12185-014-1705-9

199. Comenzo RL, Vosburgh E, Falk RH, Sanchorawala V, Reisinger J, Dubrey S, Dember LM, Berk JL, Akpek G, LaValley M, O'Hara C, Arkin CF, Wright DG, Skinner M (1998) Dose-intensive melphalan with blood stem-cell support for the treatment of AL (amyloid light-chain) amyloidosis: survival and responses in 25 patients. Blood 91(10):3662–3670

200. Dispenzieri A, Seenithamby K, Lacy MQ, Kumar SK, Buadi FK, Hayman SR, Dingli D, Litzow MR, Gastineau DA, Inwards DJ, Micallef IN, Ansell SM, Johnston PB, Porrata LF, Patnaik MM, Hogan WJ, Gertz MA (2013) Patients with immunoglobulin light chain amyloidosis undergoing autologous stem cell transplantation have superior outcomes compared with patients with multiple myeloma: a retrospective review from a tertiary referral center. Bone Marrow Transplant 48(10):1302–1307. doi:10.1038/bmt.2013.53

201. Cibeira MT, Sanchorawala V, Seldin DC, Quillen K, Berk JL, Dember LM, Segal A, Ruberg F, Meier-Ewert H, Andrea NT, Sloan JM, Finn KT, Doros G, Blade J, Skinner M (2011) Outcome of AL amyloidosis after high-dose melphalan and autologous stem cell

transplantation: long-term results in a series of 421 patients. Blood 118(16):4346–4352. doi:10.1182/blood-2011-01-330738

202. Moreau P, Milpied N, de Faucal P, Petit T, Herbouiller P, Bataille R, Harousseau JL (1996) High-dose melphalan and autologous bone marrow transplantation for systemic AL amyloidosis with cardiac involvement. Blood 87(7):3063–3064

203. Skinner M, Sanchorawala V, Seldin DC, Dember LM, Falk RH, Berk JL, Anderson JJ, O'Hara C, Finn KT, Libbey CA, Wiesman J, Quillen K, Swan N, Wright DG (2004) High-dose melphalan and autologous stem-cell transplantation in patients with AL amyloidosis: an 8-year study. Ann Intern Med 140(2):85–93

204. Vesole DH, Perez WS, Akasheh M, Boudreau C, Reece DE, Bredeson CN (2006) High-dose therapy and autologous hematopoietic stem cell transplantation for patients with primary systemic amyloidosis: a Center for International Blood and Marrow Transplant Research Study. Mayo Clin Proc 81(7):880–888

205. Comenzo RL, Gertz MA (2002) Autologous stem cell transplantation for primary systemic amyloidosis. Blood 99(12):4276–4282

206. D'Souza A, Dispenzieri A, Wirk B, Zhang MJ, Huang J, Gertz MA, Kyle RA, Kumar SK, Comenzo R, Gale RP, Lazarus HM, Savani B, Cornell R, Weiss B, Vogl DT, Freytes CO, Scott EC, Landau H, Moreb J, Costa L, Ramathan M, Callander NS, Kamble RT, Olsson R, Ganguly S, Nishihori T, Kindwall-Keller T, Wood W, Mark T, Hari P (Submitted) Improved outcomes after autologous hematopoietic cell transplantation for light chain amyloidosis: a Center for International Blood and Marrow Transplant Research Study. J Clinical Oncol

207. Moreau P, Leblond V, Bourquelot P, Facon T, Huynh A, Caillot D, Hermine O, Attal M, Hamidou M, Nedellec G, Ferrant A, Audhuy B, Bataille R, Milpied N, Harousseau JL (1998) Prognostic factors for survival and response after high-dose therapy and autologous stem cell transplantation in systemic AL amyloidosis: a report on 21 patients. Br J Haematol 101 (4):766–769

208. Goodman HJ, Gillmore JD, Lachmann HJ, Wechalekar AD, Bradwell AR, Hawkins PN (2006) Outcome of autologous stem cell transplantation for AL amyloidosis in the UK. Br J Haematol 134(4):417–425

209. Gertz MA, Blood E, Vesole DH, Abonour R, Lazarus HM, Greipp PR (2004) A multicenter phase 2 trial of stem cell transplantation for immunoglobulin light-chain amyloidosis (E4A97): an Eastern Cooperative Oncology Group Study. Bone Marrow Transplant 34 (2):149–154

210. Mollee PN, Wechalekar AD, Pereira DL, Franke N, Reece D, Chen C, Stewart AK (2004) Autologous stem cell transplantation in primary systemic amyloidosis: the impact of selection criteria on outcome. Bone Marrow Transplant 33(3):271–277. doi:10.1038/sj.bmt. 1704344

211. Perz JB, Schonland SO, Hundemer M, Kristen AV, Dengler TJ, Zeier M, Linke RP, Ho AD, Goldschmidt H (2004) High-dose melphalan with autologous stem cell transplantation after VAD induction chemotherapy for treatment of amyloid light chain amyloidosis: a single centre prospective phase II study. Br J Haematol 127(5):543–551. doi:10.1111/j.1365-2141. 2004.05232.x

212. Perfetti V, Siena S, Palladini G, Bregni M, Di Nicola M, Obici L, Magni M, Brunetti L, Gianni AM, Merlini G (2006) Long-term results of a risk-adapted approach to melphalan conditioning in autologous peripheral blood stem cell transplantation for primary (AL) amyloidosis. Haematologica 91(12):1635–1643

213. Cohen AD, Zhou P, Chou J, Teruya-Feldstein J, Reich L, Hassoun H, Levine B, Filippa DA, Riedel E, Kewalramani T, Stubblefield MD, Fleisher M, Nimer S, Comenzo RL (2007) Risk-adapted autologous stem cell transplantation with adjuvant dexamethasone ± thalidomide for systemic light-chain amyloidosis: results of a phase II trial. Br J Haematol 139(2):224–233

214. Landau H, Hassoun H, Rosenzweig MA, Maurer M, Liu J, Flombaum C, Bello C, Hoover E, Riedel E, Giralt S, Comenzo RL (2013) Bortezomib and dexamethasone consolidation

following risk-adapted melphalan and stem cell transplantation for patients with newly diagnosed light-chain amyloidosis. Leukemia 27(4):823–828. doi:10.1038/leu.2012.274

215. Kim SJ, Lee GY, Jang HR, Choi JO, Kim JS, Kim HJ, Lee SY, Min JH, Jeon ES, Kim K (2013) Autologous stem cell transplantation in light-chain amyloidosis patients: a single-center experience in Korea. Amyloid 20(4):204–211. doi:10.3109/13506129.2013. 824417

216. D'Souza A, Wirk B, Zhang MJ, Huang J, Krishnan A, Mark T, Gasparetto CJ, Hari P (2014) Improved outcomes of autologous hematopoietic cell transplantation (AHCT) for light chain (AL) amyloidosis: a Center for International Blood and Marrow Transplant Registry (CIBMTR) Study. Blood 124(21):193

217. Fadia A, Casserly LF, Sanchorawala V, Seldin DC, Wright DG, Skinner M, Dember LM (2003) Incidence and outcome of acute renal failure complicating autologous stem cell transplantation for AL amyloidosis. Kidney Int 63(5):1868–1873

218. Mereuta OM, Theis JD, Vrana JA, Law ME, Grogg KL, Dasari S, Chandan VS, Wu TT, Jimenez-Zepeda VH, Fonseca R, Dispenzieri A, Kurtin PJ, Dogan A (2014) Leukocyte cell-derived chemotaxin 2 (LECT2)-associated amyloidosis is a frequent cause of hepatic amyloidosis in the United States. Blood 123(10):1479–1482. doi:10.1182/blood-2013-07-517938

219. Huang X, Wang Q, Jiang S, Chen W, Zeng C, Liu Z (2015) The clinical features and outcomes of systemic AL amyloidosis: a cohort of 231 Chinese patients. Clin Kidney J 8 (1):120–126. doi:10.1093/ckj/sfu117

220. Sanchorawala V, Wright DG, Seldin DC, Falk RH, Finn KT, Dember LM, Berk JL, Quillen K, Anderson JJ, Comenzo RL, Skinner M (2004) High-dose intravenous melphalan and autologous stem cell transplantation as initial therapy or following two cycles of oral chemotherapy for the treatment of AL amyloidosis: results of a prospective randomized trial. Bone Marrow Transplant 33(4):381–388

221. Sanchorawala V, Brauneis D, Shelton AC, Lo S, Sun F, Sloan JM, Quillen K, Seldin DC (In press) Induction therapy with bortezomib followed by bortezomib-high dose melphalan and stem cell transplantation for AL amyloidosis: results of a prospective clinical trial. Biol Blood Marrow Transplant. doi:10.1016/j.bbmt.2015.04.001

222. Sanchorawala V, Wright DG, Quillen K, Finn KT, Dember LM, Berk JL, Doros G, Fisher C, Skinner M, Seldin DC (2007) Tandem cycles of high-dose melphalan and autologous stem cell transplantation increases the response rate in AL amyloidosis. Bone Marrow Transplant 40(6):557–562. doi:10.1038/sj.bmt.1705746

223. Sanchorawala V, Hoering A, Seldin DC, Finn KT, Fennessey SA, Sexton R, Mattar B, Safah HF, Holmberg LA, Dean RM, Orlowski RZ, Barlogie B (2013) Modified high-dose melphalan and autologous SCT for AL amyloidosis or high-risk myeloma: analysis of SWOG trial S0115. Bone Marrow Transplant 48(12):1537–1542. doi:10.1038/bmt.2013.98

224. Guillaume B, Straetmans N, Jadoul M, Cosyns JP, Ferrant A (1997) Allogeneic bone marrow transplantation for AL amyloidosis. Bone Marrow Transplant 20(10):907–908

225. Gillmore JD, Davies J, Iqbal A, Madhoo S, Russell NH, Hawkins PN (1998) Allogeneic bone marrow transplantation for systemic AL amyloidosis. Br J Haematol 100(1):226–228

226. Schonland SO, Lokhorst H, Buzyn A, Leblond V, Hegenbart U, Bandini G, Campbell A, Carreras E, Ferrant A, Grommisch L, Jacobs P, Kroger N, La Nasa G, Russell N, Zachee P, Goldschmidt H, Iacobelli S, Niederwieser D, Gahrton G (2006) Allogeneic and syngeneic hematopoietic cell transplantation in patients with amyloid light-chain amyloidosis: a report from the European Group for Blood and Marrow Transplantation. Blood 107(6):2578–2584

227. Dubrey S, Pollak A, Skinner M, Falk RH (1995) Atrial thrombi occurring during sinus rhythm in cardiac amyloidosis: evidence for atrial electromechanical dissociation. Br Heart J 74(5):541–544

228. Feng D, Syed IS, Martinez M, Oh JK, Jaffe AS, Grogan M, Edwards WD, Gertz MA, Klarich KW (2009) Intracardiac thrombosis and anticoagulation therapy in cardiac amyloidosis. Circulation 119(18):2490–2497

229. Rubinow A, Skinner M, Cohen AS (1981) Digoxin sensitivity in amyloid cardiomyopathy. Circulation 63(6):1285–1288
230. Gertz MA, Falk RH, Skinner M, Cohen AS, Kyle RA (1985) Worsening of congestive heart failure in amyloid heart disease treated by calcium channel-blocking agents. Am J Cardiol 55 (13 Pt 1):1645
231. Palladini G, Malamani G, Co F, Pistorio A, Recusani F, Anesi E, Garini P, Merlini G (2001) Holter monitoring in AL amyloidosis: prognostic implications. Pacing Clin Electrophysiol 24 (8 Pt 1):1228–1233
232. Kristen AV, Dengler TJ, Hegenbart U, Schonland SO, Goldschmidt H, Sack FU, Voss F, Becker R, Katus HA, Bauer A (2008) Prophylactic implantation of cardioverter-defibrillator in patients with severe cardiac amyloidosis and high risk for sudden cardiac death. Heart Rhythm 5(2):235–240
233. Dhoble A, Khasnis A, Olomu A, Thakur R (2009) Cardiac amyloidosis treated with an implantable cardioverter defibrillator and subcutaneous array lead system: report of a case and literature review. Clin Cardiol 32(8):E63–65. doi:10.1002/clc.20389
234. Yaoita H, Iwai-Takano M, Ogawa K, Suzuki H, Akutsu K, Noji H, Kamiyama Y, Kimura S, Ohtake H, Ishibashi T, Maruyama Y (2008) Attenuation of diastolic heart failure and life-threatening ventricular tachyarrhythmia after peripheral blood stem cell transplantation combined with cardioverter-defibrillator implantation in myeloma-associated cardiac amyloidosis. Circ J 72(2):331–334
235. Valleix S, Gillmore JD, Bridoux F, Mangione PP, Dogan A, Nedelec B, Boimard M, Touchard G, Goujon JM, Lacombe C, Lozeron P, Adams D, Lacroix C, Maisonobe T, Plante-Bordeneuve V, Vrana JA, Theis JD, Giorgetti S, Porcari R, Ricagno S, Bolognesi M, Stoppini M, Delpech M, Pepys MB, Hawkins PN, Bellotti V (2012) Hereditary systemic amyloidosis due to Asp76Asn variant beta2-microglobulin. N Engl J Med 366(24):2276–2283. doi:10.1056/NEJMoa1201356
236. Sayed RH, Rogers D, Khan F, Wechalekar AD, Lachmann HJ, Fontana M, Mahmood S, Sachchithanantham S, Patel K, Hawkins PN, Whelan CJ, Gillmore JD (2014) A study of implanted cardiac rhythm recorders in advanced cardiac AL amyloidosis. Eur Heart J. doi:10. 1093/eurheartj/ehu506
237. Pinney JH, Lachmann HJ, Bansi L, Wechalekar AD, Gilbertson JA, Rowczenio D, Sattianayagam PT, Gibbs SD, Orlandi E, Wassef NL, Bradwell AR, Hawkins PN, Gillmore JD (2011) Outcome in renal Al amyloidosis after chemotherapy. J Clinical Oncol: Off J Amer Soc Clinical Oncol 29(6):674–681. doi:10.1200/JCO.2010.30.5235
238. Singer W, Sandroni P, Opfer-Gehrking TL, Suarez GA, Klein CM, Hines S, O'Brien PC, Slezak J, Low PA (2006) Pyridostigmine treatment trial in neurogenic orthostatic hypotension. Arch Neurol 63(4):513–518
239. Sattianayagam PT, Gibbs SD, Pinney JH, Wechalekar AD, Lachmann HJ, Whelan CJ, Gilbertson JA, Hawkins PN, Gillmore JD (2010) Solid organ transplantation in AL amyloidosis. Am J Transplant 10(9):2124–2131
240. Nowak G, Westermark P, Wernerson A, Herlenius G, Sletten K, Ericzon BG (2000) Liver transplantation as rescue treatment in a patient with primary AL kappa amyloidosis. Transpl Int 13(2):92–97

Waldenstrom Macroglobulinemia: Genomic Aberrations and Treatment

Prashant Kapoor, Stephen M. Ansell and Esteban Braggio

Abstract

Waldenström macroglobulinemia (WM) is a rare, indolent, and monoclonal immunoglobulin M-associated lymphoplasmacytic disorder with unique clinicopathologic characteristics. Over the past decade, remarkable progress has occurred on both the diagnostic and therapeutic fronts in WM. A deeper understanding of the disease biology emanates from the seminal discoveries of myeloid differentiation primary response 88 (MYD88) L265P somatic mutation in the vast majority of cases and C-X-C chemokine receptor, type 4, mutations in about a third of patients. Although WM remains an incurable malignancy, and the indications to initiate treatment are largely unchanged, the therapeutic armamentarium continues to expand. Acknowledging the paucity of high-level evidence from large randomized controlled trials, herein, we evaluate the genomic aberrations and provide a strategic framework for the management in the frontline as well as the relapsed/refractory settings of symptomatic WM.

Keywords

Waldenstrom's macroglobulinemia · MYD88 · CXCR4 · IgM · BTK inhibitors

1 Definition

The first accounts of Waldenström macroglobulinemia (WM), an eponymous disease, were reported about seven decades ago in two patients who exhibited "several symptoms suggesting myelomatosis," but with "decided differences" [1].

P. Kapoor · S.M. Ansell · E. Braggio (✉)
Mayo Clinic, Scottsdale, AZ, USA
e-mail: Braggio.Esteban@mayo.edu

© Springer International Publishing Switzerland 2016
A.M. Roccaro and I.M. Ghobrial (eds.), *Plasma Cell Dyscrasias*,
Cancer Treatment and Research 169, DOI 10.1007/978-3-319-40320-5_16

Lymphadenopathy, oronasal bleeding, anemia, thrombocytopenia lymphocytoid marrow infiltration, marked increase in globulin content, and high viscosity were distinct features documented in these cases [1]. The definition of WM has evolved over time. Currently, the World Health Organization (WHO) classifies it as a subset of a low-grade, non-Hodgkin lymphoma (NHL) with unique pathologic characteristics: immunoglobulin (Ig) M monoclonal gammopathy (macroglobulinemia) of any size and infiltration of bone marrow by clonal lymphoplasmacytic cells [2]. WM represents >95 % of lymphoplasmacytic lymphoma (LPL) cases. The requirement for a minimum marrow involvement or a minimum serum IgM concentration for the diagnosis of WM was eliminated in the Second International Workshop on WM [3]. A mature dataset of 213 patients with IgM monoclonal gammopathy of undetermined significance (MGUS)-the strongest predisposing factor for WM- attempts to shed light on the controversies surrounding the definition of WM. In this study, patients who underwent bone marrow biopsy ($n = 27$) had fewer than 10 % lymphoplasmacytic cells. Only 29 patients (14 %) developed NHL, WM, chronic lymphocytic leukemia (CLL) or light chain (AL) amyloidosis with a cumulative probability of progression at 1.5 % per year [4, 5]. Therefore, the Mayo Clinic criteria adopted at least 10 % marrow involvement by clonal lymphoplasmacytic cells and a serum monoclonal protein of any size to define WM. For asymptomatic/smoldering WM, the Mayo Clinic criteria require absence of end organ damage or symptoms attributable to LPL in the setting of 10 % or more clonal lymphoplasmacytic marrow infiltration and/or IgM monoclonal protein level of ≥3 g/dL [6].

2 Epidemiology

Approximately 1,500 new cases of WM are diagnosed annually in the United States, and the incidence among octogenarians is 95-fold higher compared to patients less than 50 years of age [7]. Strong evidence exists with regard to genetic susceptibility, familial aggregation, and racial disparity in WM. Repetitive antigenic stimulation and a personal or family history of autoimmune disorders, particularly Sjögren syndrome and autoimmune hemolytic anemia, have been implicated in the development of WM [8–12]. Approximately 20 % of patients have a first-degree relative with a lymphoproliferative disorder [13]. Familial cases are generally diagnosed a decade earlier than the sporadic ones [14]. Although, the absolute risk of developing WM for family members is low, a large population-based Swedish study showed first-degree relatives having a 20-fold increased risk of developing WM [15]. This indolent malignancy is nearly twice as common in Caucasians and males [16].

The median disease-specific survival for patients with WM is estimated at 11 years [17], and in a recent analysis of the Surveillance, Epidemiology, and End Results (SEER) Data, the median overall survival (OS) for all WM patients is 6.2 (5.8–6.5) years [7]. Routine screening for this incurable malignancy is not recommended currently due to lack of effective preventative strategies [18].

3 Genomic Aberrations

3.1 Linkage Studies of the Disease

Whilst WM is mainly a sporadic disease, there are few studies showing familial linkage and predisposition to WM. In a study analyzing 1,384 cases, individuals with MGUS showed a significantly increased risk of WM (46-fold increase) [19]. Additionally, linkage reports supported familial predisposition to the disease in high-risk families, with first-degree relatives of WM showing a ~ten fold increase of IgM-MGUS [20]. Linkage analyses have suggested the existence of susceptibility genes in chromosome arms 1q, 3q, and 4q associated with development of IgM-MGUS and WM [21–25].

Several studies suggest the relationship between chronic antigenic stimulation and WM [8, 9, 11]. Paratarg-7 (P-7) is a protein of unknown function that has been associated with increased risk of WM. An antigenic analysis has shown that 11 % of WM react with anti-hyperphosphorylated P-7, compared with 2 % of controls ($P = 0.001$). Considering that the hyperphosphorylated form of the protein (pP-7) is inherited as a dominant trait [26], there is a possible indication of the association between pP-7 and WM.

3.2 Immunophenotypic Markers of the Tumor Clone

WM expresses pan B-cell markers (CD19+, CD20+, and CD22+), cytoplasmic IgM, FMC7, CD79a+, and CD38+ [27–29]. The plasma cell component of WM expresses CD19, CD45, and CD20, but also CD56 [29].

The success of molecular approaches focused on the analysis of DNA and RNA depends greatly on the isolation of the tumor population. Even though high-throughput analyses of the tumor clone can tolerate certain degree of contamination with non-tumor cells, the excess of contamination significantly affects the results. Therefore, a key aspect to be considered is the enrichment of the tumor population prior performing molecular studies.

Multiparametric sorting generates a highly purified tumor cell population; however, the approach is complex and not available in all molecular laboratories. A different option is to perform serial enrichment of B-cells (CD19+) and plasma cells (CD138+) using antibodies linked to magnetic beads. The limitation of this approach, however, is that normal B- and plasma cells and their malignant counterparts are enriched together. For FISH analysis, a purification step is not needed, as long as FISH is used in combination with immunofluorescence detection of the cytoplasmic immunoglobulin M (cIgM-FISH) [30].

3.3   Chromosomal Abnormalities in WM

Conventional cytogenetics and comprehensive array-based genomic analyses, including array-based comparative genomic hybridization (aCGH) and SNP arrays have provided the first comprehensive analyses of the WM genome [31–37]. Overall, these studies have identified a low-complexity karyotype, with a median of 2–3 chromosomal abnormalities per patient. These values are comparable to other low-grade malignancies such as CLL [38–40], and marginal zone lymphomas (MZL) [38, 41, 42], but significantly lower than more aggressive lymphomas and multiple myeloma (MM) [43–45]. Loss of heterozygosity (LOH) was also a very rare event in WM genome, only described in two cases and affecting chromosome 13 and telomeric regions in 6q and 17q [46]. Furthermore, biallelic deletions were rarely found in WM [31]. Though rare, these deletions affect important genes in cancer, including *MIRN15a-16* and *TRAF3*. *MIRN15a* and *MIRN16* are negative regulators of *BCL2* [47] and are commonly deleted in CLL [39, 40, 48]. *TRAF3* is a negative regulator of the NF-kB signaling pathway and is recurrently affected in other B-cell malignancies such as MM, diffuse large B-cell lymphoma (DLBCL) and MZL [42, 43, 45, 49].

Deletion 6q is the most common chromosomal abnormality, reported in 30–50 % of cases [31–33, 35, 37, 41, 46]. Deletion of 6q is a common abnormality across B-cell malignancies, present in DLBCL, MALT lymphomas, splenic and nodal MZL, MM and CLL [38, 41, 42]. Several studies screened 6q searching for minimal deleted regions (MDR), showing 6q21 and 6q23 as the most recurrently deleted regions [31, 35, 46]. These regions include *PRDM1* (6q21) and *TNFAIP3* (6q23). *PRDM1* down regulates PAX5, which in turn suppresses XBP1, thus acting as a cell proliferation repressor. On the other hand, *TNFAIP3* is a negative regulator of NF-kB and its inactivation leads to the constitutive activation of the pathway [31, 49, 50]. Combining copy-number and DNA sequencing data, biallelic inactivation of *TNFAIP3* was identified in 5 % of WM. Interestingly, *TNFAIP3* mRNA expression is significantly lower in cases with monoallelic deletion compared with cases without abnormalities [31]. This finding suggests the existence of *TNFAIP3* haploinsufficiency, even though additional confirmatory data is needed.

The clinical relevance of deletion 6q is still unclear. Deletion 6q was found associated with clinical parameters including low albumin, high B2M [33, 51], anemia [51] and low IgM production [52]. On the other hand, the deletion has not been associated with response rate, progression-free survival (PFS) or OS in any of these studies.

Trisomy 4 is found in 8–20 % WM and is a distinctive feature of WM compared with the remaining low-grade B-cell lymphomas and leukemias [33, 36, 41]. The implications of trisomy 4 remain to be elucidated, but a study performed in 122 from 11 families identified a linkage between cytobands 4q33–q34 and susceptibility to WM and IgM-MGUS [22].

Additional recurrent abnormalities found between 5–20 % of WM include gains of chromosomes 3, 6p, 12, and 18 and deletions 7q, 11q23 (*ATM* and others),

13q14 (*MIRN15a-16*), 17p13 (*TP53*), and Xq26 [31, 33, 38, 41, 53, 54]. Translocations involving the *IgH* locus are rare in WM, found in less than 3 % of cases [33, 36, 54, 55].

Contrarily to the extensive characterization of clonal architecture and clonal evolution that has been recently performed in most B-cell malignancies [56–61], no longitudinal genomic studies have been performed in WM to date.

3.4 Waldenström Macroglobulinemia as Paradigm of Disease with Single Causative Mutations

One of the most representative examples of a unifying single hit identified by sequencing across cancers is WM. A *MYD88* activating mutation replacing a lysine for a proline in position 265 (L265P) was found in 90 % of WM cases [62]. *MYD88* encodes an adapter protein that affects the IL-1 and Toll-like receptor pathway [63, 64]. The *MYD88* L265P promotes cell survival by spontaneously assembling a protein complex containing IRAK1 and IRAK4, leading to IRAK4 kinase activity, phosphorylation of IRAK1, dysregulation of NF-κB and JAK signaling pathways, and secretion of IL-6, IL-10, and interferon-β [65]. The same L265P activating mutation has been found in lesser extent in ABC-DLBCL (~30 %), MALT lymphomas, SMZL and CLL (<10 %), supporting the key role of *MYD88* in the pathogenesis of these neoplasias [65–67].

Additional studies using a variety of approaches confirmed the presence of *MYD88* L265P mutations in 70–100 % WM [68–75]. By using allele-specific polymerase chain reaction (AS-PCR), the *MYD88* L265P was identified in nearly 100 % of WM [68, 72], compared with ~50 % of IgM-MGUS [71, 72]. Two plausible hypotheses might explain the lower prevalence of *MYD88* L265P in IgM-MGUS compared with WM. One explanation would be that *MYD88* L265P is a universal event required for the progression from IgM-MGUS to WM. An alternative hypothesis would be the existence of different biologic subtypes of IgM-MGUS, with the *MYD88* L265P only found in the subtype evolving to WM [72, 76].

AS-PCR detection of *MYD88* L265P could be potentially used for WM detection. A comparative analysis of peripheral blood and bone marrow CD19+ populations in matched paired samples showed comparable detection values of L265P mutation in both populations (89 % in BM versus 85 % in PB) [77]. This result is very encouraging, providing a less invasive method for mutation screening and potentially eliminating the need of a bone marrow biopsy for performing molecular tests. Additionally, a recent study suggested the use of the mutation screening as a biomarker for measuring tumor burden and response assessment. Thus, it was shown that *MYD88* L265P persisted in remission cases after therapy in a comparable ratio than the observed by flow cytometry [70]. Another study showed a significant correlation between the BM involvement and levels of *MYD88* L265P measured by AS-PCR [73].

Recent studies showed that those WM patients with *MYD88* L265P presented at earlier age [78]. Furthermore, patients with *MYD88* L265P have been associated with higher bone marrow involvement, higher serum IgM, and lower IgA and IgG levels [73]. Additionally, IgM-MGUS cases with *MYD88* L265P showed a higher risk of progression to WM (OR 4.7, 95 % CI: 0.8–48.7, $p = 0.04$) [72]. Overall, these studies suggested the usage of *MYD88* L265P to potentially become a reliable tool for diagnosis, prognosis, and response assessment in WM.

MYD88 is a promising therapeutic target. The development of IRAK4 kinase inhibitors and other upstream proteins in this pathway may provide a novel therapeutic opportunity in the treatment of WM and other B-cell malignancies [62, 65]. Functional analysis performed in MYD88 and downstream targets IRAK1 and IRAK4 showed that downregulation of the pathway lead to suppression of NF-kB signaling pathway and apoptosis [68, 79]. Another key MYD88 downstream target is the Bruton tyrosine kinase (BTK). Together with IRAK1 and IRAK4, inhibition of BTK induced apoptosis in WM [79]. Interestingly, inhibition of BTK activity did not affect IRAK and vice versa, suggesting independent MYD88 signaling through IRAK and BTK pathways [80]. Thus, either the use of a therapy targeting MYD88 or the combinatorial use of BTK and IRAK inhibitors, are promising approaches in WM treatment.

Mutations in C-X-C chemokine receptor type 4 (*CXCR4*) are found in nearly 30 % of WM [75, 78, 81]. The mutations found in *CXCR4* affect the hotspot previously described in warts, hypogammaglobulinemia, infections and myelo-kathexis. (WHIM) *CXCR4* activating mutations were associated with tumor growth and propagation to extramedullary organs [81]. Using an anti-CXCR4 antibody led to tumor reduction in a C1013G/CXCR4 WM model, demonstrating its potential use as a therapeutic target [81]. Patients with mutations in both, *MYD88* and *CXCR4*, showed the highest BM involvement and serum IgM levels, compared with intermediate levels in cases with mutated *MYD88* and wild type *CXCR4*, and low levels in patients without mutations in any of those genes [78]. Moreover, patients with both mutations presented more commonly with symptomatic disease requiring therapy at diagnosis [78]. On the other hand, *CXCR4* mutations were not associated with worse OS.

Other relevant genes that have been found recurrently mutated in WM included *ARID1A* (17 %), *CD79B* (7–9 %), *TP53* (7 %), and *CD79A* (5 %) [46, 75].

3.5 Gene Expression Profiling Analyses

The WM transcriptional signature was characterized using array-based gene expression profiling [82, 83]. The most distinctive hit was the high expression level of interleukin 6 (IL6) in WM compared to related B-cell malignancies and normal B-cells [82, 83]. High IL-6 expression is associated with activation of JAK/STAT and MAPK pathways in WM [82, 84]. Furthermore, CD1c, a transmembrane glycoprotein that is structurally related to the major histocompatibility complex

(MHC) proteins, was significantly higher in WM than in MM or CLL, and could be a potential marker of WM [82].

3.6   microRNAs

A comparative miRNA profiling between CD19 + cells from WM patients and CD19 + cells from healthy donors, identified a WM-specific miRNA signature characterized by increased expression of *MIRN155, −184, −206, −363, −494*, and *−542-3p*, and decreased expression of *MIRN9* [85]. Downstream targets of these miRNAs are key pathways in WM pathogenesis, including the RAS pathway, transcription factors, cell cycle, and anti-apoptotic regulators [85]. Interestingly, the expression of those miRNAs was particularly elevated in patients with a poor outcome predicted by the International Prognostic Scoring System for WM (IPSSWM) [85].

miRNA-155 regulates proliferation and growth of WM cells through the inhibition of MAPK/ERK, PI3/AKT, and NF-κB pathways [85]. *MIRN155* knockdown was associated with decreased MDM2, resulting in an increase in p53 and CDK inhibitors [86]. The use of anti-MIRN155 inhibited in vitro and in vivo growth of WM cells, providing the rationale for miRNA targeted therapies [87]. Finally, higher *MIRN206* and lower *MIRN9* levels in WM cells have been correlated with increased expression of histone deacetylases (HDAC) and decreased expression of Histone acetyltransferases (HAT), suggesting their potential use as therapeutic targets [88].

4   Prognosis

Although typically indolent, WM can be highly heterogeneous [89]. Frequently, the cause of death is attributable to advanced age-associated comorbidities rather than WM. The IISSWM includes 5 prognostic parameters: age >65 years, hemoglobin <11.5 g/dL, platelet count <100 × 10^9/L, β2M >3 mg/L, and IgM level >7 g/dL [90]. This staging system attributes 1 point to every parameter except age, which is assigned 2 points. The total score of each patient at time of initiation of treatment prognosticates them into low (score ≤ 1), intermediate (score = 2) or high-risk categories (score ≥ 3) with significantly disparate 5-year survival rates of 87, 68, and 36 %, respectively [90]. With integration of the quality of response, the prognostic value of ISSWM is further enhanced. Patients who achieve at least a 2-month sustained partial response (PR) or a better response with the frontline therapy are able to overcome the unfavorable effects of high ISSWM. In a large Greek study, elevated lactate dehydrogenase (>250 IU/L) could further prognosticate patients with high-risk ISSWM. The median cause specific survival was 37 months (95 % CI 9.5–64.2) for those with high LDH versus 104 months (95 % CI: 89.4–118.0) for the high-risk cohort with normal LDH [91].

The Greek Myeloma Study Group reported similar survival outcomes of symptomatic WM patients treated between 1985–2000 and 2000–2010 [92]. However, a significant improvement (20-month) in median survival was evident in the United States SEER database in WM patients diagnosed after the year 2000, and the survival advantage was noticeable across all groups, except patients below 50 years of age or African Americans [7]. The 5-year relative survival estimates, defined as the ratio of the observed survival of WM patients and expected survival of the general population in a specific calendar year have increased in patients diagnosed in periods 2001–2005 and 2006–2010 in the United States [93]. Another Swedish study reported similar improvement in survival over time [94]. However, a Mayo Clinic series of patients, who were 50 years or younger at diagnosis, has reported substantial WM-associated morbidity with an estimated average years of life lost being 10.8 years, underscoring the unmet need of effective management strategies for young patients [95].

5 Clinical Features

A substantial proportion (~ 25 %) of WM patients are asymptomatic at diagnosis [96], but about 40–70 % of such patients develop symptoms within 3–10 years of diagnosis [97]. In a study of 48 patients with smoldering WM, the cumulative probability of progression was 12 % per year for the first 5 years, and declined markedly to 2 % per year for the next 5 years [97].

Initial clinical manifestations are typically vague and include nonspecific symptoms of fatigue, fever, malaise, and weight loss. With the passage of time, patients may develop symptoms/signs associated with hematopoietic tissue or organ infiltration. These include cytopenias, lymphadenopathy or hepatosplenomegaly (20–25 % cases), lung nodules, infiltrates or pleural effusion, mucosal bleeding, and diarrhea.

Osteolytic lesions (<2 %), skin plaques, Schnitzler's syndrome (presenting as chronic urticarial skin rash, a monoclonal IgM component and at least 2 of the following signs: fever, arthralgia, lymphadenopathy, hepatomegaly, splenomegaly, elevated ESR, neutrophilia, and abnormal bone imaging findings) or Bing–Neel Syndrome (central nervous system infiltration presenting with a variety of neurologic manifestations, including confusion, seizures, headache, and cranial nerve involvement) [98, 99] can rarely occur.

Normocytic, normochromic anemia is commonly encountered, and is in part, attributed to marrow B-cell infiltration compromising erythropoiesis, hyperviscosity-related reduced erythropoietin levels, mucosal bleeding, and IgM-associated hemolysis [96, 100]. Iron deficiency or overproduction of hepcidin can also be seen [101]. Hyperviscosity-related plasma volume expansion or anemia can exacerbate congestive heart failure. Bence Jones proteinuria is seen in the vast majority (80 % of patients), but rarely exceeds 1 g/24 h. The presence of nephrotic range albuminuria should heighten the clinician's suspicion for concomitant light chain (AL) amyloidosis. Up to one-third of the patients can manifest symptoms of hyperviscosity attributable to the large pentamers of IgM that are primarily confined to the intravascular compartment. Symptoms related to hyperviscosity typically occur when the serum viscosity exceeds 4 centipoise [96, 102]. Hyperviscosity syndrome (HVS) can be associated with mucocutaneous bleeding, visual disturbances, headache, dizziness, ataxia, nystagmus, tinnitus, deafness, and rarely, stroke or cognitive impairment and altered mental status. Ophthalmoscopic examination may reveal distended and tortuous retinal veins, retinal hemorrhages, and papilledema from central retinal vein thrombosis [103]. Slowly progressive, distal, symmetric, and sensory peripheral neuropathy can be encountered many patients as a result of nerve damage from specific antigenic targets of IgM such as myelin-associated glycoprotein (MAG) or endoneurial IgM deposition. Small fiber neuropathy, AL amyloidosis-associated axonal neuropathy or autonomic dysfunction and peripheral Bing–Neel syndrome from direct infiltration of the nerve are some of the other etiologies of nerve damage. Occasionally, IgM paraprotein functions as an autoantibody, and can bind to erythrocytes to cause autoimmune hemolytic anemia [98], and to platelets or von Willebrand factor to simulate immune thrombocytopenic purpura or acquired von Willebrand disease. In 10 % of cases, concomitant cryoglobulinemia and cold agglutinin syndrome have been reported. IgM precipitation can be exacerbated in cold temperatures in cryoglobulinemia and can manifest as Raynaud phenomenon, acrocyanosis, necrosis of cold-exposed body parts, or hemolytic anemia-related complications.

6   Diagnostic Evaluation

In addition to performing monoclonal protein studies at diagnosis and a unilateral bone marrow aspirate and trephine (±lymph node/involved tissue) biopsy, it is imperative to check complete blood count, liver function tests, serum creatinine, serum B2 M, lactate dehydrogenase, and a baseline computed tomographic scans of the chest, abdomen, and pelvis to aid in detection of non-palpable lymphadenopathy, hepatosplenomegaly, and other sites of extramedullary disease. The value of combined PET CT imaging has been assessed in a small prospective study that suggested a higher sensitivity of PET-CT compared to either imaging technique alone [104]. In cases of suspected lymphoplasmacytic lymphomas that are histopathologically difficult to interpret, we recommend checking bone marrow *MYD88* L265P mutation status by AS-PCR assay. Cryocrit, serum viscosity, Coombs test (cold autoantibody), electromyogram, MAG titer, and hepatitis C profile may be checked depending on the presenting signs/symptoms. If coexisting AL amyloidosis is suspected, NT-pro BNP, troponin T, echocardiogram with strain imaging, coagulation parameters and a fat aspirate to detect amyloid material should be performed. Ophthalmoscopic examination is recommended in all patients with visual disturbance, hyperviscosity symptoms, and/or IgM ≥ 3000 mg/dL.

A hypercellular marrow showing diffuse, interstitial, or nodular intertrabecular infiltrate is commonly encountered in WM. The lymphoplasmacytic infiltrate comprises a spectrum of clonal, IgM immunoglobulin-secreting B-cells, including small lymphocytes, plasmacytoid lymphocytes (showing features of both plasma cells and lymphocytes) and a small CD138 expressing plasma cell component that secrets the same light chain as the clonal lymphocytes. Dutcher bodies, representing cytoplasmic inclusions of IgM monoclonal protein invaginating into or overlying the nucleus, and reactive mast cells may be seen as well [2]. The lymphoplasmacytic cells exhibit a distinctive immunophenotypic signature, and almost universally express surface IgM and pan B-cell antigens CD19, CD20, CD22, and CD79. The phenotype of lymphoplasmacytic cells in WM is suggestive of a late stage of B-cell differentiation and probable derivation from IgM+ memory B-cells that have undergone somatic hypermutation, but not isotype switching [105].

7 Treatment

7.1 Principles of Therapy

The management of WM is guided by one basic tenet: WM is a treatable indolent malignancy, but incurable with the current therapeutic approaches. As such, the overarching goals of the management strategies are not only to provide symptomatic relief and to decrease the risk of organ damage, but to sustain long-term disease control, improve quality of life, limit therapy-related toxicities, and improve OS.

Owing to the concerns of both acute and long-term treatment-related toxicities and lack of evidence to suggest survival advantage with therapeutic intervention, earlier in the disease course, active surveillance is considered reasonable in asymptomatic patients in the absence of cytopenias [18]. Although patients with smoldering WM or IgM-MGUS do not exhibit disease-related symptoms, there is a tenfold higher risk of transformation from smoldering WM to active WM, and these patients should be monitored more closely (i.e., every 3–4 months) [97]. A quarter of patients with WM patients are asymptomatic at diagnosis, but are at an increased risk of progression to active disease within the first 5 years of diagnosis, with an annual rate of progression at 12 % [97]. The chances of progression to active WM hinge upon the serum IgM levels, hemoglobin, and the degree of marrow involvement. Within the first 5 years, over 90 % of patients with greater than 50 % marrow involvement at diagnosis progress to symptomatic WM compared to one-half of those with an infiltration of ≤50 % [97]. Survival of patients with smoldering WM is found to be similar to that of the general population of comparable age and sex, a finding that lends further credence to the approach of observation alone in asymptomatic patients. Although most patients eventually do receive treatment, approximately 10 % of those who are managed expectantly will not require therapy for over 10 years [96].

It is recommended that the treatment, in general, be reserved for patients with symptoms or signs attributable to WM. The indications for commencement of therapy include IgM-related moderate or severe neuropathy, symptomatic cryoglobulinemia or cold agglutinin disease (CAD), hyperviscosity symptoms (epistaxis, visual disturbance, dizziness), constitutional symptoms fever, weight loss, nocturnal diaphoresis severe fatigue, nocturnal diuresis, severe cytopenias associated with bone marrow infiltration (hemoglobin < 11 g/dL or platelet count < 100,000/µL), symptomatic or bulky lymphadenopathy/hepatosplenomegaly or concomitant AL amyloidosis [6, 18, 106].

Transfusion of packed red blood cells without preemptive plasma exchange is best avoided in anemic patients with hyperviscosity as it could worsen viscosity and potentially precipitate cardiac failure.

Level I evidence from randomized clinical trials in WM is sparse and there are no set standards for therapy currently. Barring, BTK inhibitor, ibrutinib, there are no agents approved by the Food and Drug Administration (FDA) specifically for newly diagnosed or relapsed refractory WM. Several agents have, however, been evaluated and used either as monotherapies or in combination regimens (Tables 1 and 2). Small sample sizes and heterogeneous patient population in clinical trials of WM (e.g., inclusion of both treatment-naïve and relapsed/refractory patients or inclusion of indolent lymphomas of various histologies in the same study) pose substantial challenges in data interpretation, comparison, and assessment of true impact of certain therapies. Moreover, trials have had to be prematurely closed as a result of under-enrollment/under participation of patients with this rare disease and lack of coordinated efforts of cancer study groups conducting clinical trials. Patients ought to be encouraged to participate in multicenter studies that have a greater likelihood to get completed and generate clinically relevant data in WM.

As the median age at diagnosis ranges from 63 to 73 years, a high proportion of patients are elderly/frail and present with comorbidities, requiring a comprehensive geriatric assessment prior to commencement of any therapy direct toward WM. Several factors have to be considered for selection of appropriate therapy including the rapidity with which disease control is desired, patient's physiologic age, performance status, severity of pre-therapy myelosuppression, presence and severity of neuropathy, or hemolytic anemia and patient's eligibility for stem cell transplantation (ASCT) in future. Stem cell toxic agents such as chlorambucil or fludarabine are best avoided in potential candidates for ASCT [106].

We recommend that all patients be evaluated at a center of excellence at least once at the time of diagnosis to confirm the diagnosis and to discuss about the prognosis, indications of therapy, evolving therapies, and the nuances associated with the management of this rare disease. All patients should be encouraged to participate in clinical trials, if available. We have outlined an off study consensus approach, practiced at Mayo Clinic for the management of patients with newly diagnosed and relapsed refractory WM in Figs. 1 and 2, respectively.

7.2 Response Assessment

Although the depth of response does not necessarily always correlate with outcome in WM, response to therapy can be easily assessed using the simple, uniform consensus panel response criteria (Table 3) that was revised in 2013 [107]. Despite

Table 1 Waldenström macroglobulinemia: schedules of commonly utilized regimens

Regimen	Agent	Dose/Route	Schedule	Cycles/Duration
Rituximab [171]	Rituximab	375 mg/m² IV	Weekly × 4 weeks; can repeat cycle at 3 months	1
Bendamustine ± Rituximab [137]	Bendamustine	90 mg/m² IV	Days 1, 2 q4 weeks	1–6
	Rituximab	375 mg/m² IV	Day 1 q4 weeks	1–6
DRC [139]	Dexamethasone	20 mg IV	Day 1 q4 weeks	1–6
	Rituximab	375 mg/m² IV	Day 1 q4 weeks	1–6
	Cyclophosphamide	100 mg/m² PO	BID day 1–5 q4 weeks	1–6
Ibrutinib [160]	Ibrutinib	420 mg PO	Daily	Until progression
Bortezomib ± Rituximab [157, 172]	Bortezomib	1.6 mg/m² IV	Days 1, 8, 15 q4 weeks	1–6
	Rituximab	375 mg/m² IV	Weekly × 4 weeks	1 and 4
Bortezomib ± Dexamethasone [173]	Bortezomib	1.3 mg/m² IV	Days 1, 4, 8, 11 q3 weeks	6
	Dexamethasone[a]	20 mg IV	Days 1,2, 4, 5,8, 9,11,12 q3 weeks	3–6
BDR [158]	Bortezomib	1.3 mg/m² IV	Days 1, 4, 8, and 11 (3 week cycle)	1
	Bortezomib	1.6 mg/m² IV	Days 1, 8, 15, and 22 q5 weeks	2–5
	Dexamethasone	40 mg IV	Days 1, 8, 15, and 22	2 and 5
	Rituximab	375 mg/m² IV	Days 1, 8, 15, and 22	2 and 5
CaRD [159] Induction therapy	Carfilzomib	20 mg/m² IV	Days 1, 2, 8, and 9 q3 weeks	1
	Carfilzomib	36 mg/m² IV	Days 1, 2, 8, and 9 q3 weeks	2–6
	Dexamethasone	20 mg IV	Days 1, 2, 8, and 9 q3 weeks	2–6
	Rituximab	375 mg/m² IV	Days 2 and 9 q3 weeks	2–6
Maintenance therapy 8 weeks after induction	Carfilzomib	36 mg/m² IV	Days 1 and 2 q8 weeks	1–8
	Dexamethasone	20 mg IV	Days 1 and 2 q8 weeks	1–8
	Rituximab	375 mg/m² IV	Day 2 q8 weeks	1–8

(continued)

Table 1 (continued)

Regimen	Agent	Dose/Route	Schedule	Cycles/Duration
R-CHOP [136]	Rituximab	375 mg/m² IV	Day 1	
	Cyclophosphamide	750 mg/m² IV	Day 1 q3 weeks	Total of 4–8
	Doxorubicin	50 mg/m² IV	Day 1 q3 weeks	Total of 4–8
	Vincristine	1.4 mg/m² (max. 2.0 mg/day) IV	Day 1 q3 weeks	Total of 4–8
	Prednisone	100 mg/m² PO	Days 1 to 5 q3 weeks	Total of 4–8
Fludarabine ± Rituximab [125]	Fludarabine	25 mg/m² IV	Days 1–5 of weeks 5, 9, 13, 19, 23, and 27	
	Rituximab	375 mg/m² IV	Day 1of weeks 1 to 4, 17, 18, and 30, 31	
Fludarabine, cyclophosphamide, Rituximab [174]	Fludarabine	25 mg/m² IV	Days 2–4 q4 weeks	1–6
	Cyclophosphamide	250 mg/m² IV	Days 2–4 q4 weeks	1–6
	Rituximab	375 mg/m² IV	Day 1q 4 weeks	1–6
Fludarabine [128]	Fludarabine	40 mg/m2/day	Daily for 5 days q4 weeks	6
Chlorambucil [128]	Chlorambucil	6–8 mg/m²/day PO	10 days q4 weeks	Max 12
Cladribine ± Rituximab [133, 175]	Cladribine	0.1 mg/kg SQ	Days 1–5 q 4 weeks	1–4
	Rituximab	375 mg/m² IV	Day 1q4 weeks	1–4
CP-R [176]	Cyclophosphamide	1000 mg/m² IV	Day 1	1–6
	Rituximab	375 mg/m² IV	Day 1	
	Prednisone	100 mg/day PO	Days 1–5	
Everolimus [162]	Everolimus	10 mg PO	Daily	Until progression
Ofatumumab [120]	Ofatumumab	300 mg IV	Week 1	1
		1000/2000 mg IV	Weeks 2–5	
Idelalisib [167]	Idelalisib	150 mg PO	BID	Until progression

Abbreviations BDR bortezomib, dexamethasone, and rituximab; *CaRD* carfilzomib, rituximab, and dexamethasone; *CP-R* cyclophosphamide, prednisone, and rituximab; DRC, dexamethasone, rituximab, and cyclophosphamide; *R-CHOP* rituximab, cyclophosphamide, doxorubicin, vincristine, and prednisone; *R/R* relapsed or refractory; *IV* Intravenous

[a]Added cycle 3 onwards for nonresponders

Table 2 Important clinical trials in waldenström macroglobulinemia

Phase	Patient Population	N	Regimens	TTP (months)	PFS (months)	OS (months)	Response rates (%) ORR	≥PR	CR
Alkylating agents									
3 [128]	Previously untreated	169	Chlorambucil versus	21	27	70	–	36	–
		170	Fludarabine	39	38	NR	–	46	–
3 [127]	Previously untreated	24	Chlorambucil continuous	–	–	65	–	–	4
		22	Chlorambucil intermittent	–	–	–	–	–	0
2 [139]	Previously untreated	72	Dexamethasone, Rituximab, Cyclophosphamide	35	67 % at 2y	95	83	74	7
3 [136]	Previously untreated	23	Rituximab-CHOP	**63 versus 22^b** (TTF)	–	NR	–	**91**	9
		25	CHOP (Cyclophosphamide, Doxorubicin, Vincristine, Prednisone)	–	–	–	–	**60**	4
3 [137]	Previously untreated	22	Bendamustine-Rituximab	–	**70**	–	95	–	–
		19	R-CHOP	–	**28**	–	95	–	–
Nucleoside analogs									
2 [177]	Previously untreated	26	Cladribine	–	–	–	–	85	12
2 [178]	Relapsed/Refractory	20	Cladribine	–	–	86 % at 4y	–	55	5
2 [179]	Relapsed/Refractory	46	Cladribine	–	–	28	–	43	2
2 [180]	Relapsed/Refractory	11	Fludarabine + Cyclophosphamide	24	–	70 % at 2y	–	55	–
2 [181]	Previously untreated	9	Cladribine	–	–	–	100	–	–
	untreated Relapsed/Refractory	20		–	–	–	40	–	–
2 [133]	Previously untreated Relapsed/Refractory	29	Cladribine + Rituximab	–	–	–	90	–	25

(continued)

Table 2 (continued)

Phase	Patient Population	N	Regimens	TTP (months)	PFS (months)	OS (months)	ORR	≥PR	CR
2 [126]	Previously untreated	27	Fludarabine + Rituximab	78	67 %	–	96	89	–
	Relapsed/Refractory	16		38	38 % at 2y		94	81	
2 [131]	Previously untreated	43	Fludarabine, Cyclophosphamide, Rituximab	–	NR	69	79	74	12
	Relapsed/Refractory								
Monoclonal antibodies									
2 [182]	Relapsed/Refractory	29	Rituximab-Extended Dose Schedule	14	–	–	66	–	0
2 [108, 115]	Previously untreated	34	Rituximab	30	51 % at 2y	85 % at 5y	53	35	0
	Relapsed/Refractory	35		32	46 % at 2y	48 % at 5y	51	20	0
2 [171]	Previously untreated	27	Rituximab	16	–	–	–	–	–
	Relapsed/Refractory								
2 [120]	Previously untreated	37	Ofatumumab	–	–	–	59	–	–
	Relapsed/Refractory								
2 [183]	Previously untreated	28	Alemtuzumab	15	–	–	75	36	4
	Relapsed/Refractory								
Proteosome inhibitors									
2 [157]	Previously untreated	26	Bortezomib + Rituximab	NR	NR	96 % at 1y	89	66	4
2 [126]	Previously untreated	23	Bortezomib, Dexamethasone, Rituximab	NR	–	–	96	83	13
2 [158]	Previously untreated	59	Bortezomib, Dexamethasone, Rituximab	–	42	82 % at 3y	85	68	3
2 [184]	Relapsed/Refractory	37	Bortezomib + Rituximab	16	16	94 % at 1y	81	51	3

(continued)

Table 2 (continued)

Phase	Patient Population	N	Regimens	TTP (months)	PFS (months)	OS (months)	Response rates (%)		
							ORR	≥PR	CR
2 [156]	Previously untreated	27	Bortezomib	NR	16	NR	–	44	0
	Relapsed/Refractory								
2 [185]	Previously untreated	27	Bortezomib	7	–	–	85	48	0
	Relapsed/Refractory								
Immunomodulatory drugs									
2 [159]	Previously untreated	31	Carfilzomib, Rituximab, Dexamethasone	NR	NR	–	87	67	3
	Relapsed/Refractory								
2 [186]	Previously untreated	20	Thalidomide	–	–	–	–	–	0
	Relapsed/Refractory								
2 [187]	Previously untreated	20	Thalidomide + Rituximab	36	–	–	80	70	5
	Relapsed/Refractory	5		15			40	40	
2 [186]	Previously untreated	16	Lenalidomide + Rituximab.	17	–	–	50	25	0
	Relapsed/Refractory								
Other newer therapies									
2 [188]	Relapsed/Refractory	60	Everolimus	25	21	NR	73	50	0
2 [170]	Relapsed/Refractory	36	Panobinostat	7	7	–	47	–	0
2 [165]	Relapsed/Refractory	37	Perifosine	13	13	–	35	11	0
2 [167]	Relapsed/Refractory	10	Idelalisib	–	–	–	80	–	–
2 [166]	Relapsed/Refractory	42	Enzasturin	11	–	–	38	–	0
2 [160][a]	Relapsed/Refractory	63	Ibrutinib	–	–	–	–	62	0

[a]Ongoing study

Abbreviations CR complete response; *NR* not reached; *ORR* overall response rate; *TTP* time to progression; *OS* overall survival; *PFS* progression-free survival; *PR* partial response; *y* years

Values in bold indicate statistically significant difference

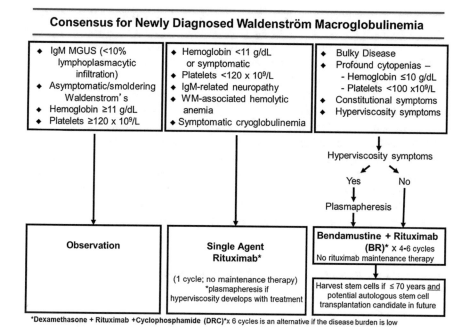

Fig. 1 Mayo Clinic off study consensus approach for the management of patients with newly diagnosed WM (www.msmart.org, version 4)

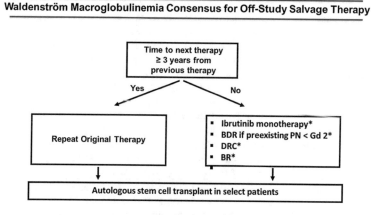

Fig. 2 Mayo Clinic off-study consensus approach for the management relapsed/refractory WM (www.msmart.org, version 4)

limitations of overreliance on IgM levels, we suggest performing SPEP and measuring serum IgM periodically in all patients. Care should be taken to perform sequential paraprotein quantification by the same methodology (total serum IgM quantitation by nephelometry and M protein quantitation by densitometry), and preferably in the same laboratory.

While a reduction in IgM levels may not always accompany symptomatic improvement and conversely improvement in symptoms may be observed in the absence of substantial IgM reduction, it remains a valuable tumor marker in most cases. Intensification of therapy for minor responders may not translate into improved survival outcomes as suggested by a study demonstrating that rituximab naïve patients who attain a minor response have similar outcomes to those achieving at least a partial response [108]. However, PFS appears to be longer with attainment of very good partial remission (VGPR), a category recently added in the uniform response criteria, or with responses deeper than VGPR attained from rituximab-based therapies [109].

Table 3 Updated response criteria from the sixth international workshop on waldenstrom macroglobulinemia [107]

Response category	Definition
Complete response (CR)	No evidence of serum monoclonal IgM protein by immunofixation and normal serum IgM level Complete resolution of extramedullary disease, i.e., lymphadenopathy and splenomegaly, if present at baseline Morphologically normal bone marrow aspirate and trephine biopsy
Very good partial response (VGPR)	Monoclonal IgM protein is detectable, but ≥90 % reduction in serum IgM level from baseline[a] Complete resolution of extramedullary disease, i.e., lymphadenopathy/splenomegaly, if present at baseline Absence of any new signs/symptoms of active disease
Partial response (PR)	Monoclonal IgM protein is detectable, but ≥50 to <90 % reduction in serum IgM level from baseline[a] Reduction in extramedullary disease, i.e., lymphadenopathy/splenomegaly if present at baseline No new signs or symptoms of active disease
Minor response (MR)	Monoclonal IgM protein is detectable, but ≥25 % to <50 % reduction in serum IgM level from baseline[a] No new signs or symptoms of active disease
Stable disease (SD)	Monoclonal IgM protein is detectable, but <25 % reduction and <25 % increase in serum IgM level from baseline[a] No progression in extramedullary disease, i.e., lymphadenopathy/splenomegaly No new signs or symptoms of active disease
Progressive disease (PD)	≥25 % increase in serum IgM level[a] from lowest nadir (requires confirmation) and/or progression in clinical features attributable the disease

[a]Sequential changes in IgM levels may be determined either by M protein quantitation by densitometry or total serum IgM quantitation by nephelometry

Although the half-life of IgM is only about 5 days, the time to maximal response can be seen over an extended period of time (5 to more than 20 months). Premature abandonment of therapies should be avoided. Clinicians should be able to appreciate the nuances involved in the assessment of response. A paradoxical initial increase of IgM or rituximab-induced "IgM flare" should not be perceived as failure of therapy [110]. A gradual decline of IgM component may be observed with monoclonal antibodies, alkylating agents and purine analogs. In contrast, a rapid and profound reduction of IgM level in the absence of significant bone marrow response can be observed with inhibitors of mTOR or BTK. As such, serial BM appraisal may be required, particularly in clinical trials, to reliably determine the response status and rule out any discordance between serum IgM and marrow findings. Moreover, the absence of clonal lymphocytes in the BM is one prerequisite for attaining complete remission (CR). Persistence of clonal CD138+ plasma cells with selective clearance of the CD20+ B-cell compartment in patients receiving certain therapies such as bendamustine has been demonstrated [1, 111, 112]. The consensus response criteria requires CT scans of chest abdomen, pelvis to determine categorical response in patients with measurable disease, and the role of PET-CT scan in conjunction with monoclonal protein response remains to be fully explored [104].

Some clinical trials are currently evaluating the prognostic impact of achieving of minimal residual disease (MRD) in WM. In *MYD88* L265P patients who achieve CR, MRD can be assessed with AS-PCR assay for *MYD88* in CD19-selected PB and BM cells.

7.3 Plasma Exchange

Hyperviscosity syndrome induced by elevated monoclonal protein is a category I indication in the American Society for Apheresis 2013 guidelines for therapeutic apheresis [113]. Circulating IgM pentamers are removed during the plasma exchange with rapid improvement in symptoms of HVS. This approach is, however, a temporizing, adjunctive measure to alleviate symptoms until substantial reduction in IgM protein from systemic therapy induced cytoreduction is achieved. The symptoms of hyperviscosity rather than the absolute serum viscosity level should dictate the need for initiating plasma exchange. Because viscosity is not linearly correlated with IgM, small volume exchanges can substantially reduce it; each session of therapeutic plasma exchange can decrease viscosity by as much as 30 % [114]. Typically saline is used as a replacement for hyperviscous plasma during each session. Some patients with multiply relapsed/refractory disease may require long-term plasma exchange as an adjunct for the management of hyperviscosity-related symptoms. Symptomatic cryoglobulinemia and IgM-related neuropathy are other recognized scenarios where this approach could be potentially utilized in addition to rituximab-based regimens. Preemptive plasma exchange can be performed in patients with high baseline viscosity or substantially elevated IgM prior to planned surgical procedures to reduce the risk of perioperative bleeding, or prior to red blood cell transfusion to reduce the risk of precipitating hypervelocity or before initiation of rituximab therapy as IgM flare associated HVS can occur.

7.4   Monoclonal Antibodies

Owing to its high efficacy in CD 20+ malignancies, good tolerability and ability of be combined with many therapies, rituximab, a chimeric, type 1 monoclonal anti-CD20 antibody, indisputably is regarded as the backbone of most regimens used for WM. Single-agent rituximab is generally reserved for patients who are unable to tolerative more aggressive options, or those with manifestations such as slowly progressive or disabling peripheral neuropathy, mild cytopenias, steroid-resistant hemolytic anemia or cold agglutinin disease (Fig. 1). The response rates observed with rituximab monotherapy are up to ~50 %, and predictably lower that those achieved with multiagent regimens [115]. Urgent plasmapheresis may be required to manage rituximab-induced flare resulting in hyperviscosity [6]. In a study, 7 patients were initially treated with 4 (cohort 1) or 8 (cohort 2) rituximab infusions that led to median PFS of 6.6 months. A phase 2 study, E3A98, conducted by the Eastern Cooperative Oncology Group (ECOG), demonstrated an overall response rate (ORR/≥ minor response) of nearly 52 % with rituximab monotherapy. In this trial of treatment naïve and previously treated patients, rituximab was administered at 375 mg/m^2, intravenously for four consecutive weeks [115]. The ORR in the two study cohorts were similar (52.9 % vs. 51.4 %). However, the trial was underpowered to determine the impact of pretreatment laboratory variables such as hemoglobin and IgM in predicting response [115]. Extended rituximab therapy, comprising a repeat 4-week course 3 months after the initial course in responders showed deeper responses in patients presenting with normal albumin or lower serum monoclonal protein (<4 g/dL) [116]. FcγIIIA polymorphisms on the effector cells, by modulating attachment of the Fc portion of rituximab, have been implicated in controlling antibody-dependent cell-mediated cytotoxicity (ADCC). Expression of valine at FcγRIIIA-158 results in patients response rates of 40 % in the homozygous and 35 % in the heterozygous forms as rituximab binds with greater avidity to such receptors. In contrast, rituximab's efficacy is found to be substantially compromised in patients whose FcγIIIA-158 receptors lack valine (~9 % RR) [109, 117, 118]. However, we currently do not routinely check for polymorphisms in Fcγ (CD16) receptors prior to initiating rituximab. Polymorphisms in FcγIIIA do not impact the efficacy of Obinutuzumab (GA 101), a glycoengineered type II CD20 antibody with enhanced cell death, increased ADCC and affinity for FcγRIIIA. Obinatuzumab has been approved in combination with chlorambucil in patients with previously untreated CLL. Its efficacy in WM remains to be elucidated.

The value of rituximab maintenance in WM remains unestablished currently, although a clinical trial of 162 newly diagnosed WM patients is ongoing to assess the value of maintenance. The trial is designed such that all patients receive uniform induction of up to six cycles of rituximab and bendamustine followed by two further cycles of rituximab every 4 weeks. Patients achieving $\geq$ PR (major response) are then assigned to either rituximab maintenance or observation. The results are awaited. A retrospective study from Dana Farber Cancer Institute evaluated the outcome of a cohort of 86 patients with WM who had responded to rituximab-based induction, and were subsequently initiated on rituximab monotherapy maintenance. Patients had received a median of eight infusions over a 2-year maintenance period. Outcomes were compared with a control group of 162 patients with similar baseline characteristics and post-induction responses that did receive any maintenance. A fourfold improvement in response rates (10 % vs. 42 %; $P < 0.0001$) was noted in the responders on rituximab maintenance compared to the nonmaintenance control population. A doubling of PFS (56.3 vs. 28.6 months; $P = 0.0001$) was noted with maintenance, and importantly, OS was also found to be better (not reached vs. 116 months; $P = 0.009$) with maintenance. However, increased toxicities, particularly grade 2 infections, were noted in prolonged rituximab use [119]. Because of paucity of data from prospective studies, and toxicities associated with long-term rituximab therapy, we currently do not advocate maintenance approach routinely.

With the differentiation of B-cells into plasma cells, downregulation of CD20 occurs and the antigen density in WM patients may become low [120]. A more potent, fully human monoclonal, type 1 anti-CD20, ofatumumab binds to an epitope on CD20 that is distinct from rituximab binding site and induces antibody complement-dependent cytotoxicity [121]. A phase II trial of 37 patients (9 treatment naïve and 28 relapsed), assigned to one of the two groups with similar patient characteristics, evaluated the efficacy of ofatumumab in WM (Table 2). A cohort of 15 patients received ofatumumab 300 mg week 1 and 1000 mg weeks 2–4 and another group ($n = 28$) received ofatumumab 300 mg week 1 followed by a higher dose of 2000 mg from weeks 2–5. Patients achieving < PR at week 16 were eligible to repeat another cycle. Two-thirds of therapy naïve patients, 57 % of relapsed patients, 52 % of rituximab pre-exposed, and 75 % of rituximab naïve patients responded. The response rate was greater in the cohort receiving the higher dose (68 % vs. 47 %). The rate of IgM flare requiring plasmapheresis was lower than that typically observed with rituximab therapy. Ofatumumab at a higher dose appeared to be more effective rituximab pre-exposed patients or those with a baseline IgM $\geq$ 4.0 g/dL [120].

Ofatumumab has been evaluated in rituximab intolerant patients (~ 10 %) to circumvent infusion-related reactions associated with rituximab. The ORR of ~ 58 % with ofatumumab in the pivotal study of fludarabine and alemtuzumab-refractory CLL is quite similar to response rates seen with this agent in WM [120, 122] (Table 2). However, a recently reported Phase 3 trial (RESONATE) that randomized patients with relapsed or refractory CLL or small lymphocytic lymphoma (SLL) to receive either ibrutinib or ofatumumab showed marked superiority of ibrutinib for the end points of response rates, PFS, and OS [123]. Although cross trial comparisons do not necessarily shed clear light, in the absence of hard data, if one were to extrapolate the results of RESONATE trial in CLL patients to WM—a malignancy known to cluster closely to CLL in the GEP studies, and in which both ofatumumab and ibrutinib are active as well the clinical setting for the use of ofatumumab outside of rituximab intolerance may be limited in WM. An ongoing phase II open label study (NCT01294579) is evaluating the safety and efficacy of ofatumumab and bendamustine followed by ofatumumab in subjects with indolent B-NHL who have relapsed after rituximab treatment.

All patients should be screened for hepatitis B prior to any anti-CD20 antibody therapy due to hepatitis B reactivation [124]. Cytopenias, infusion reactions, and IgM flare are some of the common/unique toxicities associated with the use of anti-CD20 antibodies. Rituximab-based combination therapies have led to deeper responses leading to superior PFS in some studies [109, 125, 126]. Such multidrug combinations are preferred in patients with significant constitutional symptoms and severe hematological compromise.

7.5   Alkylating Agents and Purine Analogs

Extensive use of oral alkylating agents in WM over the years has helped generate meaningful efficacy and safety data. With the passage of time chlorambucil use has fallen out of favor. Chlorambucil was one of the first agents to be evaluated in a randomized trial in WM. The patients were enrolled in the trial of continuous (0.1 mg/kg daily) versus intermittent (0.3 mg/kg/day for 7 days repeated every 6 weeks) chlorambucil over 22 years, highlighting accrual-related challenges. Response was sluggish, with a median time to response being 18–21 months from randomization. The median duration of survival was similar as was the ORR with the two schedules (75 % with continuous chlorambucil versus 64 % with intermittent therapy, $P = NS$) [127].

Purine/nucleoside analogs, fludarabine, and cladribine have been evaluated in previously untreated and relapsed WM patients. As primary therapy, single agent purine analogs show response rates of 40–100 % with responses being lower, in the range 30–50 % in the salvage setting (Table 2).

The recently published WM1 study is a large ($n = 339$) multicenter, phase III trial that randomly assigned chlorambucil or oral fludarabine (a purine analog) monotherapy as initial treatment for patients with advanced WM. The fludarabine-arm demonstrated significantly higher grade 3–4 neutropenia, but superior PFS (36.3 vs. 27.1 months; $P = 0.01$), duration of response and, most importantly, OS (not reached vs. 69.8 months; $P = 0.014$; Table 2). Furthermore, higher cumulative incidence of second malignancies was noted at 6 years, with chlorambucil (21 % versus 3.7 % with fludarabine, $P = 0.001$) [128]. Oral fludarabine is currently unavailable in the United States, and as such the clinical impact of this trial has been trivial in the US. Regardless, WM1 study is one of the key studies in advancing the field as it confirms the findings of several prior smaller studies that demonstrated the efficacy of fludarabine, and provides a yardstick to measure the activities of novel therapies in development [129]. Another randomized trial involving 92 patients with relapsed/refractory WM patients, comparing fludarabine with cyclophosphamide, doxorubicin (Adriamycin), and prednisone

(CAP) showed superior activity of fludarabine (PR 30 % with fludarabine vs. 11 % with CAP; $P = 0.019$) [130].

Preclinical data demonstrate enhancement of cytotoxicity with rituximab that sensitizes cells to alkylating agents and nucleoside analogs. Fludarabine/ cyclophosphamide/rituximab (FCR), fludarabine/cyclophosphamide (FC), and fludarabine/rituximab (FR) regimens are associated with good ORR [125]. In a study involving 43 previously untreated ($n = 28$) or relapsed/refractory patients ($n = 15$), FCR was given every 28 days for up to six courses. An ORR of 79 % (CR $\sim$ 19 %) was observed, and response rates were similar in the previously untreated and relapsed refractory patients (Table 2). A cross trial analysis suggests that although the ORR is similar to that seen with FC in a French study of 49 patients (14 untreated, 35 previously treated), evidently the response becomes deeper upon addition of rituximab, with 33 % of patients achieving at least a VGPR with FCR versus none with FC. Despite high efficacy of FCR, enthusiasm for its use has diminished owing to profound myelosuppression, particularly prolonged neutropenia in high proportion of patients (44 %) [131].

A multicenter, phase 2 trial studied a subcutaneous cladribine/rituximab regimen in 29 patients (13 previously treated and 16 untreated) with WM. The ORR was impressive at $\sim$ 90 %, and patients achieving CR (28 %) exhibited higher expression of human concentrative nucleoside transporter 1 (hCNT1) mRNA that is associated with nucleoside transportation across the plasma membrane. With a median follow-up of 43 months, the median time to treatment failure was not reached (95 % CI, 60-NR) in this study [132, 133].

Markedly high rates of transformation to high grade NHL (4.7 %) or therapy-related MDS (tMDS/AML, 1.6 %) are observed with the use of nucleoside analogs compared non-nucleoside-based regimens [134]. The median time to development of t-MDS/AML and transformation is about 5 years from initiation of nucleoside analog therapy. While effective salvage therapies are available for transformed malignancy, the median survival was a dismally low at 5 months (range: 4–5 months) with t-MDS/AMLin the series reported by Leleu et al. No predictors for the development of these complications could be identified [135]. There is evidence to suggest that is risk of transformation or development of t-MDS/AML is magnified with fludarabine–alkylator combinations compared to fludarabine monotherapy [134].

Although purine analog-based combinations exhibit substantial efficacy and produce high quality responses (CR 19–28 %), their stem cell damaging effect and myelosuppressive properties preclude their use both in fit patients with long life expectancy who are potential candidates for ASCT as well as patients at the other end of the spectrum who are frail and elderly, and therefore, at a greater risk of developing chemotherapy induced severe myelotoxicity and infectious complications.

While addition of rituximab to cyclophosphamide/doxorubicin/ vincristine/prednisone (CHOP) improved ORR and time to treatment failure compared to CHOP alone was a step forward [136], a recent phase III study promoted bendamustine/rituximab (BR) regimen as a viable, highly effective, frontline alternative in WM (Table 2). Bendamustine, a drug that was originally developed in the former East Germany, exhibits properties of an alkylating agent plus a purine analog by virtue of its unique structure. The initial fears about the difficulty in stem cell collection have not been supported by mature studies using BR in hematologic malignancies. The aforementioned noninferiority trial comparing R-CHOP to BR demonstrated high ORR with both regimens (~95 %), but better tolerability, longer PFS (~70 months versus 28 months with R-CHOP), and fewer relapses with BR [137]. Although a clear survival advantage with this doublet is yet to be reported in this indolent malignancy, it is estimated that maturation of the data will likely reveal superiority in this end point of paramount importance.

Bendamustine has also been evaluated in relapsed refractory WM patients as monotherapy or in combination with rituximab/ofatumumab, showing an ORR of 83 %, but prolonged myelosuppression in those previously exposed to a nucleoside analog [109, 138]. More recently, the therapeutic efficacy of BR salvage regimen was analyzed in an Italian retrospective study of 71 relapsed/refractory patients with WM. An ORR of 80 % observed and the median PFS was not reached after a median follow-up of 19 months. No patients were reported to have developed transformation or tMDS/AML [99].

No direct comparisons of BR regimen have been made with Dexamethasone/Rituximab/Cyclophosphamide (DRC), another commonly utilized, well-tolerated, relatively inexpensive, neuropathy- and stem cell-sparing regimen with long-term data to substantiate its efficacy. DRC showed an ORR of 83 % (7 % CR, 67 % PR, and 9 % MR) in a phase II trial enrolling 72 treatment naive patients with WM (Table 2) [139]. After a minimum follow-up of over 6 years the final analysis of this trial reported a median time to progression (TTP) of 35 months (95 % CI, 22–48 months), and the median time to next treatment of 51 months. The median OS and disease-specific survival were 95 and 104 months, respectively. Secondary myelodysplasia was not reported with this regimen. Furthermore, a majority of patients who progressed and required retreatment responded again to rituximab-based therapy [140]. Outside of clinical trials, BR and DRC remain our primary regimens of choice for the management of patients with previously untreated, symptomatic WM. For patients with bulky disease, we prefer BR over DRC regimen (Fig. 1).

7.6   Stem Cell Transplantation

Integration of ASCT in the management strategy of MM has improved survival. This modality has demonstrated encouraging outcomes with durable disease control in WM as well, albeit it remains an underutilized approach. Although the impact of ASCT reported in the retrospective studies of WM has been substantial, it falls far short of the impressive activity of this approach observed in the MM patient population and data demonstrating ASCT related survival advantage are lacking as well [141–148]. Moreover, advanced age and multiple comorbidities are not uncommon at presentation in WM, and a prospective trial comparing ASCT approach with conventional non-transplant approaches is difficult to conduct for this indolent malignancy. Therefore, the optimal timing or the subset of patients that should be offered ASCT remains to be defined. In 1999, a pilot study of 2 minimally pretreated patients with WM and 4 relapsing after purine analog-based therapy demonstrated feasibility, efficacy, and safety of high-dose therapy in WM. Two patients who had received extensive prior fludarabine therapy required two stem cell mobilization attempts. All patients were conditioned with melphalan 200 mg/m^2, barring 1 who received melphalan 140 mg/m2 + total body irradiation. One patient underwent tandem transplant. A partial remission was achieved by 5 patients, and 1 attained a CR. No treatment-related mortality (TRM) was observed. One patient with prior chlorambucil and fludarabine exposure transformed to large cell lymphoma 7 months post-ASCT. Four of the other five patients remained event-free at 2–52 months after ASCT [142]. Findings of a subsequent study highlighted the inability of ASCT to completely eradicate the disease in the vast the majority of patients [143]. However, a prolonged median PFS was 69 months and median time to retreatment of 82 months was noted after an estimated median follow-up of 69 months from ASCT [143].

Data indicate that early stem cell mobilization and harvest in the potentially ASCT-eligible patient population with an otherwise long life expectancy is a justifiable strategy. Collection of stem cells prior to exposure to multiple therapies could prevent significant damage to these cells. Many experts collect and store stem cells in first remission when the tumor burden is low (Fig. 1). Mobilizing chemotherapy or plerixafor can be avoided with such an approach as well.

The median age at ASCT was 53 years in the European Bone Marrow Transplant Registry (EBMTR) analysis of 202 patients who underwent ASCT, and the median time from diagnosis to transplantation was 18 months. BEAM (BCNU, etoposide, cytarabine, and melphalan) conditioning therapy was administered to 46 % of patients and 28 % received total body irradiation-based conditioning. One-year non-relapse mortality rate was 3.8 %, and the estimated 5-year PFS and OS rates were approximately 40 and 69 %, respectively [146]. Importantly, survival outcome depended on the number of prior therapies and disease chemosensitivity at the time of ASCT. Although, ASCT is generally not recommended as a primary consolidative approach outside of a controlled clinical trial owing to the lack survival benefit [149], cryopreserved cells could arguably be used upon first progression [6] as an early salvage approach (Fig. 2). The EBMTR data propound that ASCT is best avoided in refractory WM, heavily pretreated patients who have received more than three lines of prior therapy.

Active 'graft versus lymphoma' effect has been observed with allogeneic transplantation. However, with its prohibitively high TRM rate of up to 44 % at 1 year, it appears best to eschew allogeneic transplantation outside of controlled clinical trials [145, 149], with the possible exception of a rare fit patient with multiply relapsed/refractory disease and limited alternatives [150]. A CR rate achieved with allogeneic transplantation is high at 66 %, and OS at 3 years is shown to be 62 % for myeloablative conditioning and 66 % for reduced intensity conditioning regimens [145]. A large EBMTR series showed only a modest (10 %)

reduction in the 3-year TRM with reduced intensity conditioning approach compared to full myeloablative conditioning. Three-year relapse rates of 25 and 11 %, respectively, were documented in that series [151].

7.7   Novel Therapies

7.7.1   Immunomodulatory Drugs

Enthusiasm for the widely used anti-myeloma immunomodulatory drugs (IMiDs) has been tempered by the toxicities observed in WM patients [152]. Efficacy of both single agent thalidomide as well as thalidomide-based combinations has been evaluated in previously treated patients. Although thalidomide is not particularly myelosuppressive, disabling neuropathy observed with this drug is a dose limiting complication in patients with WM. Lenalidomide, a substantially less neurotoxic agent that was considered a promising drug until its combination with rituximab demonstrated an unexpected acute decline in hematocrit in 81 % (13/16) of patients in one of the initial studies in WM with this drug, leading to the trial's premature closure [152]. More recently, in a Mayo Clinic conducted, single arm, phase 2 trial evaluating the efficacy of combining lenalidomide (L) with the DRC regimen, the ORR and the PFS of the LDRC combination at 80 % and 25 months, respectively, appeared similar to the results evident with DRC alone. Moreover, in this study, a higher rate of anemia was observed in WM patients compared to other low-grade lymphoma histologies treated with LDRC ($\geq$ grade 3, 40 % vs. 14 %) [153].

Pomalidomide is a third generation IMiD with a substantially better neurotoxicity profile and 100-fold greater potency than thalidomide. In a phase 1 trial of relapsed and or refractory WM patients, pomalidomide was administered as a single agent for 28 days continuously per cycle. The maximum tolerated dose was substantially lower at 1 mg/day than typically used for MM patients. A schedule involving 3 weeks of continuous therapy followed by a mandatory 7-day rest period in a 28-day cycle that would allow time for recovery of cytopenias might be better tolerated, and therefore warrants further evaluation. Disappointingly, in a phase I dose-escalating trial of pomalidomide plus rituximab and dexamethasone, 3/7 patients (43 %) with a baseline IgM of >4000 mg/dL developed IgM flare with symptomatic hyperviscosity, necessitating emergent plasmapheresis and early closure of the trial [154].

7.7.2   Proteosome Inhibitors

Several regimens with proteosome inhibitors (PIs) as their backbone have proven efficacy in MM. Recently, exciting data have emerged for WM as well. However, caution should be exercised with the use of PIs as patients with WM can present with an underlying demyelinating or amyloid-related neuropathy, making use of neurotoxic agents such bortezomib challenging. Bortezomib-based therapies are highly effective, stem cell-sparing alternatives that induce rapid and durable responses within 2–3 months of initiation of therapy, and demonstrate even a greater efficacy for familial WM [155]. Development of treatment-emergent, disabling neuropathy (~ 70 % grade ≥ 2) has led to premature discontinuation of bortezomib in up to 60 % of users with a twice weekly, intravenous regimen [126, 156]. Bortezomib-based regimens can be considered for clinical situations where a rapid response is desired. These include HVS, AL amyloidosis, renal dysfunction, and symptomatic cryoglobulinemia. Bortezomib induces high (60–70 %), long lasting (up to 16 months) responses in previously untreated patients. Expectedly, the response rates decrease to approximately 40 % in the relapsed/refractory setting. Three phase 2 studies (Table 2) of bortezomib in combination with rituximab, have exhibited an ORR between 81 and 96 % in previously untreated patients [126, 157, 158]. The European Myeloma Network study omitted rituximab in the first cycle to preempt IgM flare and plasmapheresis could be avoided in all the patients, despite 44 % of patients having IgM ≥ 4000 mg/dL prior to the initiation of therapy [158]. This study introduced a unique schedule (Table 1) that transitioned patients from twice weekly intravenous administration to once a week therapy after cycle 1 in order to mitigate the risk of peripheral neuropathy. Therapy was still discontinued in 8 % of patients with weekly dosing, and the goal of attaining responses deeper than PR was compromised somewhat compared to the twice weekly schedule (Table 2). The R2 W trial is a randomized phase 2 trial evaluating subcutaneous weekly administration bortezomib to further improve upon the neurotoxicity associated with bortezomib. It remains to be seen whether changing the route and frequency of administration of bortezomib will preserve its efficacy as well.

A unique consolidative approach with 1 cycle of cladribine-cyclophosphamide-rituximab following successful stem cell harvest has been attempted in patients who completed bortezomib-rituximab therapy. Consolidation deepened the response (ORR 100 %) and led to durable remissions, with 11 of 12 patients who achieved VGPR post-consolidation upgrading their response to bortezomib-rituximab alone.

Carfilzomib, a second generation PI is an epoxyketone proteasome inhibitor that binds selectively and irreversibly to the constitutive proteasome and immunoproteasome. It is substantially less neurotoxic than bortezomib. Carfilzomib was recently evaluated in combination with rituximab and dexamethasone (CaRD regimen) in WM patient population that was unexposed to a PI or rituximab and had received ≤ 1 line of prior therapy [159]. The regimen utilized intravenous carfilzomib, 20 mg/m^2 (cycle 1) and 36 mg/m^2 (cycles 2–6), with intravenous dexamethasone, 20 mg, on days 1, 2, 8, and 9, and rituximab, 375 mg/m^2, on days 2 and 9 every 21 days. Those achieving at least stable disease received maintenance therapy 8 weeks later with intravenous carfilzomib, 36 mg/m^2, and intravenous dexamethasone, 20 mg, on days 1 and 2, and rituximab, 375 mg/m^2, on day 2 every 8 weeks for 8 cycles (Table 1). Ninety percent (28/31) of patients were previously untreated, and 11 had *CXCR* WHIM mutation. An ORR of 87.1 % (1 complete response, 10 very good partial responses, 10 partial responses, and 6 minimal responses) was observed, irrespective of *MYD88* L265P or *CXCR4* WHIM mutation status or ISSWM. Although, the median follow-up was short at 15.4 (range, 2.1–25.5) months, all patients were alive, 20 patients. Grade 2 peripheral neuropathy was observed in 1 patient (3.2 %). A single patient achieved an unprecedented molecular CR, and in no patient was the therapy discontinued for neurotoxicity. Notably, profound treatment-aggravated IgG and/or IgA hypogam-maglobulinemia was observed in the setting of recurrent sinobronchial infections, leading to intravenous immunoglobulin (IVIG) initiation and/or truncation of therapy. Carfilzomib-related asymptomatic hyperlipasemia and dexamethasone-induced hyperglycemia and were observed in 54 and 100 % of patients, respectively.

The activity of an oral, neuropathy sparing PI, oprozomib is currently being examined in WM, and studies are being planned with ixazomib, another oral PI that is further along in its development as an anti-myeloma agent. All patients on PI therapy require mandatory herpes zoster oral prophylaxis [157].

7.7.3   BTK Inhibitors

Ibrutinib (formerly PCI-32765) is an orally administered, first in class, irreversible and highly potent BTK inhibitor. BTK is an important regulator of many critical B-cell pro-survival pathways mediating cell apoptosis, adhesion, migration, and homing. Ibrutinib binds covalently to a cysteine-481 residue at the active site of BTK resulting in potent inhibition of kinase activity. It has recently been approved for patients with WM both in the frontline and relapsed setting, although no data are currently available for the previously untreated patients. Ibrutinib has previously been approved for two other hematologic malignancies: CLL and mantle cell lymphoma. The rationale for ibrutinib's use stems from the presence of *MYD88* L265P mutation that activates BTK, in the majority (>90 %) of WM patients. Its approval was based on a single arm, ongoing multicenter phase 2 trial that demonstrated durable responses in 63 patients with previously treated WM [160]. Patients received ibrutinib 420 mg orally once daily on a continuous basis. The response rate was 61.9 % (95 % CI: 48.8, 73.9). The responses consisted of very good partial remission (VGPR) (11.1 %) and PR (50.8 %) (Table 2). No patient, however, has achieved a CR so far. The median duration of response was not reached (range of 2.8–18.8 months). Ibrutinib appears to be a well-tolerated drug demonstrating rapid improvements in serum IgM (median drop from 3,610 to 915 mg/dL) and hemoglobin (median time to response was 1.2 months) levels. It primarily reduces IgM secretion, evidently showing a lack of major improvement in the marrow burden tumor despite profound and rapid decline in the IgM levels. *CXCR4* WHIM (response rate 30 % in mutants vs. 77 % in wild type) and *MYD88* WT status were determinants of response. About two-thirds of patients with extramedullary disease experienced a reduction in lymphadenopathy, and ibrutinib-associated lymphocytosis served as a marker of superior response. Common adverse events included thrombocytopenia (Grade ≥ 2, 14.3 %) and neutropenia (Grade ≥ 2, 25.4 %), seen primarily in the heavily pretreated patients. Atrial fibrillation in patients with a prior history (4.8 %), procedure-related bleeding (3.2 %), and recurrent epistaxis associated with marine oil supplements (3.2 %), were other notable adverse effects.

Preclinical data suggest that concomitant use of inhibitors of CXCR4 may be instrumental in overcoming ibrutinib-mediated resistance [81]. An ongoing randomized double-blind, placebo-controlled, phase III study (NCT02165397) is currently examining the efficacy of ibrutinib plus rituximab in patients with previously treated WM. Other ongoing studies include a phase I study of ibrutinib in combination with lenalidomide and a study of ibrutinib plus bendamustine and rituximab in patients with relapsed refractory B-cell NHL, including WM.

7.8   Emerging Therapies

Extensive basic research over the past two decade has unraveled many critical pathways and identified several effective targeted therapies in WM.

7.8.1   Phosphoinositide-3-Kinase (PI3 K), AKT, and Mammalian Target of Rapamycin (MTOR) Inhibitors

The constitutively activated PI3K/AKT/mTOR pathway regulates proliferation, survival, angiogenesis, and cell metabolism in WM [161]. Ghobrial et al. recently updated the results of a phase II trial of everolimus, an oral, raptor, mTORC1 inhibitor that were administered until progression, or unacceptable toxicity [162]. The trial allowed sequential dose de-escalation of everolimus for toxicity. Responses were rapid (median time to achieve response was 2 months; range: 1–26 in those attaining PR (50 %)), and the median duration of response was not reached. Unfortunately, substantial toxicities were encountered with two-thirds of patients experiencing grade 3 or higher toxicities, or requiring dose reduction or treatment delays. Twenty-five percent of the patients died of progressive WM. Everolimus has also been combined with bortezomib and rituximab (Table 2) [163]. Discordance between serological and marrow response has been observed with everolimus, as suggested by a decline in serum IgM levels, but persistent or increased bone marrow disease. With continuous everolimus therapy, drug resistance develops from incomplete TORC2 inhibition. An exciting approach that warrants further evaluation utilizes NVP-BEZ235, a dual inhibitor of the PI3 K/AKT/mTOR (both rictor and raptor) pathway [164].

A phase II trial of 37 relapsed/refractory WM patients evaluated novel oral Akt inhibitor, perfosine [165]. A vast of majority of patients had received prior rituximab therapy. Perifosine was given at a dose of 150 mg for six 28-day cycles after which those achieving stable disease or a better response could be continued on perifosine until progression. Responses were rapid and appeared durable (Table 2).

Enzastaurin is an investigational oral serine/threonine kinase inhibitor that targets the PKC and PI3 K/AKT pathways and has been evaluated in a phase 2 trial of 42 patients. It demonstrated an ORR of 38 % (Table 2) and was well tolerated. Grade 3 toxicities were rare [166]. The development of enzastaurin has, however, hit a roadblock due to absence of meaningful activity in a recent phase III trial of diffuse large B-cell lymphoma in which enzastaurin was being evaluated in the maintenance setting.

Another enzyme playing a critical role in normal B-cell development is PI3K, delta isoform. It transduces signals from the B-cell receptor (BCR), toll-like receptors, and several other receptors, including CD40, and cytokine receptors. Hyperactivation of this pathway has been observed in WM cells. Idelalisib is a selective oral inhibitor of PI3K delta with remarkable efficacy. It has been granted accelerated approval for patients with relapsed follicular lymphoma and SLL that have received at least two prior systemic therapies, and is also approved in combination with rituximab for relapsed CLL patients who are deemed unfit to undergo additional chemotherapy due to comorbidities. Overall survival improvement has not yet been demonstrated, and continued approval for these indications may be contingent upon verification of clinical benefit in confirmatory trials.

A single arm phase II trial of 125 patients with indolent lymphomas, refractory to both rituximab and an alkylating agent examined the efficacy of oral idelalisib monotherapy. The trial included ten WM/LPL patients who received 125 mg twice daily until disease progression or unacceptable toxicity [167]. An impressive ORR of 80 % was noted in WM/LPL (Table 2) and further studies evaluating the efficacy of this agent in WM are ongoing. Diarrhea, pneumonitis, elevation in aminotransferases, pyrexia, rash, colitis, intestinal perforation, and neutropenia are some of the toxicities encountered with idelalisib use.

7.8.2 Histone Deacetylase Inhibitors

Histone deacetylase inhibitors (HDAC) epigenetically modify the chromatin structure by acetylating diverse substrates. Vorinostat, an HDAC inhibitor causes apoptosis of WM cells via downregulation of the cytoprotective MAPK ERK1/2 and inhibitors of apoptosis (IAP) family of proteins. It also activates multiple caspases, proapoptotic MAPKs, and JNK [168]. Promising preclinical activity has been observed with Panobinostat (LBH589) in WM. It is the first in class HDAC inhibitor to be recently approved for relapsed refractory MM [169]. It has been shown to inhibit bone marrow stromal cell-triggered or IL-6- and IGF-1-induced proliferation of WM cell lines. Single-agent panobinostat administered at a dose of 30 mg orally, 3 days a week was evaluated in a small phase II trial of 36 patients with relapsed and/or refractory WM [170]. Poor response rates, short duration of response in conjunction with high rates of quality of life-altering toxicities including fatigue (83 %), diarrhea (58 %), nausea (44 %), anorexia (42 %), and taste disturbance (28 %) have dampened enthusiasm for its use.

Although major therapeutic advances have occurred in the therapeutics of WM, it remains an incurable disease. The recent discovery of the presence of MYD88 L265 mutation in the vast majority of WM patients has undoubtedly given an impetus to the development of several targeted agents. In the foreseeable future, the therapeutic landscape of WM will continue to expand as additional novel classes of agents are evaluated (Table 4) and more effective therapies with better toxicity profiles become available for this rare malignancy.

Table 4 Novel classes of agents currently being evaluated in clinical trials of WM

Phase		Identifier	Drugs
1	Selective phosphodiesterase 4 inhibitor	NCT01888952	Roflumilast and prednisone
1	Bromodomain (BET) inhibitor	NCT02238522	ZEN003365
1	Anti-Endosialin/TEM1 Monoclonal Antibody	NCT01748721	MORAb-004
1	Glutaminase inhibitor	NCT02071888	CB-839
1	Aurora A kinase inhibitor	NCT01812005	Alisertib with or without rituximab
1		NCT01567709	Alisertib plus vorinostat
1		NCT01695941	Alisertib, bortezomib and rituximab
1	Anti-CTLA-4 Ab	NCT01729806	Ipilimumab and rituximab
1,2	TLR7, 8 and 9 antagonist	NCT02092909	IMO-8400
1	Autologous CD19 CAR T cells	NCT02153580	Cellular immunotherapy (autologous CD19 CAR T cells)
1,2		NCT01865617	autologous anti-CD19CAR-4-1BB-CD3zeta-EGFRt-expressing T lymphocytes
1,2		NCT00466531	19-28z CAR expressing autologous T cells
1,2	Antifolate Agent	NCT01947140	Pralatrexate plus romidepsin (Histone deacetylase inhibitor)
1,2	Hypomethylating Agent	NCT01998035	Romidepsin plus oral 5-Azacytidine
1,2	Poly ADP ribose polymerase inhibitor	NCT01326702	Veliparib plus bendamustine and rituximab
2	Tetracycline	NCT02086591	Doxycycline
2	Selective Syk inhibitor	NCT01796470	GS-9973 plus idelalisib (selective oral PI3 K delta inhibitor)
2		NCT01799889	GS-9973

Please refer to www.clinicaltrials.gov for current status of these trials
TLR toll-like receptor; *CAR* chimeric antigen receptor; *ADP* adenosine diphosphate

References

1. Waldenström J (1944) Incipient myelomatosis or 'essential' hyperglobulinemia with fibrinogenopenia a new syndrome?. Acta Medica Scandinaviva CXVII:217–246
2. Swerdlow S et al (ed) (2008) WHO Classification of tumors of haematopoietic and lymphoid tissues, Page 194, International Agency for Research on Cancer 2008
3. Owen RG et al (2003) Clinicopathological definition of Waldenstrom's macroglobulinemia: consensus panel recommendations from the second international workshop on waldenstrom's macroglobulinemia. Semin Oncol 30(2):110–115
4. Kyle RA et al (2011) IgM monoclonal gammopathy of undetermined significance (MGUS) and smoldering Waldenstrom's macroglobulinemia (SWM). Clin Lymphoma Myeloma Leuk 11(1):74–76
5. Kyle RA et al (2003) Long-term follow-up of IgM monoclonal gammopathy of undetermined significance. Blood 102(10):3759–3764
6. Ansell SM et al (2010) Diagnosis and management of Waldenstrom macroglobulinemia: Mayo stratification of macroglobulinemia and risk-adapted therapy (mSMART) guidelines. Mayo Clinic Proc Mayo Clinic 85(9):824–833
7. Nelson S. et al (2013) Changing epidemiology and improved survival in patients with waldenstrom macroglobulinemia: review of surveillance, epidemiology, and end results (SEER). Data122:3135-3135
8. Aoki H et al (1995) Frequent somatic mutations in D and/or JH segments of Ig gene in Waldenstrom's macroglobulinemia and chronic lymphocytic leukemia (CLL) with Richter's syndrome but not in common CLL. Blood 85(7):1913–1919
9. Martin-Jimenez P et al (2007) Molecular characterization of heavy chain immunoglobulin gene rearrangements in Waldenstrom's macroglobulinemia and IgM monoclonal gammopathy of undetermined significance. Haematologica 92(5):635–642
10. Royer RH et al (2010) Differential characteristics of Waldenstrom macroglobulinemia according to patterns of familial aggregation. Blood 115(22):4464–4471
11. Wagner SD, Martinelli V, Luzzatto L (1994) Similar patterns of V kappa gene usage but different degrees of somatic mutation in hairy cell leukemia, prolymphocytic leukemia, Waldenstrom's macroglobulinemia, and myeloma. Blood 83(12):3647–3653
12. Kristinsson SY et al (2012) Familial aggregation of lymphoplasmacytic lymphoma/Waldenstrom macroglobulinemia with solid tumors and myeloid malignancies. Acta Haematol 127(3):173–177
13. Treon SP et al (2006) Characterization of familial Waldenstrom's macroglobulinemia. Ann Oncol Official J Eur Soc Med Oncol ESMO 17(3):488–494
14. McMaster ML (2003) Familial Waldenstrom's macroglobulinemia. Semin Oncol 30 (2):146–152
15. Kristinsson SY et al (2008) Risk of lymphoproliferative disorders among first-degree relatives of lymphoplasmacytic lymphoma/Waldenstrom macroglobulinemia patients: a population-based study in Sweden. Blood 112(8):3052–3056
16. Wang H et al (2012) Temporal and geographic variations of Waldenstrom macroglobulinemia incidence: a large population-based study. Cancer 118(15):3793–3800
17. Ghobrial IM et al (2006) Prognostic model for disease-specific and overall mortality in newly diagnosed symptomatic patients with Waldenstrom macroglobulinaemia. Br J Haematol 133 (2):158–164
18. Kyle RA et al (2003) Prognostic markers and criteria to initiate therapy in Waldenstrom's macroglobulinemia: consensus panel recommendations from the Second International Workshop on Waldenstrom's Macroglobulinemia. Semin Oncol 30(2):116–120
19. Kyle RA et al (2002) A long-term study of prognosis in monoclonal gammopathy of undetermined significance. N Engl J Med 346(8):564–569
20. McMaster ML (2003) Familial Waldenstrom's macroglobulinemia. Semin Oncol 30(2): 146–152

21. McMaster ML (2003) Familial Waldenstrom's macroglobulinemia. Semin Oncol 30(2): 146–152
22. McMaster ML et al (2006) Genomewide linkage screen for Waldenstrom macroglobulinemia susceptibility loci in high-risk families. Am J Hum Genet 79(4):695–701
23. Treon SP et al (2006) Characterization of familial Waldenstrom's macroglobulinemia. Ann Oncol 17(3):488–494
24. Treon SP et al (2012) Familial disease predisposition impacts treatment outcome in patients with Waldenstrom macroglobulinemia. Clin Lymphoma Myeloma Leuk 12(6):433–437
25. Royer RH et al (2010) Differential characteristics of Waldenstrom macroglobulinemia according to patterns of familial aggregation. Blood 115(22):4464–4471
26. Grass S et al (2011) Hyperphosphorylated paratarg-7: a new molecularly defined risk factor for monoclonal gammopathy of undetermined significance of the IgM type and Waldenstrom macroglobulinemia. Blood 117(10):2918–2923
27. Owen RG et al (2001) Waldenstrom macroglobulinemia. Development of diagnostic criteria and identification of prognostic factors. Am J Clin Pathol 116(3):420–428
28. Owen RG et al (2003) Clinicopathological definition of Waldenstrom's macroglobulinemia: consensus panel recommendations from the second international workshop on waldenstrom's macroglobulinemia. Semin Oncol 30(2):110–115
29. San Miguel JF (2003) Immunophenotypic analysis of Waldenstrom's macroglobulinemia. Semin Oncol 30(2):187–195
30. Ahmann GJ et al (1998) A novel three-color, clone-specific fluorescence in situ hybridization procedure for monoclonal gammopathies. Cancer Genet Cytogenet 101(1):7–11
31. Braggio E et al (2009) Identification of copy number abnormalities and inactivating mutations in two negative regulators of nuclear factor-kappaB signaling pathways in Waldenstrom's macroglobulinemia. Cancer Res 69(8):3579–3588
32. Braggio E et al (2009) High-resolution genomic analysis in Waldenstrom's macroglobulinemia identifies disease-specific and common abnormalities with marginal zone lymphomas. Clin Lymphoma Myeloma 9(1):39–42
33. Nguyen-Khac F et al (2013) Chromosomal aberrations and their prognostic value in a series of 174 untreated patients with Waldenstrom's macroglobulinemia. Haematologica 98 (4):649–654
34. Poulain S et al (2011) High-throughput genomic analysis in Waldenstrom's macroglobulinemia. Clin Lymphoma Myeloma Leuk 11(1):106–108
35. Schop RF et al (2006) 6q deletion discriminates Waldenstrom macroglobulinemia from IgM monoclonal gammopathy of undetermined significance. Cancer Genet Cytogenet 169 (2):150–153
36. Terre C et al (2006) Trisomy 4, a new chromosomal abnormality in Waldenstrom's macroglobulinemia: a study of 39 cases. Leukemia 20(9):1634–1636
37. Mansoor A et al (2001) Cytogenetic findings in lymphoplasmacytic lymphoma/Waldenstrom macroglobulinemia. Chromosomal abnormalities are associated with the polymorphous subtype and an aggressive clinical course. Am J Clin Pathol 116(4):543–549
38. Ferreira BI et al (2008) Comparative genome profiling across subtypes of low-grade B-cell lymphoma identifies type-specific and common aberrations that target genes with a role in B-cell neoplasia. Haematologica 93(5):670–679
39. Kay NE et al (2011) Progressive but previously untreated CLL patients with greater array CGH complexity exhibit a less durable response to chemoimmunotherapy. Cancer Genet Cytogenet 203(2):161–168
40. Ouillette P et al (2011) Acquired genomic copy number aberrations and survival in chronic lymphocytic leukemia. Blood 118(11):3051–3061
41. Braggio E et al (2012) Genomic analysis of marginal zone and lymphoplasmacytic lymphomas identified common and disease-specific abnormalities. Mod Pathol 25(5): 651–660

42. Rinaldi A et al (2011) Genome-wide DNA profiling of marginal zone lymphomas identifies subtype-specific lesions with an impact on the clinical outcome. Blood 117(5):1595–1604
43. Annunziata CM et al (2007) Frequent engagement of the classical and alternative NF-kappaB pathways by diverse genetic abnormalities in multiple myeloma. Cancer Cell 12(2):115–130
44. Carrasco DR et al (2006) High-resolution genomic profiles define distinct clinico-pathogenetic subgroups of multiple myeloma patients. Cancer Cell 9(4):313–325
45. Keats JJ et al (2007) Promiscuous mutations activate the noncanonical NF-kappaB pathway in multiple myeloma. Cancer Cell 12(2):131–144
46. Poulain S et al (2013) Genome wide SNP array identified multiple mechanisms of genetic changes in Waldenstrom macroglobulinemia. Am J Hematol 88(11):948–954
47. Cimmino A et al (2005) miR-15 and miR-16 induce apoptosis by targeting BCL2. Proc Natl Acad Sci U S A 102(39):13944–13949
48. Calin GA et al (2002) Frequent deletions and down-regulation of micro- RNA genes miR15 and miR16 at 13q14 in chronic lymphocytic leukemia. Proc Natl Acad Sci U S A 99 (24):15524–15529
49. Compagno M et al (2009) Mutations of multiple genes cause deregulation of NF-kappaB in diffuse large B-cell lymphoma. Nature 459(7247):717–721
50. Novak U et al (2009) The NF-{kappa}B negative regulator TNFAIP3 (A20) is inactivated by somatic mutations and genomic deletions in marginal zone lymphomas. Blood 113 (20):4918–4921
51. Ocio EM et al (2007) 6q deletion in Waldenstrom macroglobulinemia is associated with features of adverse prognosis. Br J Haematol 136(1):80–86
52. Chang H et al (2007) Analysis of 6q deletion in Waldenstrom macroglobulinemia. Eur J Haematol 79(3):244–247
53. Schop RF et al (2002) Deletions of 17p13.1 and 13q14 are uncommon in Waldenstrom macroglobulinemia clonal cells and mostly seen at the time of disease progression. Cancer Genet Cytogenet 132(1):55–60
54. Schop RF et al (2002) Waldenström macroglobulinemia neoplastic cells lack immunoglobulin heavy chain locus translocations but have frequent 6q deletions. Blood 100(8):2996–3001
55. Chang H et al (2004) Analysis of IgH translocations, chromosome 13q14 and 17p13.1(p53) deletions by fluorescence in situ hybridization in Waldenstrom's macroglobulinemia: a single center study of 22 cases. Leukemia 18(6):1160–1162
56. Braggio E et al (2012) Longitudinal genome-wide analysis of patients with chronic lymphocytic leukemia reveals complex evolution of clonal architecture at disease progression and at the time of relapse. Leukemia 26(7):1698–1701
57. Keats JJ et al (2012) Clonal competition with alternating dominance in multiple myeloma. Blood 120(5):1067-1076
58. Knight SJ et al (2012) Quantification of subclonal distributions of recurrent genomic aberrations in paired pre-treatment and relapse samples from patients with B-cell chronic lymphocytic leukemia. Leukemia 26(7):1564–1575
59. Landau D et al (2013) The evolution and impact of sublconal mutations in chronic lymphocytic leukemia. Cell 152(4):714–726
60. Schuh A et al (2012) Monitoring chronic lymphocytic leukemia progression by whole genome sequencing reveals heterogeneous clonal evolution patterns. Blood 120(20): 4191–4196
61. Ouillette P et al (2013) Clonal evolution, genomic drivers, and effects of therapy in chronic lymphocytic leukemia. Clin Cancer Res 19(11):2893–2904
62. Treon SP et al (2012) MYD88 L265P somatic mutation in Waldenstrom's macroglobulinemia. N Engl J Med 367(9):826–833
63. Muzio M et al (1997) IRAK (Pelle) family member IRAK-2 and MyD88 as proximal mediators of IL-1 signaling. Science 278(5343):1612–1615

64. Wesche H et al (1997) MyD88: an adapter that recruits IRAK to the IL-1 receptor complex. Immunity 7(6):837–847
65. Ngo VN et al (2011) Oncogenically active MYD88 mutations in human lymphoma. Nature 470(7332):115–119
66. Morin RD et al (2011) Frequent mutation of histone-modifying genes in non-Hodgkin lymphoma. Nature 476(7360):298–303
67. Pasqualucci L et al (2011) Analysis of the coding genome of diffuse large B-cell lymphoma. Nat Genet 43(9):830–837
68. Ansell SM et al (2014) Activation of TAK1 by MYD88 L265P drives malignant B-cell Growth in non-Hodgkin lymphoma. Blood Cancer J 4:e183
69. Gachard N et al (2013) IGHV gene features and MYD88 L265P mutation separate the three marginal zone lymphoma entities and Waldenstrom macroglobulinemia/lymphoplasmacytic lymphomas. Leukemia 27(1):183–189
70. Jimenez C et al (2013) MYD88 L265P is a marker highly characteristic of, but not restricted to. Waldenstrom's macroglobulinemia. Leukemia 27(8):1722–1728
71. Landgren O, Staudt L (2012) MYD88 L265P somatic mutation in IgM MGUS. N Engl J Med 367(23): 2255–2256; author reply 2256–2257
72. Varettoni M et al (2013) Prevalence and clinical significance of the MYD88 (L265P) somatic mutation in Waldenstrom's macroglobulinemia and related lymphoid neoplasms. Blood 121 (13):2522–2528
73. Xu L et al (2013) MYD88 L265P in Waldenstrom macroglobulinemia, immunoglobulin M monoclonal gammopathy, and other B-cell lymphoproliferative disorders using conventional and quantitative allele-specific polymerase chain reaction. Blood 121(11):2051–2058
74. Poulain S et al (2013) MYD88 L265P mutation in Waldenstrom macroglobulinemia. Blood 121(22):4504–4511
75. Hunter ZR et al (2014) The genomic landscape of Waldenstrom macroglobulinemia is characterized by highly recurring MYD88 and WHIM-like CXCR4 mutations, and small somatic deletions associated with B-cell lymphomagenesis. Blood 123(11):1637–1646
76. Fonseca R, Braggio E (2013) The MYDas touch of next-gen sequencing. Blood 121 (13):2373–2374
77. Xu L et al (2014) Detection of MYD88 L265P in peripheral blood of patients with Waldenstrom's Macroglobulinemia and IgM monoclonal gammopathy of undetermined significance. Leukemia 28(8):1698–1704
78. Treon SP et al (2014) Somatic mutations in MYD88 and CXCR4 are determinants of clinical presentation and overall survival in Waldenstrom macroglobulinemia. Blood 123(18): 2791–2796
79. Yang G et al (2013) A mutation in MYD88 (L265P) supports the survival of lymphoplasmacytic cells by activation of Bruton tyrosine kinase in Waldenstrom macroglobulinemia. Blood 122(7):1222–1232
80. Advani RH et al (2013) Bruton tyrosine kinase inhibitor ibrutinib (PCI-32765) has significant activity in patients with relapsed/refractory B-cell malignancies. J Clin Oncol 31(1):88–94
81. Roccaro AM et al (2014) C1013G/CXCR4 acts as a driver mutation of tumor progression and modulator of drug resistance in lymphoplasmacytic lymphoma. Blood 123(26):4120–4131
82. Chng WJ et al (2006) Gene-expression profiling of Waldenstrom macroglobulinemia reveals a phenotype more similar to chronic lymphocytic leukemia than multiple myeloma. Blood 108(8):2755–2763
83. Gutierrez NC et al (2007) Gene expression profiling of B lymphocytes and plasma cells from Waldenstrom's macroglobulinemia: comparison with expression patterns of the same cell counterparts from chronic lymphocytic leukemia, multiple myeloma and normal individuals. Leukemia 21(3):541–549
84. Hodge LS, Ansell SM (2011) Jak/Stat pathway in Waldenstrom's macroglobulinemia. Clin Lymphoma Myeloma Leuk 11(1):112–114

85. Roccaro AM et al (2009) microRNA expression in the biology, prognosis, and therapy of Waldenstrom macroglobulinemia. Blood 113(18):4391–4402
86. Sacco A et al (2010) Epigenetic modifications as key regulators of Waldenstrom's Macroglobulinemia biology. J Hematol Oncol 3:38
87. Sacco A et al (2013) microRNA Aberrations in Waldenstrom Macroglobulinemia. Clin Lymphoma Myeloma Leuk
88. Roccaro AM et al (2010) microRNA-dependent modulation of histone acetylation in Waldenstrom macroglobulinemia. Blood 116(9):1506–1514
89. Dhodapkar MV et al (2003) Prognostic factors and response to fludarabine therapy in Waldenstrom's macroglobulinemia: an update of a US intergroup trial (SW0G S9003). Semin Oncol 30(2):220–225
90. Morel P et al (2009) International prognostic scoring system for Waldenstrom macroglobulinemia. Blood 113(18):4163–4170
91. Kastritis E et al (2010) Validation of the International prognostic scoring system (IPSS) for Waldenstrom's macroglobulinemia (WM) and the importance of serum lactate dehydrogenase (LDH). Leuk Res 34(10):1340–1343
92. Kastritis E et al (2011) No significant improvement in the outcome of patients with Waldenstrom's macroglobulinemia treated over the last 25 years. Am J Hematol 86(6): 479–483
93. Castillo JJ et al (2014) Survival trends in Waldenstrom macroglobulinemia: an analysis of the Surveillance, Epidemiology and End Results database. Blood 123(25):3999–4000
94. Kristinsson SY et al (2013) Patterns of survival in lymphoplasmacytic lymphoma/Waldenstrom macroglobulinemia: a population-based study of 1,555 patients diagnosed in Sweden from 1980 to 2005. Am J Hematol 88(1):60–65
95. Vallumsetla N et al (2014) Outcomes of young patients with Waldenstrom macroglobulinemia (WM). J Clin Oncol 32(15_suppl)
96. Garcia-Sanz R et al (2001) Waldenstrom macroglobulinaemia: presenting features and outcome in a series with 217 cases. Br J Haematol 115(3):575–582
97. Kyle RA et al (2012) Progression in smoldering Waldenstrom macroglobulinemia: long-term results. Blood 119(19):4462–4466
98. Baehring JM et al (2008) Neurological manifestations of Waldenstrom macroglobulinemia. Nature clinical practice. Neurology 4(10):547–556
99. Bing JAN (1936) Two Cases of Hyperglobulinaemia with affection of the central nervous system on a toxi-infectious basis. Acta Medica Scand 88:492–506
100. Singh A et al (1993) Increased plasma viscosity as a reason for inappropriate erythropoietin formation. J Clin Investig 91(1):251–256
101. Ciccarelli BT et al (2011) Hepcidin is produced by lymphoplasmacytic cells and is associated with anemia in Waldenström's macroglobulinemia. Clin Lymphoma Myeloma Leuk 11 (1):160–163
102. Stone MJ, Pascual V (2010) Pathophysiology of Waldenstrom's macroglobulinemia. Haematologica-the Hematology Journal 95(3):359–364
103. Menke MN et al (2006) Hyperviscosity-related retinopathy in waldenstrom macroglobulinemia. Arch Ophthalmol 124(11):1601–1606
104. Banwait R et al (2011) The role of 18F-FDG PET/CT imaging in Waldenstrom macroglobulinemia. Am J Hematol 86(7):567–572
105. Kriangkum J et al (2004) Clonotypic IgM V/D/J sequence analysis in Waldenstrom macroglobulinemia suggests an unusual B-cell origin and an expansion of polyclonal B cells in peripheral blood. Blood 104(7):2134–2142
106. Dimopoulos MA et al (2009) Update on treatment recommendations from the fourth international workshop on Waldenstrom's Macroglobulinemia. J Clin Oncol Official J Am Soc Clin Oncol 27(1):120–126
107. Owen RG et al (2013) Response assessment in Waldenstrom macroglobulinaemia: update from the VIth international workshop. Br J Haematol 160(2):171–176

108. Gertz MA et al (2009) Clinical value of minor responses after 4 doses of rituximab in Waldenstrom macroglobulinaemia: a follow-up of the eastern cooperative oncology group E3A98 trial. Br J Haematol 147(5):677–680

109. Treon SP et al (2011) Attainment of complete/very good partial response following rituximab-based therapy is an important determinant to progression-free survival, and is impacted by polymorphisms in FCGR3A in Waldenstrom macroglobulinaemia. Br J Haematol 154(2):223–228

110. Ghobrial IM et al (2004) Initial immunoglobulin M 'Flare' after rituximab therapy in patients diagnosed with Waldenstrom macroglobulinemia an eastern cooperative oncology group study. Cancer 101(11):2593–2598

111. Varghese AM et al (2009) Assessment of bone marrow response in Waldenstrom's macroglobulinemia. Clin Lymphoma Myeloma 9(1):53–55

112. Barakat FH et al (2011) Residual monotypic plasma cells in patients with waldenstrom macroglobulinemia after therapy. Am J Clin Pathol 135(3):365–373

113. Schwartz J et al (2013) Guidelines on the use of therapeutic apheresis in clinical practice-evidence-based approach from the Writing Committee of the American Society for Apheresis: the sixth special issue. J Clin Apheresis 28(3):145–284

114. Ballestri M et al (2007) Plasma exchange in acute and chronic hyperviscosity syndrome: a rheological approach and guidelines study. Annali dell'Istituto superiore di sanita 43(2):171–175

115. Gertz MA et al (2004) Multicenter phase 2 trial of rituximab for Waldenstrom macroglobulinemia (WM): an eastern cooperative oncology group study (E3A98). Leukemia Lymphoma 45(10):2047–2055

116. Dimopoulos MA et al (2005) Predictive factors for response to rituximab in Waldenstrom's macroglobulinemia. Clin Lymphoma 5(4):270–272

117. Treon SP (2010) Fcgamma receptor predictive genomic testing and the treatment of indolent non-Hodgkin lymphoma. Clin Lymphoma Myeloma Leuk 10(5):321–322

118. Treon SP et al (2005) Polymorphisms in FcgammaRIIIA (CD16) receptor expression are associated with clinical response to rituximab in Waldenstrom's macroglobulinemia. J Clin Oncol Official J Am Soc Clin Oncol 23(3):474–481

119. Treon SP et al (2011) Maintenance Rituximab is associated with improved clinical outcome in rituximab naive patients with Waldenstrom Macroglobulinaemia who respond to a rituximab-containing regimen. Br J Haematol 154(3):357–362

120. Furman RR et al (2011) A phase II trial of atumumab in subjects with Waldenstrom's macroglobulinemia. Blood 118(21):1581

121. Cheson BD (2010) Ofatumumab, a novel anti-CD20 monoclonal antibody for the treatment of B-cell malignancies. J Clin Oncol J Am Soc Clin Oncol 28(21):3525–3530

122. Wierda WG et al (2010) Ofatumumab as single-agent CD20 immunotherapy in fludarabine-refractory chronic lymphocytic leukemia. J Clin Oncol J Am Soc Clin Oncol 28(10):1749–1755

123. Byrd JC et al (2014) Ibrutinib versus ofatumumab in previously treated chronic lymphoid leukemia. N Engl J Med 371(3):213–223

124. Kapoor P et al (2008) Anti-CD20 monoclonal antibody therapy in multiple myeloma. Br J Haematol 141(2):135–148

125. Treon SP et al (2009) Long-term outcomes to fludarabine and rituximab in Waldenstrom macroglobulinemia. Blood 113(16):3673–3678

126. Treon SP et al (2009) Primary therapy of Waldenstrom macroglobulinemia with bortezomib, dexamethasone, and rituximab: WMCTG clinical trial 05-180. J Clin Oncol J Am Soc Clin Oncol 27(23):3830–3835

127. Kyle RA et al (1998) Waldenstrom's macroglobulinemia: A prospective study comparing daily oral versus intermittent chlorambucil. Br J Haematol 102(1):244

128. Leblond V et al (2013) Results of a randomized trial of chlorambucil versus fludarabine for patients with untreated Waldenstrom macroglobulinemia, marginal zone lymphoma, or lymphoplasmacytic lymphoma. J Clin Oncol J Am Soc Clin Oncol 31(3):301–307

129. Ghobrial IM (2013) Choice of therapy for patients with Waldenstrom macroglobulinemia. J Clin Oncol J Am Soc Clin Oncol 31(3):291–293

130. Leblond V et al (2001) Multicenter, randomized comparative trial of fludarabine and the combination of cyclophosphamide-doxorubicin-prednisone in 92 patients with Waldenstrom macroglobulinemia in first relapse or with primary refractory disease. Blood 98(9): 2640–2644

131. Tedeschi A et al (2012) Fludarabine plus cyclophosphamide and rituximab in Waldenstrom macroglobulinemia: an effective but myelosuppressive regimen to be offered to patients with advanced disease. Cancer 118(2):434–443

132. Laszlo D et al (2010) Rituximab and subcutaneous 2-chloro-2'-deoxyadenosine combination treatment for patients with Waldenstrom macroglobulinemia: clinical and biologic results of a phase II multicenter study. J Clin Oncol J Am Soc Clin Oncol 28(13):2233–2238

133. Laszlo D et al (2011) Rituximab and Subcutaneous 2-Chloro-2'-Deoxyadenosine as Therapy in Untreated and Relapsed Waldenstrom's Macroglobulinemia. Clin Lymphoma Myeloma Leuk 11(1):130–132

134. Leleu X et al (2009) increased incidence of transformation and myelodysplasia/acute leukemia in patients With Waldenstrom macroglobulinemia treated with nucleoside analogs. J Clin Oncol 27(2):250–255

135. Leleu X et al (2009) Balancing risk versus benefit in the treatment of Waldenstrom's Macroglobulinemia patients with nucleoside analogue-based therapy. Clin Lymphoma Myeloma 9(1):71–73

136. Buske C et al (2009) The addition of rituximab to front-line therapy with CHOP (R-CHOP) results in a higher response rate and longer time to treatment failure in patients with lymphoplasmacytic lymphoma: results of a randomized trial of the German Low-Grade Lymphoma Study Group (GLSG). Leukemia 23(1):153–161

137. Rummel MJ et al (2013) Bendamustine plus rituximab versus CHOP plus rituximab as first-line treatment for patients with indolent and mantle-cell lymphomas: an open-label, multicentre, randomised, phase 3 non-inferiority trial. Lancet 381(9873):1203–1210

138. Treon SP et al (2011) Bendamustine alone and in combination with Cd20-directed monoclonal antibody therapy is active in patients with relapsed or refractory Waldenstrom's macroglobulinemia. Ann Oncol 22:189

139. Dimopoulos MA et al (2007) Primary treatment of Waldenstrom macroglobulinemia with dexamethasone, rituximab, and cyclophosphamide. J Clin Oncol 25(22):3344–3349

140. Dimopoulos MA et al (2012) primary treatment of waldenstrom's macroglobulinemia with dexamethasone, rituximab and cyclophosphamide (DRC): final analysis of a phase II study. ASH Ann Meeting Abs 120(21):438

141. Anagnostopoulos A et al (2006) Autologous or allogeneic stem cell transplantation in patients with Waldenstrom's macroglobulinemia. Biology of blood and marrow transplantation: J Am Soc Blood Marrow Transplant 12(8):845–854

142. Desikan R et al (1999) High-dose therapy with autologous haemopoietic stem cell support for Waldenstrom's macroglobulinaemia. Br J Haematol 105(4):993–996

143. Dreger P et al (1999) Myeloablative radiochemotherapy followed by reinfusion of purged autologous stem cells for Waldenstrom's macroglobulinaemia. Br J Haematol 106(1): 115–118

144. Dreger P, Schmitz N (2007) Autologous stem cell transplantation as part of first-line treatment of Waldenstrom's macroglobulinemia. Biology of blood and marrow transplantation: J Am Soc Blood Marrow Transplant 13(5):623–624

145. Gilleece MH et al (2008) The outcome of haemopoietic stem cell transplantation in the treatment of lymphoplasmacytic lymphoma in the UK: a British Society Bone Marrow Transplantation study. Hematology 13(2):119–127

146. Kyriakou C et al (2010) High-dose therapy and autologous stem-cell transplantation in Waldenstrom macroglobulinemia: the Lymphoma working party of the European Group for blood and marrow transplantation. J Clin Oncol Official J Am Soc Clin Oncol 28(13): 2227–2232

147. Munshi NC, Barlogie B (2003) Role for high-dose therapy with autologous hematopoietic stem cell support in Waldenstrom's macroglobulinemia. Semin Oncol 30(2):282–285

148. Tournilhac O et al (2003) Transplantation in Waldenstrom's macroglobulinemia–the French experience. Semin Oncol 30(2):291–296

149. Bachanova V, Burns LJ (2012) Hematopoietic cell transplantation for Waldenstrom macroglobulinemia. Bone Marrow Transplant 47(3):330–336

150. Gertz MA et al (2012) Stem cell transplant for Waldenstrom macroglobulinemia: an underutilized technique. Bone Marrow Transplant 47(9):1147–1153

151. Kyriakou C et al (2010) Allogeneic stem-cell transplantation in patients with Waldenstrom macroglobulinemia: report from the Lymphoma Working Party of the European Group for Blood and Marrow Transplantation. J Clin Oncol Official J Am Soc Clin Oncol 28(33): 4926–4934

152. Treon SP et al (2009) Lenalidomide and rituximab in Waidenstrom's macroglobulinemia. Clin Cancer Res 15(1):355–360

153. Rosenthal et al A Phase 2 Study of Lenalidomide, Rituximab, Cyclophosphamide and Dexamethasone (LR-CD) for Untreated Low Grade Non-Hodgkin Lymphoma Requiring Therapy: Waldenström's Macroglobulinemia Cohort Results Blood 122(21): p. 4352

154. Treon SP, Tripsas C, Warren D. Phase I Study of Pomalidomide, Dexamethasone and Rituximab (PDR) in Patients with Relapsed or Refractory Waldenstrom's Macroglobulenima. Hematological Oncology. 31(S1): p. 536

155. Treon SP et al (2012) Familial disease predisposition impacts treatment outcome in patients with Waldenstrom macroglobulinemia. Clin Lymphoma Myeloma Leuk 12(6):433–437

156. Chen CI et al (2007) Bortezomib is active in patients with untreated or relapsed Waldenstrom's macroglobulinemia: a phase II study of the National Cancer Institute of Canada Clinical Trials Group. J Clin Oncol 25(12):1570–1575

157. Ghobrial IM et al (2010) Phase II trial of weekly bortezomib in combination with rituximab in untreated patients with Waldenstrom Macroglobulinemia. Am J Hematol 85(9):670–674

158. Dimopoulos MA et al (2013) Primary therapy of Waldenstrom macroglobulinemia (WM) with weekly bortezomib, low-dose dexamethasone, and rituximab (BDR): long-term results of a phase 2 study of the European Myeloma Network (EMN). Blood 122(19):3276–3282

159. Treon SP et al (2014) Carfilzomib, rituximab and dexamethasone (CaRD) is highly active and offers a neuropathy sparing approach for proteasome-inhibitor based therapy in waldenstrom's macroglobulinemia. Blood 124(4):503-510

160. Treon SP et al (2015) Ibrutinib in previously treated Waldenström's macroglobulinemia. N Engl J Med 372(15):1430-1440.

161. Leleu X et al (2007) The Akt pathway regulates survival and homing in Waldenstrom macroglobulinemia. Blood 110(13):4417–4426

162. Ghobrial IM et al (2014) Long-term results of the phase II trial of the oral mTOR inhibitor everolimus (RAD001) in relapsed or refractory Waldenstrom Macroglobulinemia. Am J Hematol 89(3):237–242

163. Ghobrial IM et al (2013) Phase I/II trial of everolimus, bortezomib and rituximab in relapsed or relapsed/refractory Waldenstrom's Macroglobulinemia. Blood 122(21):4402

164. Roccaro AM et al (2010) Dual targeting of the PI3K/Akt/mTOR pathway as an antitumor strategy in Waldenstrom macroglobulinemia. Blood 115(3):559–569

165. Ghobrial IM et al (2010) Clinical and translational studies of a phase II trial of the novel oral Akt inhibitor perifosine in relapsed or relapsed/refractory Waldenstrom's macroglobulinemia. Clin Cancer Res 16(3):1033–1041

166. Ghobrial IM et al (2012) A multicenter phase II study of single-agent enzastaurin in previously treated Waldenstrom macroglobulinemia. J Clin Oncol Official J Am Soc Clin Oncol 18(18):5043–5050

167. Gopal AK et al (2014) PI3 K delta inhibition by idelalisib in patients with relapsed indolent lymphoma. N Engl J Med 370(11):1008–1018

168. Sun JY et al (2011) Vorinostat induced cellular stress disrupts the p38 mitogen activated protein kinase and extracellular signal regulated kinase pathways leading to apoptosis in Waldenstrom macroglobulinemia cells. Leukemia Lymphoma 52(9):1777–1786

169. San-Miguel JF et al (2014) Panobinostat plus bortezomib and dexamethasone versus placebo plus bortezomib and dexamethasone in patients with relapsed or relapsed and refractory multiple myeloma: a multicentre, randomised, double-blind phase 3 trial. Lancet Oncol 15 (11):1195–1206

170. Ghobrial IM et al (2013) Results of a phase 2 trial of the single-agent histone deacetylase inhibitor panobinostat in patients with relapsed/refractory Waldenstrom macroglobulinemia. Blood 121(8):1296–1303

171. Dimopoulos MA et al (2002) Treatment of Waldenstrom's macroglobulinemia with rituximab. J Clin Oncol Official J Am Soc Clin Oncol 20(9):2327–2333

172. Ghobrial IM et al (2009) Phase II Trial of Weekly bortezomib in combination with rituximab in relapsed or relapsed/refractory Waldenstrom's Macroglobulinemia. Blood 114(22):1067

173. Veronique L et al (2013) Phase II Trial In advanced waldenstrom macroglobulinemia (WM) patients with bortezomib: interest of addition of dexamethasone to bortezomib on behalf of the french CLL/WM intergroup (NCT 00777738) 122:4359–4359

174. Tedeschi A et al (2013) Fludarabine, cyclophosphamide, and rituximab in salvage therapy of Waldenstrom's macroglobulinemia. Clin Lymphoma Myeloma Leuk 13(2):231–234

175. Nguyen-Khac F et al (2013) Chromosomal aberrations and their prognostic value in a series of 174 untreated patients with Waldenstrom's macroglobulinemia. Haematologica 98 (4):649–654

176. Ioakimidis L et al (2009) Comparative Outcomes Following CP-R, CVP-R, and CHOP-R in Waldenstrom's Macroglobulinemia. Clinical Lymphoma & Myeloma 9(1):62–66

177. Dimopoulos MA et al (1994) Primary therapy of waldenstroms macroglobulinemia with 2-chlorodeoxyadenosine. J Clin Oncol 12(12):2694–2698

178. Liu ES et al (1998) Bolus administration of cladribine in the treatment of Waldenstrom macroglobulinaemia. Br J Haematol 103(3):690–695

179. Dimopoulos MA et al (1995) Treatment of waldenstroms macroglobulinemia resistant to standard therapy with 2-chlorodeoxyadenosine - identification of prognostic factors. Ann Oncol 6(1):49–52

180. Dimopoulos MA et al (2003) Treatment of Waldenstrom's macroglobulinemia with the combination of fludarabine and cyclophosphamide. Leukemia Lymphoma 44(6):993–996

181. Dimopoulos MA et al (1993) Treatment of Waldenstrom Macroglobulinemia with 2-Chlorodeoxyadenosine. Ann Intern Med 118(3):195–198

182. Treon SP et al (2005) Extended rituximab therapy in Waldenstrom's macroglobulinemia. Ann Oncol 16(1):132–138

183. Treon SP et al (2011) Long-term follow-up of symptomatic patients with lymphoplasmacytic lymphoma/Waldenstrom macroglobulinemia treated with the anti-CD52 monoclonal antibody alemtuzumab. Blood 118(2):276–281

184. Ghobrial IM et al (2010) Phase II trial of weekly bortezomib in combination with rituximab in relapsed or relapsed and refractory Waldenstrom macroglobulinemia. J Clin Oncol 28 (8):1422–1428

185. Treon SP et al (2007) Multicenter clinical trial of bortezomib in relapsed/refractory Waldenstrom's macroglobulinemia: Results of WMCTG trial 03-248. Clin Cancer Res 13 (11):3320–3325

186. Dimopoulos MA et al (2001) Treatment of Waldenstrom's macroglobulinemia with thalidomide. Journal of clinical oncology: official journal of the American Society of Clinical Oncology 19(16):3596–3601
187. Treon SP et al (2008) Thalidomide and rituximab in Waldenstrom macroglobulinemia. Blood 112(12):4452–4457
188. Ghobrial IM et al (2010) Phase II trial of the oral mammalian target of rapamycin inhibitor everolimus in relapsed or refractory Waldenstrom macroglobulinemia. J Clin Oncol 28 (8):1408–1414

Printed in the United States
By Bookmasters